Praise for
THE END OF VIOLENCE

"Dr. Slutkin's revelation of violence as a disease is nothing short of a paradigm shift. Violence has been misdiagnosed and mismanaged for too long. The science and movement in this book will move us forward as a species."
— **Peter Piot, MD, PhD, founding executive director of UNAIDS, co-discoverer of the Ebola virus**

"Science sometimes totally upends our view of the world. From our revolving around the sun, to invisible disease-causing germs, and now to understanding violence differently than we had: as something to treat as if it were an infectious disease — and cure with a new approach. This is the type of discovery that can change the course of human health, and even human history."
— **Dr. Al Sommer, Dean Emeritus, Johns Hopkins University Bloomberg School of Public Health**

"*The End of Violence* is a visionary work. At the same time, it is grounded in real stories, science, and experience. Dr. Slutkin's book is a must-read, not only for practitioners but also for everyday people who care about their families, their futures, and those around them."
— **Dr. Susan L. Bissell, founding director, Global Partnership to End Violence Against Children; formerly, global chief for child protection, UNICEF**

"Twenty-five years ago I sought out Gary Slutkin while searching for a solution to the gun violence we experienced in Los Angeles. I got far more than I hoped for. The methods he describes in his groundbreaking new book helped reduce our gun violence to new historic lows and save thousands of lives."

— **Charlie Beck, former chief, LA Police Department**

"*The End of Violence* shows how urgent it is to see and manage violence in an entirely new way. For leaders responsible for public safety, and *all* of us — we need to wake up fast to these innovative insights about all forms of violence — community violence, police violence, political violence — if this country is to have a chance."

— **Khalil Gibran Muhammad; professor, Princeton University; founder and director of the Institutional Antiracism and Accountability Project; and author of *The Condemnation of Blackness***

"Dr. Gary Slutkin's ideas and evidence are having as profound an effect on how violence is seen and reduced as antibiotics did for infectious disease. People are desperately looking for solutions at the global, national, local, and even household level. This book will be in demand by concerned individuals, students, journalists, and policymakers around the world."

— **Dan Ratner, founder of Public Good and author of *Nanotechnology***

"Gary Slutkin is an inspiring pioneer of both ideas and action. He has rethought violence as a contagious disease and been a pathbreaker for how to treat it. *The End of Violence* reports on his journey of understanding and action, and encapsulates his wisdom and accumulated knowledge in a wonderfully readable account."

— **Dan Smith, former director of the Stockholm International Peace Research Institute and secretary general of International Alert**

"In a country driven by violence, it's difficult to see our carnage for what it is: a disease. Pay close attention to the work Slutkin has done to separate violence from politics, poverty, and morality and you will never see it the same way again.

— **Rafael Alvarez, author of *The Fountain of Highlandtown* and former staff writer for *The Wire***

"Dr. Slutkin is the person who illuminated, in both theory and practice, the science about how violence acts as a contagious disease. This book shows how he came to that realization, how it works, and what we need to do now. The results that have been documented in the United States, Latin America, and beyond are truly remarkable. Dr. Slutkin gives us hope by providing a new path for us all.

— **James Mercy, former director of the Division of Violence Prevention at the CDC**

"This book does more than explain Dr. Slutkin's discovery that violence is a communicable disease — it also offers extremely practical applications. We're overdue to take its lessons and apply them everywhere: in our neighborhoods, in our cities, and around the world. The world needs this book now to change the tide of violence and build a world of peace.

— **Rima Salah, former assistant secretary-general of the United Nations**

"Dr. Slutkin sees things differently than most of us and the result is that violence has a new diagnosis and is now in a new category — a health epidemic. I have no doubt that Dr. Slutkin's discovery and practical applications will result in a global campaign to stop violence and that it will succeed. This book takes us on his path to discovery and gives us the science and the way forward."

— **Céline Gounder; senior fellow at the Kaiser Family Foundation; internist, infectious disease specialist, and epidemiologist at NYU Grossman School of Medicine and Bellevue Hospital**

"As the longest-serving director of the US Department of Justice's programs and research agency and co-chair of President Obama's task force on twenty-first century policing, I have come across many approaches to reducing violence and improving life in our communities. Dr. Slutkin's approach changed the way we see things and much of what we do in a more fundamental way. This book shows us something brand new — something we didn't know before about violence, and how our future may be more hopeful than we thought."
— **Laurie Robinson, former assistant attorney general, US Department of Justice**

"We have been needing a new solution to violence and to our forced displacement problem for decades if not more. Now, we have a breakthrough. *The End of Violence* gives us a whole new way of seeing and helping solve these previously intractable problems. An urgent read."
— **Mark Connolly, senior advisor, UNICEF Latin America and Caribbean**

"A book that will help each of us feel safer and more able to protect the people around us. To read this book is to have hope as well as tools to be safe — and help change the way things are now."
— **Leon Andrews, president and CEO of Equal Measure; formerly director of race, equity and leadership, National League of Cities**

THE END OF VIOLENCE

www.penguin.co.uk

THE END OF VIOLENCE

Eliminating the World's Most Dangerous Epidemic

GARY SLUTKIN, MD

torva

TRANSWORLD PUBLISHERS

UK | USA | Canada | Ireland | Australia
India | New Zealand | South Africa

Transworld is part of the Penguin Random House group of companies
whose addresses can be found at global.penguinrandomhouse.com.

Penguin Random House UK, One Embassy Gardens,
8 Viaduct Gardens, London SW11 7BW

penguin.co.uk

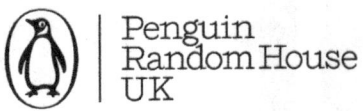

First published in Great Britain in 2026 by Torva
an imprint of Transworld Publishers

001

Copyright © Gary Slutkin 2026

The moral right of the author has been asserted.

Every effort has been made to obtain the necessary permissions with
reference to copyright material, both illustrative and quoted. We apologize
for any omissions in this respect and will be pleased to make the
appropriate acknowledgements in any future edition.

As of the time of initial publication, the URLs displayed in this book link or refer to
existing websites on the internet. Transworld Publishers is not responsible for, and
should not be deemed to endorse or recommend, any website other than its own or
any content available on the internet (including without limitation at any website,
blog page, information page) that is not created by Transworld Publishers.

No part of this book may be used or reproduced in any manner for the purpose of
training artificial intelligence technologies or systems. In accordance with Article 4(3)
of the DSM Directive 2019/790, Penguin Random House expressly reserves this work
from the text and data mining exception.

Printed and bound in Great Britain by Clays Ltd, Elcograf S.p.A.

The authorized representative in the EEA is Penguin Random House Ireland,
Morrison Chambers, 32 Nassau Street, Dublin D02 YH68.

A CIP catalogue record for this book is available from the British Library

ISBNs:
9781911709121 (hb)
9781911709138 (tpb)

Penguin Random House is committed to a sustainable future
for our business, our readers and our planet. This book is made
from Forest Stewardship Council® certified paper.

CONTENTS

Introduction   1

Part One: Infection

   Chapter One: Assessment and Diagnosis   11

   Chapter Two: Making Sense of "Senseless Violence"   21

Part Two: Transmission

   Chapter Three: Your Brain on Violence   41

   Chapter Four: Exposure   59

   Chapter Five: Susceptibility   83

Part Three: Interruption and Elimination

   Chapter Six: Interrupting Spread   111

   Chapter Seven: Norms and Systems   149

   Chapter Eight: Infections of the State   191

Epilogue: A World Without Fear   241

Acknowledgments   255
Glossary   269
Action Plan   275
   What You Can Do to End Violence Now:
   Action Plan for Individuals, Families, and Communities

CONTENTS

Notes   283
Solutions by Violence Syndrome   301
Additional References by City and Country   311
    What's Happening in These Places Now: 2025 Updates
Bibliography and Further Reading   315
Index   323

INTRODUCTION

The beginning is the end, and the end is the beginning.
— Early Kabbalah text

It was in 1979, while serving as chief resident in medicine at San Francisco General Hospital, that I was first tasked with reversing an epidemic.

Tuberculosis was back, and San Francisco was dealing with the worst outbreak in the country. Every week, dozens of new patients were stricken with this ancient but still present sickness — a disease that had killed hundreds of millions through history.

In the nineteenth century, people called TB "consumption" for the way it seemed to consume its victims from the inside, devouring them until they were pale emaciated husks, racked by hacking coughs. The English writer John Bunyan called it "the Master of Death."

The process for treating this outbreak was slow and methodical. We would identify the sick, start them on medication, then trace their contacts so we could examine every person they regularly encountered who might have been exposed. TB is airborne and spreads quickly, so when one person staggered into SF General coughing up blood, we knew that others weren't far behind.

While leading this effort, I was invited to Somalia, where TB was rampant in the refugee camps. I spent the next ten years in

Somalia, Uganda, Malawi, Tanzania, Kenya, Zaire, Thailand, and more than a dozen other countries, treating not just TB but other infectious diseases that were devastating the cities, villages, and, especially, the camps of displaced people running from oppression and civil war. TB, cholera, and eventually HIV/AIDS were my main areas of focus in those years.

What I saw then still haunts me: the distended bellies of bone-thin, starving children suffering from pneumonia, diarrheal diseases, and malaria; refugee mothers and children wasting away in huts in the desert; the boats of Lake Victoria piled high with the coffins of Tanzanians lost to AIDS; ghost towns where so many people had died.

It was a textbook example of epidemic disease: How they begin, how they spread, and, most importantly, how they are controlled and eliminated. In 1990, I was brought to Geneva to form and run WHO's intervention development unit, a cross-departmental team tasked with designing, testing, and implementing interventions to prevent and manage infectious outbreaks. In my time at WHO,* in studying past epidemics, I learned two important lessons.

The first was that humanity's approaches to ending epidemics had become "stuck," with years, decades, centuries, and, in some cases, almost all of human history passing with no progress being made.

The second lesson was that this lack of progress was usually not due to a lack of will or even resources. It was because we had fundamentally misdiagnosed the problem.

When we misdiagnose an epidemic disease, millions of lives can be lost.

This is what has happened with violence and why I am writing this book.

---

* My assignments at WHO were field epidemiologist, deputy director for Central and East African country programs under Dr. Tarantola, coordinator for the joint AIDS-TB program, lead on sentinel surveillance methods, and chief of intervention, development, and support for the Global Programme on HIV/AIDS (1987–1994).

In 1994, after fifteen years abroad, I was exhausted. Although I was only in my early forties, years of constant travel and emotionally draining work had left me depleted, lonely, and isolated. Somalia had been arduous, due not only to the sheer scale of the suffering but also to the strain of working in a dictatorship. Years in the epicenter of AIDS in Africa, where death was ubiquitous, had been equally draining.

I needed a break. I needed to go home.

I wasn't sure where home was anymore, but my parents, who lived in Chicago, were getting older and I wanted to see them. I drafted a letter of resignation to WHO, put my stuff in storage, and booked a one-way ticket from Geneva to O'Hare with no clear plan for what I'd do next.

In Chicago, I rented the top floor of a Lithuanian couple's home. I had left all my medical textbooks in Geneva, but I always kept one book around: *The Tibetan Book of Living and Dying*, which I read and reread constantly. On most mornings, I'd meditate and then go for a walk, sometimes watching the sun come up over the lake. I spent a lot of time alone. The only thing I took out of my years-old storage unit in Oak Park was my bike, which I rode through the city, along the lake, through the neighborhoods and run-down industrial zones, and past deserted baseball fields.

I had been away more than a decade, and the culture shock was profound. I had gotten used to jerry-rigged or nonexistent plumbing, but here in the States, clean water was taken for granted, piped hot and cold into multiple rooms in each home. I had grown accustomed to being without electricity and sweating through clothes in hot climates. Here, everyone left the lights on all day long and turned their thermostats up or down one or two degrees to optimize comfort. In the refugee camps, daily food rations were limited. Here, the endless array of fresh and packaged foods available in the grocery stores initially made me dizzy. In Somalia, the people celebrated when it rained, as it watered the crops needed to feed chronically underweight camels, goats, and children. Back in downtown Chicago, people complained when their shoes got wet.

I was so out of touch with American popular culture that when a friend referred to Michael Jordan, I had no idea who he was.

Still, I was gradually adjusting to a more stable, easier life. No more cross-country treks by Land Cruiser on deeply rutted roads chasing cholera to determine where to deploy urgently needed health workers, fluids for rehydration, and tents. I didn't know what I wanted to do next, but I figured that whatever it was, I wouldn't face a daily epidemic crisis. Even the AIDS epidemic was beginning to stabilize in the United States at the time.

However, within a few weeks, I noticed something disturbing. Chicago was experiencing one of the worst violent-crime waves in decades. Every time I picked up a copy of the *Chicago Tribune*, there were stories of children and young people losing their lives to violence: A thirteen-year-old killing his twelve-year-old brother. A sixteen-year-old robbing a neighborhood store, shooting the clerk in the face. Another kid so young that when he was arrested for a killing, he cried and asked for his mother.

The story of Yummy Sandifer hit me especially hard.

Robert Sandifer was an eleven-year-old boy nicknamed "Yummy" because of his love of candy. His body was found under a viaduct beneath railroad tracks at East 108th Street — he had been shot twice in the back of the head, execution-style.

The day before his murder, as part of a required gang initiation, Yummy had opened fire on a group of teenagers, killing a fourteen-year-old girl. The kids who killed Yummy were avenging the girl's death. They were fourteen and sixteen.

A child killer killed by other *children*, his body left beneath a railroad overpass.

I had witnessed violence in Chicago before — or, more accurately, witnessed its effects. When I was in medical school living on the South

Side and working shifts at the University of Chicago's emergency department as part of my rotations, I'd regularly see people with gunshot wounds and stabbings rushed in on stretchers.

In those years in the ER, I'd sometimes wondered if maybe violence could be treated in some way that went beyond surgeries, sutures, and bandages. But then the next patient would fly into triage, and I was snapping on gloves with no time to think about anything beyond the procedure to be performed right then, the individual life to be saved. Emergency medicine was minute to minute, hour to hour, day to day. The priority was to stop the bleeding. Immediately.

In those days, I lived on the South Side, at Fifty-Third and Harper, in a basement apartment that smelled like wet paint. I'd ride my bicycle to the University of Chicago campus for classes, to study in the library, or to do clinical rotations on the wards. On the way home, I'd stop off at a newsstand on Fifty-Fifth Street for a paper.

One evening in the mid-1970s, a story in the paper caught my eye. It was just below the fold: "Man Stabbed on 54th and Harper" — a block from my apartment. As I pedaled home, I saw a man spraying down the sidewalk with a hose, washing away the blood.

At the time, I saw these events as senseless tragedies, with no clear reason behind them.

But twenty years later, when I read about Yummy, something changed for me. In my time overseas, I'd seen heavily armed men walk through the streets of Nairobi, had been waved through checkpoints by men with semiautomatic weapons in Rwanda, had stared down the barrels of big guns drawn on me at night in the desert in Somalia. I'd watched children in the refugee camps run in terror from truckloads of armed men coming to "recruit" them to be soldiers. But learning of Yummy being killed in that way, in my hometown, felt different.

It wasn't just that he'd been so young or that the killing had been so brutal. It was also that his murder wasn't random; it was part of an established ritual, one that demanded initiation by violence. Yummy had shot people because it was what he had to do to belong. And the rules that dictated he shoot people were the same rules that dictated he would be shot. In a way, no one involved had a choice.

And this was not an isolated case.

In the days after Yummy's death, I found myself asking a lot of questions:

How had the violence gotten this bad?

Why were there so many senseless killings in Chicago and across the whole country?

And was anyone doing anything about it that was working?

The more questions I asked, the less sense it made.

But if you ask enough questions and dig deeply enough into the data, eventually, some insights will reveal themselves. That's what happened for me. The more people I talked to, the more statistics I read, the more maps I pored over, plotting murders with red pushpins, the clearer it became: The patterns of violence I was seeing in Chicago were not all that different from the patterns I had observed with TB or other epidemics in Somalia, Uganda, Thailand, and San Francisco.

When I came back to the United States, I thought I had left infectious diseases behind. But what I found upon returning was yet another epidemic, one that was still spreading — in fact, spreading constantly all across the country.

I was witnessing a disease outbreak that seemed deeply misunderstood and that did not yet have a clear diagnosis or cure.

CURING VIOLENCE

I am a scientist by training, an internal medicine and infectious disease physician and then an epidemiologist.

I have spent a large portion of my career working to contain epidemic outbreaks in many areas of the world, from tuberculosis in San Francisco to cholera in Somalia to AIDS in Africa and Asia, and I have seen many diseases up close in city ERs, rural clinics, and makeshift field hospitals. I've had the opportunity to lead teams to stop the spread of disease in refugee camps, villages, and cities and even helped design some strategies for global containment at the World Health Organization.

And what I began to see that summer of Yummy's killing in Chicago and what I can tell you now with certainty is this: *Violence is a contagious disease.* I don't mean that metaphorically. I mean that violence infects a population via the same rules and processes as other infectious diseases: *Exposure* leads to *infection*, which progresses to *disease*, which leads to *transmission* and *further exposure.*

Violence is often thought of as a social disorder or a moral problem. Some people believe it is inherent in human nature, that it has always been with us and always will be.

I do not see it that way at all. It makes sense that in trying to better understand violence, we would focus on the morality of those engaging in it or the social context that might make someone more likely to do so. But these discussions obscure the scientific reality that violence is a disease state, one that infects our brains and bodies, impairs and alters their functions, and spreads on exposure from one person to another. Like other infections, those who come into contact with violence are at risk of contracting it. And in the absence of the right care, those who contract it are at risk of progressing to severe disease.

Current versions of the International Classification of Diseases include violence, and there are over a hundred studies showing that violence is contagious like TB, influenza, smallpox, polio, cholera, and COVID. It can spread just as rapidly and be just as devastating — if not more — for individuals, families, and communities. Like many diseases, it strikes every person and community differently and exacerbates existing inequalities. And all too often, it completely overwhelms attempts to contain it.

Through the organization I founded — originally called CeaseFire and now Cure Violence Global — we have spent the past twenty-five years trying to end violence using the same approaches public health workers use to contain and stop the spread of any contagious disease. And this basic epidemic-control approach has proven remarkably adaptable to all the forms violence takes in our world, from gang violence in Chicago to civil war in Syria; from domestic abuse in private households to nuclear war prevented via talks in hushed conference rooms; from bullying to hate speech to school shootings. It is even adaptable to the state violence we see on the world stage today and to the brutal wars being fought in Ukraine and the Middle East. Each syndrome of violence has its characteristic signs and symptoms, but it's all the same disease.

This is good news. It means that we don't need to solve all our social problems or fix human nature before we can stop violence. Violence is not something we can police, punish, or moralize our way out of. Instead, we need to diagnose, understand, and treat *the disease*, just as societies have done for countless other diseases throughout history.

Ending a disease that's been with us for all of human history might seem too big a task to undertake. But it has been done many times before. Smallpox and plague devastated us for millennia; today smallpox is totally gone and plague is rare. In just the past fifty or so years, we have not only rid the earth of millennia-old contagions, we've immunized billions of children, reduced child deaths by 50 percent, dramatically turned the corner on AIDS, TB, and malaria, and almost eradicated polio. Some of the greatest killers of all time are either gone or on their way out. Of course, there is no vaccine for violence the way there is for polio and smallpox. But as we will see throughout this book, there are effective and proven strategies for containing and interrupting its spread, resulting in large reductions and long streaks of elimination.

We know how to end pandemics. That means we know how to create a world nearly free of violence — by using the time-tested and proven epidemic-control playbook that has rid the planet of so many other lethal and pernicious contagions.

That's our goal.

And I have good reasons to believe it is one within our grasp.

PART ONE

INFECTION

CHAPTER ONE

ASSESSMENT AND DIAGNOSIS

The knowledge about man is still in its infancy.

— Albert Einstein

At WHO, we were frequently asked to do quick assessments of an epidemic situation, often after having been in a country for just a few days or a week. Sometimes it was an entirely new disease; sometimes it was a new form or mutation of a disease; sometimes it was new to that country; and sometimes a situation we'd thought we understood had changed. Regardless, we needed to learn as much as we could as quickly as we could.

One of medicine's flaws is its practitioners' certainty in diagnosis with insufficient investigation. When time is of the essence, it's easy to be swayed by what the previous doctor said or what the patient or family member in the waiting room reported as a diagnosis. But if physicians don't keep asking questions, diseases can be misdiagnosed and incorrect treatments applied. One has to look only at the history of other diseases to see the counterproductive approaches doctors have taken when they tried to treat things they did not understand. This is true for an individual patient as well as for a disease.

In medicine and public health, we have to keep an open mind, ask broad questions, listen carefully, then narrow our inquiries in response to what we hear.

To help a patient, we need to know:

> How they feel
> What their symptoms are
> When and where those symptoms occur
> What treatments they have tried
> Whether any of those treatments have worked

In 1994, I felt I needed to adopt this diagnostic approach with my hometown as we had for other diseases in other cities and countries. I had to take a kind of medical history of the city of Chicago and the violence occurring there. I collected information, opinions, and data from as many sources as possible. I spoke with community leaders, parents, young people, formerly incarcerated people, local clergy, foundation representatives, police, government officials in health, justice, and schools, and researchers in many fields. I read every report on violence I could find. I studied statistics about all forms of violence and pored over maps, graphs, and charts.

I treated the city like a patient but also the way I treated any epidemic in any new place. I asked almost everyone I met what they thought was going on.

> How does the situation of violence in the city look to you?
> What do you hear and see in the news or other sources?
> What is being done?
> Is anything working?

Most people agreed that violence was a very serious and important problem. But no one could agree on how to solve it, and the majority thought there was nothing anyone could do about it.

A lot of them advocated harsher penalties and more punishment. One business leader I met told me, "We know what to do with them."

"What?" I asked.

"Lock all of them up," he replied.

I didn't ask who *them* referred to. I didn't have to.

His racism (as it seemed to me) aside, the science showed that as an approach to violence, punitive measures were counterproductive and only created more harm. I asked people more specific questions: Okay, so what should we do? What can be done to stop the shootings? A lot of them brought up many important social issues that needed solutions, but so many people just shrugged their shoulders or threw up their hands. The problem was hopeless, too big, too complex, too difficult to even bother trying to fix.

I'd seen this attitude before in other countries with other epidemics. In fact, this was common. When people become too overwhelmed by a problem, they give up.

One day, I ran into a police officer in a bookstore and asked him what he thought of the violence in his city.

"We do what we can," he said. "But we know the violence is always going to be there."

These responses enraged me. I think it was because, in my decade or so with WHO and other organizations abroad, I'd been part of many teams tasked with solving seemingly unsolvable problems on local, national, and even global levels, so I wasn't used to being still while people were dying by the hundreds every year. Especially in my home city.

At WHO, if we had been fighting an epidemic that caused deaths on the scale Chicago was experiencing, we would have mobilized teams of epidemiologists, doctors, nurses, and educators, raced to the scene, and set up procedures to rid the area of disease as quickly as possible. But when it came to violence, even the leaders charged with protecting residents' health and safety — including officials in the city's health department at the time — told me: "It's none of our business," "It's not our problem," and "We don't have any money."

Essentially: *We don't know what to do.*

I quickly learned that people who didn't live in neighborhoods with high rates of violence — those who weren't hearing gunshots every night, who weren't losing children, parents, friends, and neighbors — responded to my questions mostly with the shrugs. That's when it became even more obvious that if I wanted to understand violence in Chicago, I needed to talk to the people who were experiencing it and, of course, those who were committing it.

So I spent a lot of time that fall and winter driving across the city attending community meetings in the neighborhoods where violence was a daily reality.

The Westside Health Authority (WHA) was the first community organization I spent significant time with. Located in the Austin neighborhood, it had been founded by an impressive woman named Jackie Reed with the original goal of keeping area hospitals (which were severely underfunded and understaffed) from closing. Over time, however, Jackie and her colleagues had broadened their mission to include reducing illegal drug sales, increasing access to employment, and preventing violence. All of which she rightly saw as important factors in her community's health.

At first, I attended the meetings just to get the lay of the land. Typically, they were held in the evenings in the back room of Jackie's office. It was a typical community-event space: chairs arranged in a loose rectangle, coffee in a metal urn in the back, a small table holding doughnuts, sugar, and cream.

Most meetings at the WHA were contentious. Representatives from four or more other organizations were usually there, and they often disagreed — loudly, frequently, and passionately — about the best way to reduce violence in their community. Some, including Jackie, wanted to focus on jobs. Others wanted to "root out" drugs, as they put it. At the time, crack cocaine and heroin were major problems, and community members had seen their neighborhoods hollowed out by the attendant crime.

Others thought the focus should be on youth initiatives. The schools in the area were not good, and they argued that kids were violent because they had "nothing better to do." Some believed the main focus of the center should be on addiction services; some thought the focus should be on getting more aid for pregnant mothers; still others thought the focus should be on helping people get food.

Everyone seemed to agree on the problems. Where they disagreed was on which problem to tackle first, and how.

I met many wonderful people at WHA — passionate, dedicated, and smart people. Sitting in my folding chair in the back of the room, I listened to their pleas for funds and sometimes for new ideas. I heard frustration and idealism and a deep love for their communities that had nurtured them and their families.

What I didn't hear a lot of was data. No one seemed to have any. Decisions were being made based on feelings or intuitions or something that had happened last week. This lack of data coupled with the differing viewpoints and, as is often the case for community organizations, a lack of funds made it very difficult for them to establish a strategy, especially a scalable, long-term one, for reducing violence in the neighborhood.

Case in point: midnight basketball.* A local pastor had instituted these late-night games because most of the shootings in his neighborhood happened late at night. His church had a small gymnasium, and he opened it up during those hours and hosted three-on-three tournaments with free Gatorade and pizza for anyone who showed up.

And show up they did. Dozens of teenagers, some of them gang-affiliated, began joining teams. The pastor told me that a lot of people

---

* Even these activities were highly controversial then. Many thought that teenagers were beyond help, that past a certain age, it was too late for them. This was also the time of the "crime bill"; people were less focused on prevention and more focused on being "tough on crime." I was in HHS in DC then and was aware there was an alternative bill, a thirty-three-city crime-prevention bill that was proposed by three agency heads. It was refused by the administration.

were helped, and he thought there seemed to be a drop in shootings and fewer kids getting into trouble.

"How many fewer shootings have we seen so far?" I asked him. "Did you keep track?"

The pastor looked at me like I had two heads. "I'm not running an experiment," he said, smiling. "I'm running a church."

Like many of the Chicagoans I'd spoken to since my return to the States, the pastor cared deeply about the way violence was affecting his community, and he did a lot of great work. But neither he nor anyone on the ground had data showing whether all that great work was actually working.

BRINGING THE INVISIBLE TO LIGHT

In the mid-1990s, there were anecdotal success stories about after-school programs and late-night basketball games keeping kids out of trouble or inspiring them to go back to high school or community college instead of joining gangs. But science runs on data. And unfortunately, there was no quantifiable data correlating these programs with a reduction in shootings or killings in a neighborhood.*

Programs like midnight basketball surely made a big difference for some individuals, but they had little impact at the community level.

It reminded me of the early days of the TB epidemic in San Francisco. Patients would arrive at San Francisco General very sick and in desperate need of help. But although it was essential we treat each individual, we knew they were coming from the community, where many had been infected, where they had likely infected others, and where new infections might still be occurring.

We knew curing one person or even a few people would not be

---

* I performed a review of prior studies with input from the DOJ and the CDC. These studies showed behavioral help for young people, but there was insufficient data specific to community-wide violence reduction.

enough to reverse the course of the outbreak. These diseases must be cured on two levels — the individual level and the epidemic level in the community.

San Francisco needed a community-level strategy for TB control, and that needed to be implemented citywide.

The same was true for violence in Chicago. But we didn't realize it, because at the time, the problem didn't have a coherent theory or diagnosis. We were treating a bunch of recognizable symptoms without understanding the underlying sickness or the contagion that was keeping it going.

FOLLOWING THE DATA

That summer in Chicago, as both the temperature and the murder rate crept up, I found myself thinking about how I could understand and address the problem in a new way. Leaning on my epidemiological training, I asked myself: *Are we looking at killings scientifically? And if so, what are we not seeing?*

While I was attending meetings and talking to anyone who was familiar with the problem of violence in the city, I was also researching in archives and organizing the data. Through contacts at the CDC and several local, national, and international research groups, I collected as much data as I could about violence in Chicago, the United States, and other countries. I looked at the statistics neighborhood by neighborhood, city by city, year by year, searching for patterns and correlations related to rates of violence over the course of the twentieth century and as far back as I could find records.

The first time I saw a graph plotting the rates of killings in Chicago and in the United States going back to 1900, I saw an unmistakable series of waves rising and falling in an extremely familiar pattern.

The graph I was looking at was unambiguous.

The numbers and rates of killings over time looked exactly like an epidemic curve.

Epidemic Waves[*]

Smallpox *(World)*   **Violence** *(US)*

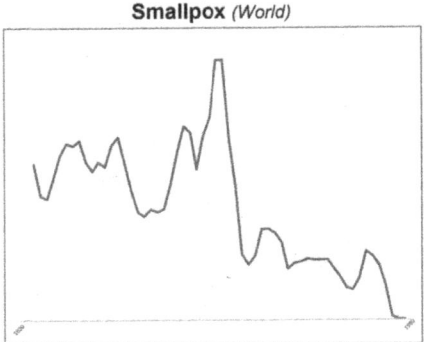
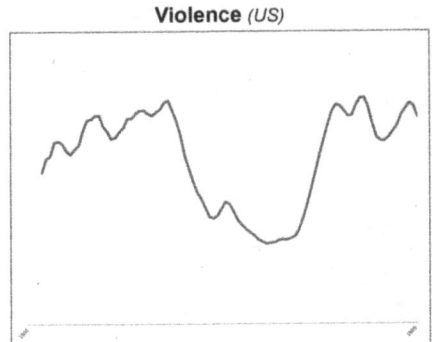

All epidemics are really multiple epidemics in time and space — a cluster of overlapping hot spots occurring simultaneously and feeding each other through contagion.[†]

At the most basic level, the pattern for epidemics looks something like this: A contagious disease comes into a community and spreads, often exponentially, infecting new people, new homes, new neighborhoods, sometimes even new countries. Then — either because the disease runs out of susceptible people or because the community takes the right measures to stop the spread — the disease level falls to a new baseline, possibly to rise again with subsequent outbreaks. This process continues until the disease is controlled or locally eliminated. I had seen this pattern play out dozens of times in Africa and Asia with TB, cholera, malaria, and AIDS, and now I was seeing it play out with violence in my hometown.

When I looked at the maps of violence across Chicago, I also saw the characteristic clustering of epidemic disease, just as we'd see for outbreaks of cholera or meningitis or AIDS. Small dots on a map were outbreaks clustering in certain areas, sometimes merging with

---

[*] Smallpox fell to zero in 1977 after a global campaign.
[†] Epidemics can plateau or dip depending on the math of exposure and susceptibility (discussed later). Plateaus show up in epidemic diseases when the balance between exposure and susceptibility remains steady, when there is continued spread but no discernible or major peak.

one another to form larger clusters. Clustering in time and clustering in space. Where there was one red marker (representing a case or a death), there would likely be many others.

A shooting commonly led to more shootings. Incident would follow incident, after which there could be relative quiet for a period of days. Then new outbreaks would occur, one area after another, in waves.

Waves are the defining pattern by which epidemics spread. And the more data on violence I looked at, the more waves I saw.

I saw these characteristic waves and clustering in the charts and graphs for Atlanta, Washington, DC, and Detroit.

Then for Los Angeles and New York City.

And for the United States as a whole.

Epidemic Clustering

Cholera *(Bangladesh)*

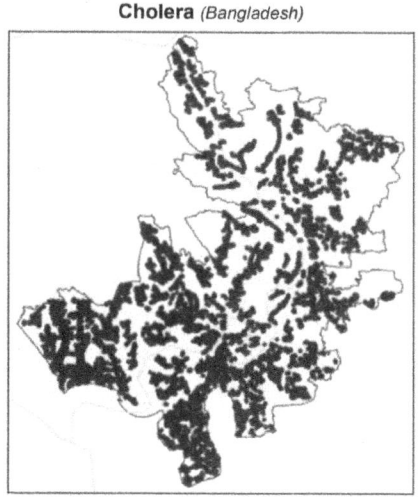

Violence *(Chicago)*

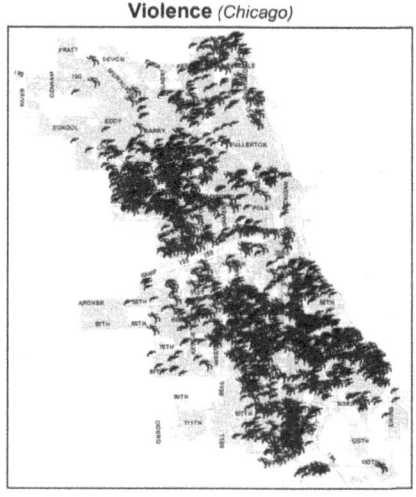

For most of my life, I had been following breadcrumbs, trying to figure out what to do next. This had taken me from Chicago to San Francisco and from there to Tunis, Mombasa, Mogadishu, the Bo'o camp of the Hiran region of Somalia, Kampala, Bujumbura, Blantyre, multiple countries in Africa, Bangkok, Chiang Mai, Thailand, Geneva, and, finally, back to Chicago. And it had taken me from internal medicine to infectious diseases, from being a resident to being a hospital doc, from working as a field epidemiologist to working as a chief at WHO. And it had taken me from TB to cholera and malaria to HIV/AIDS.

I hadn't thought much about where the breadcrumbs might be leading. I saw life as being like continuous ER triage: You treated the sickest or most urgent patient in front of you, then, once things stabilized, you moved on to the next. You thought about the future in terms of minutes and hours, not years and decades.

I couldn't have predicted that the patients, communities, and outbreaks I had treated and learned from were preparing me to examine and then take on the disease I feared the most.

CHAPTER TWO

MAKING SENSE OF "SENSELESS VIOLENCE"

Man will become better when you show him what he is like.
— Anton Chekhov,
Note-Book of Anton Chekhov

Science makes the invisible visible — it illuminates what we can't ordinarily see or understand. Humankind did not begin to win the centuries-long battle against the devastating epidemics of plague, leprosy, and typhoid fever and the more recent epidemics of malaria, cholera, HIV, and COVID until scientists were willing to look beyond myths and moralism and develop new approaches based on scientific data and discoveries.

My time at WHO was a master class in how to approach epidemics in a systematic, reliable, and scalable fashion. We would look at the data of an epidemic and what had and had not worked in the past and adapt the basic epidemic playbook to investigate, diagnose, and control a contagion to the epidemic at hand. The international epidemic-control community applies the following methods to one epidemic disease after another.*

1. **Educating the public about the disease:** Creating widespread awareness and understanding of the disease through public education campaigns utilizing media and social media; billboards, posters, flyers, and leaflets; public speaking, influencers; and institutions of all types, including government, nongovernment, schools, and community organizations.
2. **Active case finding:** Proactively identifying and reaching out to the most active cases as well as people at highest risk of developing a disease via public health workers, community members, social media and other sources, then providing support and care to stop the progression and spread of disease.
3. **Creating outreach systems and networks:** Recruiting, selecting, training, and supporting a network of locally hired health workers or messengers who have access, credibility, and trust in the most affected communities and then ensuring conversations are conducted confidentially, nonjudgmentally, and safely.
4. **Reducing further exposure:** Ensuring follow-up by the trained and trusted messengers of both active cases and their contacts, reducing exposure to other contacts, managing the most active cases, and instituting temporary containment only if necessary for public safety.
5. **Shifting norms and behaviors:** Encouraging behaviors that reduce spread and exposure via individual support, community-level discussions and decisions on desired norms and expectations, and, sometimes, legislation, if helpful and acceptable.

---

* This is why epidemiologists can deal with many diseases, from malaria to Ebola to COVID to whatever other diseases show up in communities, cities, and countries around the globe.

This is the playbook we used to halt transmission of tuberculosis in San Francisco, to stop the spread of AIDS in Uganda, and to eliminate cholera in Somalia. And that summer in Chicago in the mid-1990s, I began to wonder: Since violence seemed to spread with the same pattern as contagious disease, could we contain and control violence the same way we did for all other contagious diseases and adapt the epidemic-control playbook to this and other epidemics of violence?

That would mean focusing on community-level impact — treating entire communities, not just individuals. It would mean working with and studying neighborhoods as a whole, one by one, to see where the most transmission was occurring. It would mean recruiting people from the community to be its health workers, then training them to detect where spread was occurring and intervene before, during, and after outbreaks. It would require a laser focus on a single objective: the violence itself.*

This was to be my and my colleagues' working theory, the city of Chicago our test case. I didn't know at the time if the theory was correct. What I did know was that there was only one way to find out.

But first, to effectively treat disease of any kind, you need to diagnose it correctly — not just name it but deeply *understand it* and the mechanisms by which it operates. This is especially true for a new disease or for a disease that is not responding to the current approaches. And with violence, we were still in the dark.

A TERRIBLE HALLOWEEN

One Halloween evening about fifteen years ago, I was watching children trick-or-treating on my block in Chicago when one of our community-outreach workers called me from the Back of the Yards neighborhood, on the southwest side of the city.

---

* This is a critical matter in epidemic control. There are other factors, and they can be dealt with as well, but it is crucial to focus directly on the disease and show how it is spread as soon as you know.

"Doc," she said. Her voice was shaking. "Get down here. It's bad. We need you."

I didn't need to hear more. I raced out and drove there fast.

Back of the Yards had become an established hub for Cease-Fire, the organization I founded in the early 2000s to apply the epidemic-control approach to combating violence. By this point, we had spent years making connections, hosting community events, and selecting and training violence interrupters — people whose job was to detect the possibility of a violent event before it happened and head it off. Our efforts had paid off: Back of the Yards was not one of our areas of focus at the time, but we were working in the nearby neighborhoods of Brighton Park and Gage Park and we had a good record of success there.

But that Halloween night was a terrible setback.

On an evening when the sidewalks should have been filled with kids in cute costumes, the street was instead crowded with ambulances, police officers, and shocked residents standing frozen, their eyes wide in horror. Yellow police tape surrounded an area the size of a small swimming pool. In the center of it, on the sidewalk, was a pool of blood.

"Thirty-two-year-old mom, shot straight in the head," our outreach worker informed me. "Seven months pregnant. Trick-or-treating with her three little daughters. They saw it happen."

Within minutes, state representative Susana Mendoza, one of our organization's biggest champions in the state legislature, called me, enraged, *demanding* to know how this had happened. Other state reps and state senators had gotten in the habit of calling me whenever there was a shooting in or near neighborhoods where CeaseFire was operating. They saw it as a failure on our part.

"What was the reason for the killing?" she asked.

Her question was simple, but there was no easy answer. All we knew was that there had been a shooting and the mom hadn't been the target.

"Wrong place, wrong time," the outreach worker told me after I'd hung up with the state representative. Her voice was shaking and she was holding her head. "People in cars shooting at each other just missed and hit her."

This wasn't comforting to hear. It wasn't comforting to me, and it certainly wouldn't be a comfort to the woman's young daughters, seven, five, and two years old. There are no comforting explanations when a mother of three with a fourth on the way is gunned down on the sidewalk.

There's a very common phrase that people use to describe this kind of tragedy. Even today. You've probably heard it in the aftermath of school and other mass shootings. I've even heard it in reference to wars.

Mayors use it. Police chiefs use it. Reporters use it. Community activists use it.

Senseless violence:

I heard this phrase commonly during those early days working in Chicago. And every time I did, I got a little more frustrated. It seemed like just another way for people to justify throwing up their hands and moving on. It suggests that violence is beyond our ability to understand. And if it is beyond our ability to understand, then it must be beyond our ability to do anything about. It's just a random unexplainable phenomenon that we all have to make our peace with.

Did anyone actually believe this? I didn't. Calling violence *senseless* didn't satisfy the scientist part of me, a guy addicted to problem-solving trained to have an almost obsessive need to understand an underlying process.

Shootings like the ones that killed Yummy Sandifer and that mother on Halloween should of course be seen as devastating, unacceptable, and shocking.

But *senseless*??

The more I connected the dots of violence and infectious diseases, the less I could accept a language that cloaked violence in mystery. The term *senseless violence* placed the problem beyond the realm of human understanding, and I couldn't believe or accept that. Not when so many people were dying.

When you get the flu, your doctor doesn't throw up her hands and declare it senseless. You never hear people speak of "senseless cholera" or "senseless polio." There is a logical explanation, albeit invisible, debilitating, and lethal, for these diseases.

Take malaria. As a disease process, it's now well known. Mosquitoes carrying single-cell parasites, called plasmodia, in their salivary glands bite human or animal hosts and transmit the parasite to the blood. The plasmodia make their way to the liver, reproduce, burst out, and invade red blood cells; these rupture sequentially and infect the blood. The infecting agent, the plasmodia, can now be picked up by another mosquito, and the sequence repeats itself in another host. The complex process operates invisibly inside, outside, and between people and mosquitoes. (In this case, as we can see, the process is between people and mosquitoes, but for TB, AIDS, COVID, and many other diseases, transmission is just among humans!)

We understand the logic and science of this disease. We understand how an infecting agent enters the body, how it replicates, how it does its damage; we understand how it is transmitted to others. The spread of disease follows a series of logical steps we can understand.

From the start, I believed that there had to be an underlying *logic* to violence too. But we weren't looking for it, or we were looking in the wrong places. Or we weren't thinking very scientifically.

Faced with a diagnostic uncertainty, we have collectively classified violence as everything from a moral problem to spiritual malaise to an inborn character trait. Then, as now, it was common to cite poverty, drugs, poor schools, inadequate housing, and many other social and environmental issues as primary explanations for violence. All of them were (and are) grave problems that must be addressed as soon as possible. But as explanations for violence, they seemed insufficient and not specific. And none of these hypotheses explained or predicted the processes of contagion.

None of them explained, for example, why one person is more likely to abuse his spouse or children while another person from the same community is less likely. They didn't explain why one person with certain beliefs committed a violent hate crime while another person with the same beliefs did not, or why one person with a grievance might do a mass shooting while another person would never dream of doing that.

Nor does it explain why so many poor countries around the world have low rates of violence or why, as Paul Collier, a former lead economist for the World Bank, wrote in *The Bottom Billion*, that economic development has failed to bring decreases in violence.

"We failed at economically developing our way out of violence in these countries for forty years," he told me.

The more I read and thought about violence, the more convinced I became that explaining violence the way we were fails to grasp what is really going on. If we were going to make sense of violence, we needed to look deeper and differently. Not through the moral lens or the social-dysfunction lens — we'd tried that already, with little success — but through the same system of inquiry we use to understand other health problems:

What are the mechanisms? What is going on *inside*?

I now understand that we had a lot of this backward — fixing poverty, drugs, bad schools, and inadequate housing won't get rid of violence. Actually, addressing those problems is impossible while the violence is going on. Businesses can't flourish, kids can't learn, and poverty can't be reduced until the violence stops.* Reducing violence is therefore the most urgent task and clears a path to make many of the other changes we need.

---

* This was why, in the mid-2010s, the World Bank started a violence-prevention initiative for the first time in its history. I gave annual presentations at its headquarters. Their leaders told me the only reason they hadn't done this sooner was that their board was "risk averse." At the time, the president of the World Bank was a physician, but when they returned to having economists run the organization, they didn't keep up the programs.

Put another way, inadequate schools do not cause children to bully or beat up their classmates, but kids who fear being bullied or beat up at school will not be able to learn. Most people don't commit violent crimes because their businesses fail or because they live in low-income housing. But businesses fail because violent crime deters customers and raises security costs, and people get stuck in low-income housing because violent crime prevents property values from rising.

Violence can be termed an *everything problem* because it exacerbates all existing problems. Almost all serious epidemics do the same thing. They overwhelm life. And as with all serious epidemics, it is not enough to treat the symptoms. We need to understand and interrupt the underlying disease process.

THE LOGIC OF DISEASE

In San Francisco in 1981, while we were fighting the TB epidemic, signs of a new disease appeared.

Patients who were otherwise completely healthy young men showed up at SF General with extremely rare infections of the brain, eyes, lungs, heart, and other organs. Even as an infectious disease fellow, I had not seen most of these diseases before. My fellow doctors and I were at a loss to explain what we were seeing. Toxoplasmosis of the brain, *Pneumocystis carinii* infections of the lung, cytomegalovirus of the eye — it was unusual to see a patient with any of these diseases, let alone all of them simultaneously. And more and more of these patients were showing up every day.

And those patients were dying.

We were scared. We didn't know what was going on or what to do about it. We didn't know if we were looking at a new disease or just one we hadn't seen before. And, scarier still, we didn't know for sure but we feared it was contagious.

When my teacher and mentor in TB control, Dr. Phil Hopewell, got stuck with a needle while caring for a patient in the ICU, he feared he would get sick and die. (He didn't.) An orthopedic surgeon at SFGH was so terrified of this new and deadly illness, she refused to operate on people she believed might have it.

What to do?

All learning about a disease occurs through observation, characterization, analysis, and classification. Scientists, physicians, and epidemiologists are trained to describe a disease's characteristics, consider its causes (its etiology), observe how it develops or progresses within specific organs or systems of the body (its pathogenesis), and determine the underlying mechanisms that cause the symptoms.

And if the disease is contagious, we are taught to investigate how the infection spreads from one person to another. There are many different possibilities, and some diseases have more than one mode of transmission.

When I moved into a new role as assistant director of communicable diseases for San Francisco, I met daily with city officials, other epidemiologists, and infectious disease experts working to figure out the cause of this new epidemic. But I was also an assistant clinical professor at San Francisco General, so I still made regular rounds on the wards, and I saw the new disease up close. It had become clear to us that the disease was contagious because of the clusters in time and space and among people in close contact with each other. Patients had begun arriving in San Francisco from other parts of the country, seeking care that had been refused them in most of the nation's hospitals, so we also understood that this scourge was spreading well beyond the Bay Area and in dozens of other cities and states. And as our experience and the data made clear, it was spreading mostly among gay men,* especially those who had multiple partners and who did not use protection.

---

* This was not the case in Africa and in other areas of the world, where the spread was overwhelmingly among the *heterosexual* population. Several estimates suggest 80 percent of HIV/AIDS in Africa was heterosexually transmitted and 10 to 15 percent transmitted from mother to child. See P. R. Lamptey, "Reducing Heterosexual Transmission of HIV in Poor Countries," *British Medical Journal* 324 (2002): 207–11, DOI: 10.1136/bmj.324.7331.207.

This presented San Francisco city officials with a serious public health conundrum: How could we help the most heavily afflicted populations change the behaviors shown to be major contributors to the spread of this epidemic?*

We were all aware of how much violence, discrimination, and hatred the gay community faced, and we did not want to add to it. Even San Francisco, one of the largest havens for gay men in the country, had been roiled by homophobic violence in the recent past with the 1978 assassination of Harvey Milk, the first openly gay person elected to citywide office. The mayor, George Moscone, had been killed in the same shooting, paving the way for Dianne Feinstein — my new boss — to assume the office.

As a longtime city official — and the person who found Milk dead on the floor of an office in city hall — Feinstein was well aware of public health and safety issues. She was also an advocate for gay rights. She went back and forth with Mervin Silverman, the city's head of public health, about whether to close San Francisco's bathhouses, which were centers of gay life but also of unprotected sex. Closing them might slow the transmission of this new disease that was wreaking havoc on its hosts' otherwise healthy immune systems — but it also might further stigmatize gay men.

Mayor Feinstein eventually made the call to close the bathhouses in an attempt to reduce exposure. Still, this was only a temporary stopgap. I thought — we all thought — that it was just a matter of time before AIDS began to affect the general population. To prevent this from happening and to reduce further spread of the disease in the gay community, we had to understand it completely.

But even with this urgency and the full support of the city, understanding, diagnosing, and, eventually, stemming the tide of AIDS was slow work. It took two years to discover that it was caused by an

---

* Specific behaviors associated with this disorder included the use of IV needles, and it was particularly common among hemophiliac patients. However, the largest risk factor seemed to be a high frequency of sexual contact with other men.

infectious virus and two more to develop a test for it. During that time — and for many years to come — there was so much death and suffering, grief and mourning.

But all those thousands of hours researchers spent in exam rooms, emergency departments, ICUs, operating rooms, and research labs attempting to understand the disease, racing against time to treat the symptoms it caused — none of it was wasted. Because arising from the terror and tragedy of those years came a new understanding of what we eventually came to call HIV and AIDS: We learned how the infecting agent, HIV, spread and how it killed immune system cells, making the infected person susceptible to so many other infections.

Although there is still no cure, we now know what to do to prevent, treat, and control the contagion. We have come to make sense of this brutal disease and its biology and we can explain to people what it is, how it is transmitted, and what to do to avoid getting and spreading it. And in the years since, public health officials have gotten better and better at applying these methods, even in Africa, where the rates of infection were massively higher (as high as 30 percent of the population in some major cities) than they were in the United States.

Violence, like other devastating diseases such as TB and AIDS, has a variety of syndromes. Violence can present as bullying, domestic abuse, sexual assault, or gangland executions. It can range in severity from a schoolyard fight to a war. Yet, regardless of the form it takes, violence, like other diseases, follows the same predictable pattern.

Once we understand a disease's invisible logic, we can begin to make sense of how to fight it. And we have a set of strategies we can replicate.

DISEASE THINKING

My father was a research chemist. Listening to him talk about his work when I was young, I was captivated by the spirit of inquiry driving all science. I trusted science as a means to access and understand the invisible world.

I still recall the excitement of going with my father to his laboratory when I was seven or eight years old. Alongside children's-version biographies of Babe Ruth, Joe DiMaggio, and Jackie Robinson that I borrowed from the public library, I had begun reading about scientists like van Leeuwenhoek, Pasteur, Edison, Copernicus, Galileo, and Darwin. And now I was finally going to *see* science in action. I imagined a kind of magical workshop full of billowing fumes, vapors, and unusual visual marvels.

Instead, I mostly saw equipment — test tubes, beakers, and Bunsen burners. At first I was disappointed. Then my dad showed me that the microscopes and vials were the tools that made it possible for scientists to explore what was invisible to the naked eye.

It thrilled me, this realization that there was another world beneath our world, one that was invisible but completely real. It became my obsession and soon grew into a fascination with understanding the human body and how it worked.

Every Saturday morning, my mother took me and my brother to the public library, and I'd check out books about cells and germs. On my desk, instead of model cars or airplanes, I had a see-through model of the human body with removable organs and muscles, bright red arteries and blue veins, and nerves to and from the brain.

Often throughout my career as a physician and an epidemiologist, I have found my mind wandering back to those childhood visits to my father's lab, to the wonder I felt learning about the basic methods by which science makes the invisible world known to us. Even when technologies are crude, methods imprecise, and conclusions inaccurate, this quest to better understand is one of the most awesome things about science. It is a relentless attempt to make sense of what's going on in the body, and by doing this, science turns helplessness into hope and care and, in many cases, cure.

Tuberculosis is a powerful example of the progression from a disease's diagnosis to its near elimination. Scientists began to make sense of this most devastating of diseases, the world's oldest pandemic, only very recently. Ancient texts and bones show that TB has been with us for at least nine thousand years, and in fact, molecular studies have led some scientists to believe that it's been around for close to forty thousand years. And for essentially *all* that time, disability or death was the almost inevitable outcome for those infected.

No one really understood the disease correctly. It was thought for many years to be hereditary, sometimes with a supernatural twist. In the sixteenth century, the Swiss physician Paracelsus thought it was due to an internal organ not fulfilling its alchemical duties. In the early nineteenth century, New Englanders blamed the disease on vampirism, believing that family members who passed away from tuberculosis returned from the dead to suck the life from and infect the living. They were so confident of this theory that groups of villagers often dug up the corpses of those who had died from TB so they could perform rituals intended to neutralize the threat.

It wasn't until the 1880s, when German physician Robert Koch developed new methods to study the disease, that the true cause of TB began to crystallize.

Dr. Koch examined tuberculosis systematically, then designed a culture medium to grow the bacteria so he could test his theory. He infected guinea pigs with his culture, an extract grown from humans and animals with TB. All the guinea pigs died of TB, and the agent was found in them postmortem.

These results allowed Koch to determine that this mass killer was not hereditary, supernatural, or, as some believed, a moral failing. The agent causing TB was an airborne microorganism, a specific type of bacteria we now call mycobacteria. That the disease often showed up in the children of infected parents was a result of contagion, not genetics, not morality.

This was a seismic discovery. It meant that TB was not a curse, an inheritance, or evidence of God's wrath. And it was not unavoidable. Koch later won the Nobel Prize for solving the centuries-old mystery of tuberculosis, possibly the greatest killer of all time.

Thanks to his research, doctors and public health workers knew how it was transmitted, how infectious it was, and how it made people sick. They had a clear path forward to stop it, and some steps could be taken right away.

Things were starting to make sense.

STUCK THINKING

In the mid-1980s, when I was working in Somalia with the Ministry of Health's Refugee Health Unit to stem a cholera outbreak, the military commander under President Barre and the most powerful person in northern Somalia was General Gani. Concerned that the sickness could spread from Gannet, the first camp infected and the primary hot zone, to his military, he approached the medical team with a solution:

"We could kill the people with cholera," he proposed.

Our team was shocked and horrified. Of course we did not take General Gani's suggestion, but in a short time, I saw that, in his own way, he was following a certain logic: eliminate everyone with the disease, and you eliminate the disease. What General Gani didn't realize was that for every one person with the disease, there were many more *carriers* — people in a latent, presymptomatic phase of the disease, what's called the incubation period. These people were not yet sick but were still capable of spreading cholera invisibly.

Too often, given the limited understanding of how violence works, many people have been a bit like General Gani — they come up with solutions they believe are "tough," "clear cut," and "definitive" but that actually make things worse.

One could argue that America's criminal justice system has historically been predicated on a failed strategy of fighting violence with more violence. Prisons do not contain violence; if anything, they are incubators* of the disease, as they are for many other diseases. The threat of incarceration or, in some states, execution does not seem to deter it. And excessive force in policing escalates it. Punitive measures like these don't stop the disease from spreading; they accelerate the transmission.

The Somali Refugee Health Unit trained health workers from the camps themselves to fight the epidemic. They were taught to find people with early cases of the disease, isolate them and rehydrate them, provide clean water to the community, and support behavior change, and after weeks and months of tireless effort, we got the cholera outbreak under control in that region. And in just a year, we eliminated it completely from the whole country.

The old way of thinking is not working for violence. But as physician Harry F. Dowling wrote in *Fighting Infection*, "The proper direction and control of public health measures are impossible unless the leaders know what they are fighting against." And that starts with getting the diagnosis right.

DISEASE IN PRACTICE

Diagnosing a disease correctly requires a deep well of knowledge, training, and experience. But it also requires an openness and willingness to challenge preconceptions and biases. It requires being able to look anew at a patient or a problem while also evaluating everything the last doctor or even the last group of specialists said or saw. Sometimes we need to *rethink* a diagnosis, especially if a patient or community situation is not getting better.

---

* In prisons, exposure to disease is high, quarters are close, and access to medical care is intermittent at best. At the SF TB center, we regularly tested incarcerated persons for TB and contact-traced within the facilities. Later, testing programs and contact tracing were set up for HIV as well. Violence should be treated the same way as other diseases in our prison systems. Cure Violence conducted a pilot program of violence interruption in the UK's Cookham Wood Prison in 2015 and 2016 and found a 95 percent reduction in group attacks and a 50 percent reduction in all violence. Still, this only helped an already misguided societal response.

As a young physician, I saw many times how easy it was to cling to an incorrect diagnosis, accept a flawed premise, and just keep doing the same thing even if it wasn't working.

In the ER, the objective is to save the patient's life and reduce the suffering. First, doctors and nurses stabilize the patient: They stop the bleeding, provide respiratory support, and rush the patient to surgery if needed. Often, these measures are enough. But sometimes, these necessities can lead to a kind of myopia or tunnel vision. You can focus so much on stopping the bleeding that you don't look closely enough at the cause of it or at what is going on inside.

Some physicians did not see evidence of TB on X-rays in San Francisco in the early 1980s, but it was not because they were not competent or because they hadn't examined the patient and X-rays closely — it was because they had not *considered* the diagnosis of tuberculosis, a disease that some believed had basically been eliminated. They might have been looking for chronic lung disease or lung cancer, so even when TB was staring them in the face, they couldn't see it clearly.

People who work in public health, epidemiology, and disease control must think further — beyond individual patient care, and beyond the hospital. We need to see beyond the apparent and immediate presentation of symptoms to the illness's underlying processes as well as the broader canvas of disease in the community.

In the 1980s, it did not occur to me to apply the usual disease-diagnosis thinking to patients who came into the ER with injuries caused by violence. I thought — we all thought — that the cause of the injury was rather obvious: Someone had been shot, stabbed, or beaten, and that was pretty much the end of the story. Instead of trying to understand the disease processes underlying and surrounding the injury, we focused on the disease's immediate symptoms and outcomes — blood loss, tissue damage, death. We didn't zoom out to consider prior events or potential subsequent events surrounding the violence: Was this an isolated shooting or a retaliation? How did it connect to other shootings? And was the condition recurring — had the patient been treated for similar injuries before, and was he at risk of sustaining new ones in the future?

If we had taken the time to step back a little and approach beatings, stabbings, and shootings with more curiosity, openness, and care, we might have begun to think about violence as not merely an event but a disease and contagious disease state.

We might have asked ourselves: What happens next for this patient? What is the natural life cycle of this specific disease? What are all the other syndromes of violence we're seeing in him or others? How might this disease present differently in different people and places and settings? What does it look like in its earlier stages? Its middle stages? Its late stages?

And, most important, how does it spread and what do we do to stop it from spreading further?

PART TWO

TRANSMISSION

CHAPTER THREE

YOUR BRAIN ON VIOLENCE

The mind is a tool; the question is, do you use the tool or does the tool use you?

— Zen proverb

We aren't born violent. Violence is not innate, congenital, or inherent to an individual or group.* Nor is it a universal human urge. It is an *acquired* illness. And contagious.

It is understood that with every contagious disease, there is some agent that enters the body and replicates. In clinical medicine and epidemiology, this is called an etiologic agent, and it is commonly a virus or a bacterium or even a parasite. (Another etiologic agent of disease is the prion, which is not a living agent at all but an abnormal protein that replicates in the brain.)

People who have objected to the formulation of violence as a contagious disease sometimes say that violence can't be contagious because

---

* There are rare seizure disorders associated with violence. There are also variations in neurotransmitters, but these are not thought to play a part in the violence destroying our communities, countries, and world.

there is no single particle to cause spread, no specific collection of cells, or exogenous matter that sets off the chain reaction of new infections.

And yet, for other epidemic diseases in history, isolating the infectious agent had not been the primary diagnostic criterion. If you had the hacking cough of tuberculosis, the painful boils of bubonic plague, or the sweaty forehead and rosy cheeks of scarlet fever, you were diagnosed with that condition. The contagion seemed observable, even if the mode of transmission could not yet be explained.

We now know that cholera begins in the GI tract and small intestines when a person ingests *Vibrio cholerae*, usually by drinking contaminated water or by eating food that has been prepared by unclean hands. To become infected with TB, a person has to breathe in *Mycobacterium tuberculosis* after another person has coughed nearby; it then begins its course in the upper respiratory tract and lungs. HIV infects a person when the human immunodeficiency virus gains entrance to the bloodstream through unprotected sex, maternal-child transmission, or contact with contaminated blood from a transfusion or a needle.*
With violence, the infection begins in the brain when people experience or are exposed to violence — when they see it, participate in it, are victims of it, and, we learned, even when they *hear* about it.†

TB, malaria, and cholera are caused by "bugs" — small organisms that gain entrance to the body and then change the functioning of one or more organ systems. Although the infectious agent of violence is not visible under a microscope in the same way germs are, it still causes changes in how the brain and body *function*. The functional or structural change doesn't show up on routine X-rays or in blood work, but it is visible in the symptoms of people's behavior, sometimes years or decades after they were exposed.

---

* Most countries now screen all blood products for HIV; that was a priority among the African Ministries of Health I worked with.

† As we will get to later, the amount of exposure determines if there is an infection. For some diseases, we can test for infection; for others we either cannot or it is very difficult. In the next chapter we will learn about vicarious exposure.

And although there may not be a living particle that "infects" people with violence, the absence of a traditionally understood agent makes violence *more* dangerous than these other diseases.

TB is airborne. AIDS is transmitted via bodily fluids. With violence, there isn't a single infectious agent to avoid. It enters through a more efficient and infectious pathway than bacteria and viruses use. The closest that research studies have come to determining an etiologic agent is the *visual experience* of violence. In other words, we catch violence by primarily *seeing* it.

HIJACKING THE BRAIN

Dorland's Illustrated Medical Dictionary defines *disease* as "any deviation or interruption of structure or function of a part, organ, or system of the body, as manifested by characteristic symptoms and signs causing morbidity and mortality."

Take cholera.* Once the infectious agent enters the body, it can "hijack" the intestines, replicate there, and subtly change how the intestines work. One of the organ's chief functions is to absorb water from what we eat and drink, but the toxin shuts that ability down. Infected persons experience severe diarrhea, which can lead to acute dehydration, a life-threatening drop in blood pressure, and death — sometimes in just a few hours.

But this doesn't happen because their intestines have been damaged; it's because their intestines have *changed their function*. They have been commandeered — *hijacked* — and used as a site for further replication and transmission, rather than for normal healthy water and mineral absorption. The symptoms are caused by these changes in function of an organ system.

---

* As we will see with violence, most infectious diseases have complex pathways that work with or through existing physiological systems. Cholera produces a toxin that binds to cells lining the intestinal wall and activates an enzyme called *adenylate cyclase*. This increases the production of cyclic AMP (cAMP), which stimulates intestinal cells to secrete large amounts of water and electrolytes into the intestinal lumen.

This is what a contagious disease does. Upon infecting a host, it copies itself, and that replication allows it to spread to others.

This is the main story of a contagious disease: It replicates, resulting in changes in function with, symptoms of disease, disability, and, in some cases, death.

Violence is no different. But the organ whose function it changes isn't the gut or the lungs.

It's the brain.

Exposure to violence involves many parts of the brain. It begins with the brain's visual-processing center: You are exposed to violence when you witness it. You become infected when a neural system essentially makes a copy of the behavior you witnessed and encodes that script into your brain, where it may lie dormant for days, weeks, or even years. That infection turns into full-blown symptomatic disease when something causes you to consciously or, more commonly, unconsciously activate that violence script to provide "relief" from physical, social, or emotional pain.

In short: Violence changes the brain's functioning.

Exposure to violence changes how people think and, in turn, how they act.

THE VISUAL EXPERIENCE OF VIOLENCE

The experience of violence is processed visually. The optic nerve, which starts at the back of the eye, is actually *part of the brain* and an automatic port of entry into it. The journey from eye to brain is direct and immediate. Once you see something, it's in your brain.

This is especially problematic because it means there are no initial physical barriers to the intake of violence. The body has at least some defense mechanisms at entry for fighting off diseases that are encountered from the outside — it can repel flu, cold, and COVID viruses at the level of the mucosa and defuse intestinal pathogens like *Vibrio cholerae*, *E. coli*, and salmonella through the normally present stomach acid.

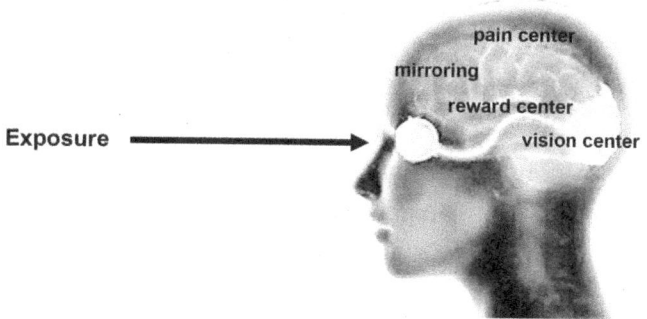

However, with violence, there is nothing standing between exposure and infection. As you see an act of violence, the image hits your retinas. Photoreceptors turn that image into electrical signals, which are carried through the optic nerve to the relevant areas of the brain. These signals imprint on the visual cortex and other brain areas.

This is your brain acquiring an initial infection or imprint of violence. Even if you have no conscious intention of acting violent, violence can be coded into your brain. If so, it remains there, latent, until possible moments of activation.

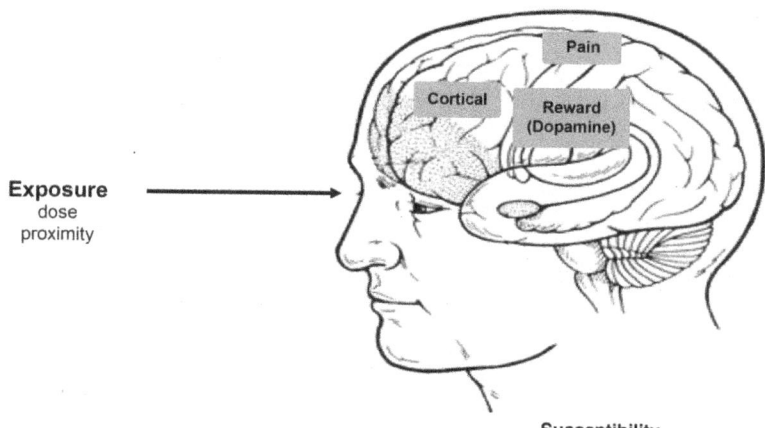

BOBO ON THE BRAIN

In 1961, the influential psychologist Albert Bandura ran a study with two- and three-year-olds, children who were old enough to speak but not advanced enough yet to have formed a full repertoire of conversational gestures. They were still learning how to move through the world — how to act, how to interact, and how to describe actions to others.

Children at this age are constantly learning, but not everything they learn is purposely *taught*. Three-year-olds are less like pupils sitting at school desks and more like sponges soaking up what goes on around them.

Bandura suspected that this "sponge-y" style of learning was far more powerful than people realized, and he set out to prove it. In his lab at Stanford, he established a playroom with a variety of toys, including Bobo, an inflatable clown with a weight at the bottom; if you hit the clown, it would go down and then rocket back up. Bandura brought a group of three-year-olds into the room and observed them from behind one-way glass. Most played contentedly with many of the toys with no clear preference for any in particular. Then an adult came in, walked up to Bobo, punched the toy in the face, threw it in the air, and said things like "Sock him in the nose!" and "Pow!" He did this multiple times, then left the room.

After this event, with no prompting, almost all of the thirty-six kids in the experiment walked up to the clown and punched it. Many of them yelled what they'd heard the adult say: "Sock him in the nose!" and "Pow!" No one had told the children to do these things; they just did them.

Why?

Bandura's relatively simple experiment is often cited as a critical turning point in the scientific literature of observational learning. In a way, his work shows us what we already knew: So much of how we learn to be in the world comes from observing others and unconsciously copying their behaviors; it's the starting point for how behaviors are formed. Some of the earliest things children learn to do is smile in response to a smile and make a face in response to someone making a face. When you stick out your tongue at children, they'll stick out theirs. When you laugh, they laugh.

When I give presentations, I sometimes show this photo:

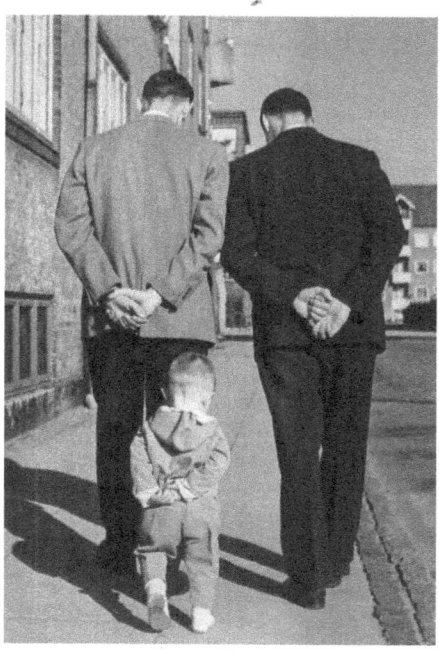

It's a slightly humorous scene: Two men are walking with their hands clasped behind their backs, and the toddler between them is doing the exact same thing. No one had to sit this child down and tell him: *This is how adults walk in the world.* He just did it.

Whether it's toddlers imitating how grown men walk, children learning to speak, musicians watching each other's hands on the piano keys, or dancers picking up new moves in real time on the dance floor, the neurological mechanism is the same. All of these behaviors proceed through copying (also known as mirroring). This is one of the brain's most efficient and powerful mechanisms to acquire new behaviors and skills at any age.

We are constantly copying, mimicking, and mirroring the people around us, usually without even noticing it. Have you ever moved to a different part of the country and found yourself slowly acquiring the regional accent? Or adopted the mannerisms of a friend, a partner, or even a TV personality?

A neuroscientist colleague, Charles Frith, once described an experience he had while strolling with a colleague of his who had a limp from childhood polio. "When we walk together," he told me, "I can't help but find myself limping as well." Like so many other processes in the brain, this imitation goes on behind the curtain of awareness.

MIRROR, MIRROR

In 1992, Italian neuroscientist Giacomo Rizzolatti and his graduate students were studying the brains of macaque monkeys, specifically the premotor cortex — the part of the brain where preparation for movement occurs. Located just in front of the motor cortex, the premotor cortex selects a complex set of movements to achieve a certain goal, then puts the whole process in motion. You might say it codes these specific motions. For example, in the case of eating a piece of food, one moves one's hand over the object, grasps it, lifts it, and puts it in one's mouth.

Electrodes were inserted in the premotor cortex of the monkey's brain, and a laboratory technician would stand across the room, pick something up, then put it back down, signaling the monkey to do the same. Eventually, Dr. Rizzolatti and his team were able to successfully locate the specific premotor neurons that fired when the monkey performed this sequence of actions. In the process, he and his team found something else — something they hadn't been looking for.

As the story goes, while eating lunch in the lab one day, a scientist on Rizzolatti's team heard the sound of increased electrical activity coming from the apparatus attached to the monkey's brain, even though no experiments were taking place. All the scientist was doing was eating lunch — in front of a plate-glass window, right in the monkey's line of sight.

Click, click, click — the machine was recording the neurons' activity.

The monkey wasn't moving. He didn't have anything to pick up. But as he watched the scientist pick up a spoon and lift it to his mouth, his brain — specifically the part of his brain related to motor activity — reacted as though the monkey were performing that same act.

In other words, the monkey didn't have to perform an action for the neurons in the premotor cortex of his brain to fire — *he just had to see it being performed.* Those brain cells have come to be known as *mirror neurons,* and they were subsequently found in humans as well. Mirror neurons may be present across the brain, but so far, scientists have located them primarily in the premotor cortex, where movement is planned and regulated. When you observe others, mirror neurons activate your motor system — this is one of the ways imitation works.

Prior to Rizzolatti's research, scientists believed that the brain was like a switchboard, receiving sensory inputs toward the back and middle of the cortex and directing them to various regions of the brain for integration, synthesis, and analysis. According to this model, if you performed an action such as picking up a spoon in response to smelling a hearty bowl of soup, the action was actually the last step in a long chain of communication among neurons. First, the brain registered the odor and classified it as something desirable. After that, neurons in your prefrontal cortex (the area that governs what we think of as decision-making) directed your body to eat and sent signals to the premotor and then motor areas to instruct your arm, hand, and fingers to pick up the spoon. After you dipped it into the soup and brought it to your lips, the mouth, throat, and swallowing mechanisms went through their own complicated maneuvers. All executed in milliseconds.

This switchboard model was orderly. Everything happened quickly but sequentially — from neuron to neuron, brain area to brain area.

But Rizzolatti's research — and the research of other neuroscientists, such as Marco Iacoboni — revealed a key shortcut: *The same neuron* that codes for *seeing* an action also codes for *doing* the action.

Essentially, these neurons condensed what scientists once believed were multistep pathways into a single type of cell, allowing perception and action to take place almost simultaneously.

Mirroring

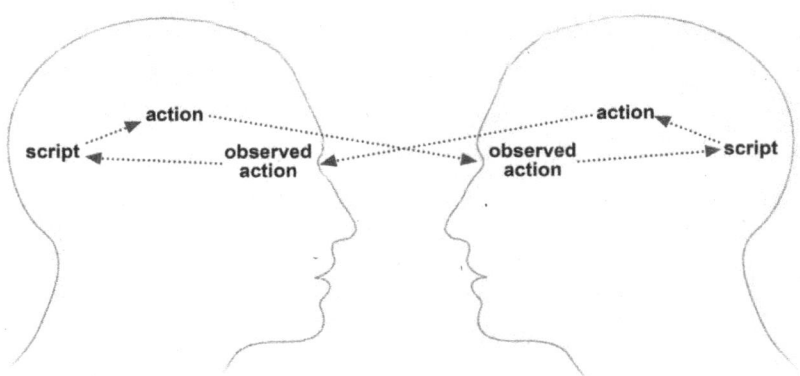

Though scientists had models for imitation for decades, the discovery of neuron types that both see and do can help us understand how *seeing and copying* happens.

Mirroring is a remarkably efficient process that helps the brain learn new behaviors. The problem is that mirror neurons don't differentiate between right and wrong, good and bad, helpful and harmful.

In *Contagion of Violence*, a landmark Institute of Medicine and National Research Council workshop report published in 2013,* Dr. Iacoboni suggested that the presence of this mirroring mechanism in the brain explains why we are "automatically influenced by what we perceive, thus proposing a plausible neurobiological mechanism for contagion of violent behavior." Mirror neurons, Dr. Iacoboni continued, "provide an important missing link between the social science

---

* I was on the planning committee of this historic workshop, which was attended by some of the leading scientists and clinicians from the United States and around the world, including researchers who studied several different syndromes of violence. This workshop was key to the scientific acceptance and validation of the epidemic nature of violence.

data on contagion of violence and the model that draws similarities between contagious mechanisms in infectious diseases and contagion of violence."

Newer research is beginning to uncover the role this mechanism may play specifically in priming the brain for violence. In one study, Stanford University researchers found that when mice watched other mice fight, the neurons in their brains fired as though they themselves were fighting, and when those neurons were subsequently activated, the mice became three times more aggressive. Although these experiments were done on mice, we know that in humans, too, seeing violence causes more violence. The fact that the human brain contains mirror neurons "indicates they may have been conserved across evolution," wrote Nirao Shah, a professor of neurobiology at Stanford and the lead author of the study.*

Rizzolatti's experiments showed that once you see an action performed, the action can be coded in your brain whether you mirror it or not at the time, a finding that helps explain the long latency period that violence often has in the body. Imagine a man who witnessed domestic abuse as a child and vowed never to repeat the violence he saw his father inflict on his mother but then, *decades* later, found himself doing exactly that. The script for violence was latent, or inactive, in his brain for all those years, existing on a cellular level without his conscious knowledge.

When you see an act of violence, your brain doesn't simply store it away in the memory areas. It acquires it as a set of complex actions, behaviors, and, perhaps, felt experiences.

Engaging in acts of violence is, of course, much more complex than grasping and lifting an object. But mirror neurons are not the only mechanism by which complex behaviors are imprinted on the brain. Another is the acquisition of what the social psychologist Rowell Huesmann calls scripts — that is, preloaded complex responses to common events. Dr. Huesmann's research has shown that people

---

* In this study, the mirror neurons not only mimicked but controlled the behavior, as the neurons were in more primitive parts of the brain, including the hypothalamus.

who see or encounter violence often encode a unique response script: A child sees his father insulted by his mother, and in response, his dad yells at and beats up his mom; the child talks back to his mother and is slapped in response. The more we're exposed to a violent script, the more our minds replay and rehearse it. And the more likely we are to respond violently later when an inciting situation arises.

This is analogous to the way TB symptoms can appear long after the infection entered the body. In a typical case, TB settles in the lung and replicates, but not to the stage of producing clinical symptoms. First it lies dormant.

A dormant infection can persist for decades. But if there is a shock or change in your immune system — in your *susceptibility* — the disease can rise to the surface. This is what we saw in Uganda (and globally) with HIV. The virus was that shock to the system, damaging people's T cells. With their immune systems thereby weakened, dormant tuberculosis became active disease.*

Infection occurs when violent scripts are copied and replicated in the brain. Yet these scripts can lie latent for years or even decades,

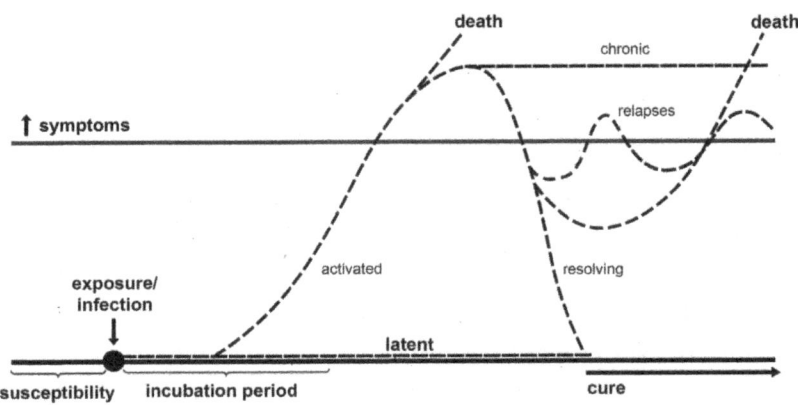

Possible Courses of Contagious Disease

---

* This shock to the system or effect of HIV/AIDS on tuberculosis happened globally. I reported on this and the mechanisms to WHO's first Global Meeting of Ministers of Health, First International Conference on the Global Impact of AIDS, March 8–10, 1988.

invisible, just as a case of shingles doesn't emerge for half a century after a childhood bout of chicken pox. The violent scripts remain latent until some trigger in the body activates them to symptomatic disease.

THE BRAIN ON DOPAMINE

The brain on violence uses the *same neural pathways* that govern our most basic human needs: food, sex, belonging, and relief from pain.

These are the neural pathways for dopamine, a neurotransmitter primarily found in parts of the midbrain. Although dopamine was discovered in 1910, it wasn't until the late 1950s that Swedish neuropharmacologist Arvid Carlsson and his colleagues revealed dopamine as the key player in the brain's reward system.

Since then, a lot has been written about dopamine pathways — specific routes that are activated in the brain in response to outside stimuli. These roads run through deeper and more primitive levels of the brain than the cortex, and they are where dopamine mediates experiences of motivation, reward, and pleasure. When you see something that you like or want or need or that excites you, your brain releases dopamine. Broadly put, humans are wired to engage in dopamine-releasing behaviors, because dopamine makes us feel good.

Everyone has a typical dopamine baseline — an amount usually present in the brain. But when you experience something pleasurable — or, more precisely, when you *expect to* — there is an increase in the amount of dopamine released; it floods those brain pathways and motivates behavior toward a goal. After you achieve that goal, however, and return to your baseline, that baseline might be lower, which means you need to engage in even more of the behavior to experience the same amount of pleasure you did before.

It's no coincidence that we get dopamine boosts from the anticipation of food and sex as well as from social connection, approval, and belonging. Survival requires that we eat, that we compete for mates, that we reproduce, and that we gain acceptance within groups. So over time, the brain evolved to reward these activities.

Reward Network

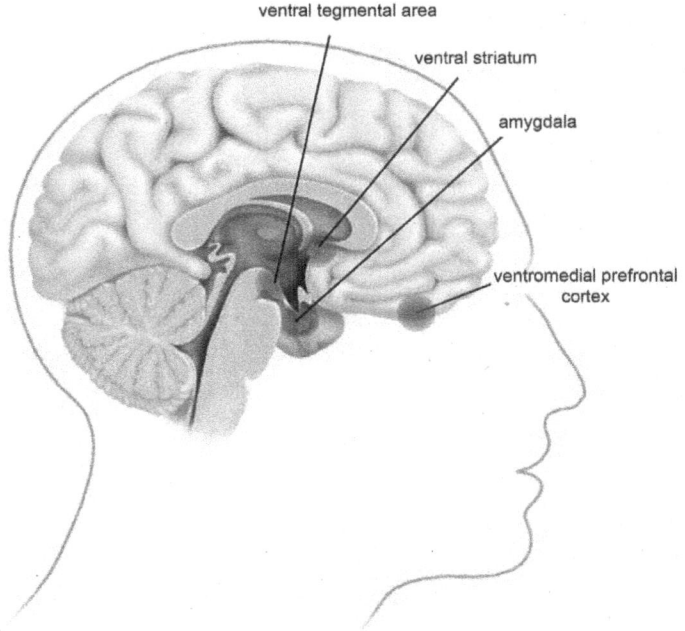

Physical reward, food, sex
Social reward, belonging, influence

The same goes for violence.

Of course, when it is inflicted on us, violence does not usually cause a dopamine release. But when committing violence provides relief from emotional pain (for example, if a person hurts someone against whom he has a grievance), increases social standing (or prevents it from falling), or otherwise leads to a physical or social reward, the brain may be flooded with this motivating neurotransmitter. What's more, the anticipatory nature of the dopamine pathway means that the relief or pleasure you feel is derived not from the actual behavior but from the expectation of relief or pleasure that you believe the behavior will bring.

In other words, the dopamine rush might come not from the first bite of the steak but from the sizzle on the grill, not from the pizza but from the delivery person ringing the doorbell, and not from the sex itself as much as from the anticipation of how the romantic evening will culminate.

Imagine the brain as a forest, a dense, complex ecosystem with acres of trees, vegetation, and rocks. The foliage is unremitting; branches and brambles make it hard to see very far on either side.

Then you notice a clear path running through these woods, twisting and turning in the thickets of greenery. You know that if you follow the path, you'll end up somewhere good — someplace bright, someplace airy, someplace where you will find relief or joy. Maybe the beach.

Dopamine is like that path to the beach. Along and at the end of that path are things that you believe will make you feel good or bring relief. The *anticipatory* nature of dopamine release is what makes violence so extraordinarily seductive. Under the right circumstances, violence feels good. But you don't have to engage in violence to get that feeling; you simply have to anticipate the hit of dopamine that violence will bring when it is rewarded by social acceptance from your peers or others you want to impress. The script was already in your brain.

SOCIAL PAIN IS REAL PAIN

But it isn't just the anticipation of social reward that motivates violence. Sometimes, the motivation is the other side of the coin — the avoidance of pain. Anyone who has ever suffered from a relentless toothache or a dislocated shoulder or any number of other injuries or diseases knows that pain narrows the world. We will do almost anything to avoid or escape it.

Too often, people think of pain as being physical only, something that happens to your actual body. Touching a hot stove, hitting your thumb with a hammer — that is what we think of as "real" pain, whereas the psychological pain of loss, of grief, of ostracization is considered different in type and seen as perhaps less real.

But the brain, of course, is not just a part of the body. It is *an integrated system*. And research indicates that social pain — from rejection, disapproval, humiliation — is just as real and often just as painful as if from a physical wound.

The science is clear that rejection by a romantic partner or social exclusion from a workplace community, a group of friends at school, or even a stranger is *real* pain and registers in the brain as such. Neuroimaging research shows that feelings of social exclusion activate the dorsal anterior cingulate cortex and the anterior insula* — the same areas and pathways that are activated by physical pain.

Although physical pain feels like a single, unified experience, pain

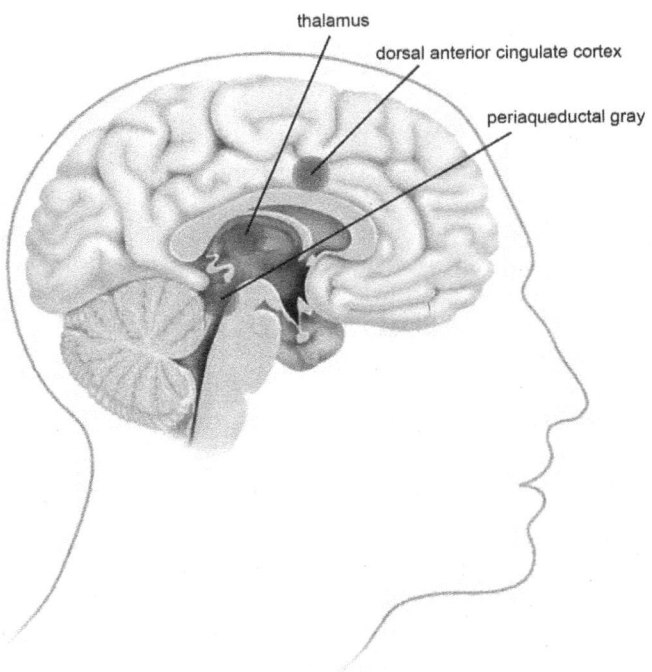

Pain Network

Physical pain, injury, sore
Social pain, exclusion, rejection, grievance

---

* The anterior insula is located laterally in the brain, and not shown in this medial brain view.

researchers have found that physical pain has two components. One is the sensory process that tells you where the pain is and what it feels like (whether it's burning, sharp, dull, et cetera); the other is the affective process that tells you that the pain is unpleasant and a source of great distress.

Even though being excluded, mocked, or dumped isn't a physical injury (there is no fresh wound or broken bone), your brain processes the event using the *same affective component* of the neural network that processes the feeling of the wound or broken bone — the part of the brain that tells you, *This really hurts and I can't stand it.*

And that's enough. You do not need both components — sensory and affective — for a feeling to qualify as pain; you can feel its depth and understand it emotionally even though there is no localized injury.

Social pain is real and terrible. Naomi Eisenberger, a researcher at UCLA, has proposed that the brain evolved to process social pain in this way because, historically, rejection and disconnection were just as threatening to our species' health as physical injury. When people are separated from the group, they are vulnerable. Humans are social creatures and depend on others for survival.

Sometimes the desire to experience the pleasure or potential reward of social acceptance and avoid the pain of social exclusion can be useful and foster norms that benefit the majority — for instance, it might lead people to vote or quit smoking. But when the social pressure of your group encourages or requires violence, as was the case for Yummy, it can be lethal. The dopamine system does not distinguish between good and bad, right and wrong. It simply moves toward the likelihood of social acceptance and away from the likelihood of exclusion. This is why doing everything you can to avoid pain might lead to more of it. And if you're in need of relief from pain of prior violence, you may cause more of it.

CHAPTER FOUR

EXPOSURE

When people are free to do as they please, they usually imitate each other.

— Eric Hoffer, *The Passionate State of Mind*

All contagious diseases are different. But every contagious disease follows the same epidemic sequence, whether it spreads within a family, a community, a country, or across the world.

Exposure
↓
Infection
↓
Disease
↓
Transmission
↓
Exposure to more people
↓
Epidemic

Imagine for a moment that it is once again March 2020. You've seen news reports about COVID in China and about the growing number of cases in the United States, but the disease doesn't seem to have come to your community yet. You go to a Starbucks. It's pretty empty, so you don't even think about a mask; no one is wearing one. You figure you're safe. Or maybe you don't think about it at all. As you wait in line, the man in front of you turns around and begins talking to you. He's a little close, you think.

He laughs.

Then he coughs.

If he has active Covid, this is **exposure**. But unless the man looks visibly sick, you have no way of knowing you've been exposed. Latte in hand, you walk home. That night you eat dinner, read a book, then go to sleep as usual, feeling fine. On the invisible level, however, coronavirus has begun to take hold. The cough delivered a viral load large enough to get past your body's first defenses: your nasal hairs, moist mucosa, some local antibodies from similar past infections in the nose and mouth. Already, the virus is beginning to replicate in your nose and throat.

This is **infection**.

You might not have any symptoms yet. But two days later, you're coughing. You try to wait it out, but the cough doesn't go away, and you're starting to feel very sick. Your body aches. You have a high fever. Soon you have trouble breathing.

This is **disease**.

What is true for COVID is true for all contagious diseases, including violence:

The greater the exposure, the greater your risk of catching the disease.

PREDICTING ITSELF

Soon after arriving at the conclusion that violence as I was seeing it in Chicago was an epidemic disease, I assembled a group of physicians and local and national researchers who were investigating violence and related topics as part of a larger scientific advisory group. I was still digging into the data and beginning to think more deeply about how violence fit into the basic infectious disease framework. I'd been working on a graphic representation of sorts, a chart I could use to explain this new way of thinking to people without scientific backgrounds — politicians, community leaders, the public.

It looked something like this:

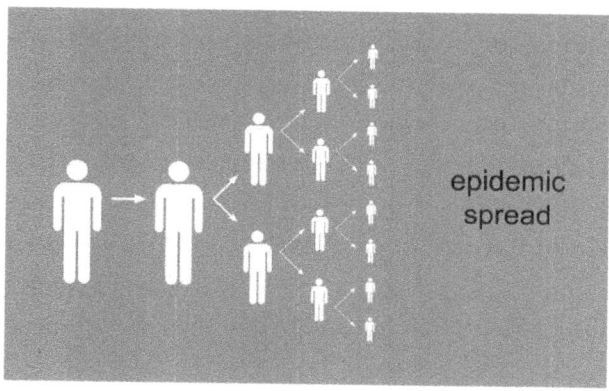

At this point, I was beginning to understand the logic of how violence spread and I could see its epidemic characteristics on maps and graphs, but I still hadn't worked out why it spread to some people and not others or how we could predict where it would spread next.

One afternoon, I was talking through some of these questions with Kathy Christoffel, a pediatrician and researcher at the Lurie Children's Hospital of Chicago and a professor at Northwestern University's Feinberg School of Medicine.

We were sitting in a corner booth at the diner down the street from her office finishing lunch, and I was sketching diagrams on a paper tablecloth and pointing at a chart I'd brought. I needed clarity on one particular issue: "What is the greatest predictor of a violent event?" I asked.

In medicine, we always want to know this sort of thing. Understanding that, for example, untreated hypertension is the greatest predictor of a stroke and a long history of smoking is the greatest predictor of lung cancer is crucial for both preventive and diagnostic purposes.

Kathy peered over her plate at my tablecloth notes.

"That's easy," she said. "The greatest predictor of a violent event is a previous violent event."

Sitting across from her in the diner that day, I wanted to smack myself on the head. It really was that simple.

One act of violence follows another. It predicts *itself*.

Kathy knew this from literature and practice. She'd seen it her whole career in pediatrics. When a patient came into the ER injured from a shooting, others would inevitably follow. I'd seen this myself in San Francisco, although I hadn't put the pieces together. And the community knew it too. Everyone said that violence begets violence.

I had already seen the typical epidemic-shaped waves on graphs of killings in Chicago, Los Angeles, New York City, Memphis, Detroit, and the country as a whole. I had already seen the hot-spot-like clustering of violent events on the maps of Chicago. But I had missed something basic.

If something is a risk factor for itself, you are dealing with not just disease but *contagious* disease.

The logic of disease, in its most basic form, is straightforward: cause and effect.

The logic of contagious diseases is that *cause and effect are one and the same.*

The greatest predictor of a case of flu are other cases of flu. The greatest predictor of a case of TB are other cases of TB. The same goes for meningococcal meningitis, measles, mumps, syphilis, gonorrhea, chlamydia, and AIDS.

Disease leads to more of the same disease anytime and anywhere there is contact and proximity — in homes, workplaces, schools, kindergartens, and prisons.

Communities do not suffer outbreaks of tuberculosis randomly. They suffer outbreaks of TB because someone with TB infected

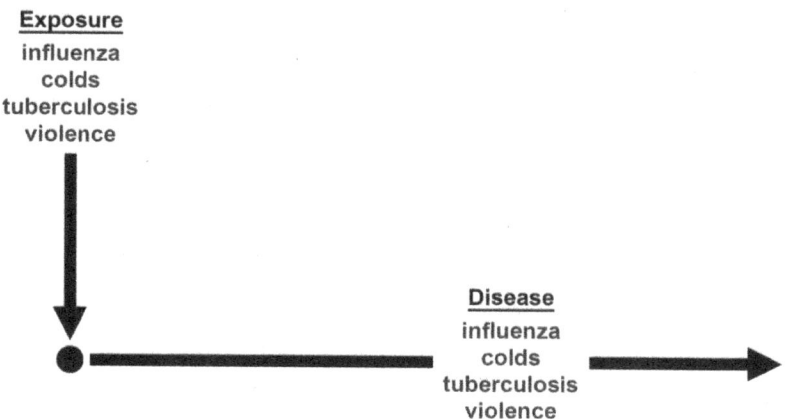

someone else in the community. (This is one of the reasons epidemiologists do active case finding and contact tracing — to see who else has been exposed and might need medical attention. And it's why we test family members and close contacts of patients with active TB.) The same is true with violence.

Of course, there are many factors, such as prior trauma and susceptibility, that contribute to how and why violence shows up in some people and not in others, just as there are many contributing factors that lead to developing (or not developing) other diseases. But the *necessary* element is specific: exposure. *Without exposure to violence, there is no violence.**

Our world is awash in images and depictions of violence — they're in the media, in films, in video games. Given this level of exposure, you'd think we would all be infected.

The good news is that the human brain can distinguish between different contexts — it can differentiate between the image of violence and the actual real-world analogue. While violent films and video games are often blamed for increasing levels of violence, extensive research has revealed no convincing evidence that they cause

---

* Completely eliminating exposure is almost impossible, of course. But by understanding the link between exposure and disease, we can take steps to limit the amount of exposure to infection.

real-world acts of violence. The brain is able to recognize when violence is fiction and when it is real — at least to a certain degree. This is perhaps one reason of many why youth violence rates in Japan are so low despite the high prevalence and popularity of extremely violent video games.

Social media, however, exposes users to real violence every day, reaching exponentially larger numbers of people faster than ever before. Not only does it allow the spread of violent images and videos of actual events, it can threaten, incite, or humiliate others into engaging in violence. And that violence is not fictional. It is very real.

The high visibility of violence across social media platforms has inspired copycat actions such as school shootings, mass terror attacks, and self-harm. It is likely that countless violent acts, ranging from bullying to insurrection, are related in some way to social media activity. And the integration of humanlike AI chatbots on these social media platforms and elsewhere is making the situation worse. Some chatbots have been characterized by social scientists as psychopathic and sadistic, and they can play a role in normalizing violent scripts of all kinds, including suicides.

But the fundamental question remains: Given that everyone has some level of exposure to violence, why is it that some go through life acting violently while others don't? Once exposed, what makes some of us more likely to be infected or "catch" violence than others?

That's what I wanted to explore more in Chicago in the late 1990s. I just needed a place to start. There was so much to do, and we were so obviously behind.

REDUCING EXPOSURE

Once I decided to use public health principles to fight this disease the same way we'd fought TB in San Francisco, cholera in Somalia, and HIV/AIDS in Central and East Africa, I realized there was no better place to start than my hometown of Chicago, a city with an extremely high exposure to violence and therefore a high level of transmission, disease, and mortality.

The problem was that I was a free agent now. I no longer had the backing of WHO or any institution. And fighting an infectious disease takes organization — strategy, management, political will.

Without those things, I would be seen by the local folks as nothing more than a guy with an idea, maybe a crazy one. I wasn't sure if I should start a new organization, something I'd never done before, or join an existing one. Neither option seemed right, but I knew I couldn't do this work alone.

Luckily, while considering all this, I got a call from a former colleague from my days at WHO. Wayne Wiebel is an epidemiologist and anthropologist and a very cool character, a freewheeling guy with a graying ponytail who rode around Chicago on a black-and-gold Harley just as he'd ridden across Southeast Asia in the 1970s.

Wayne and I had met in 1991 when I was asked by headquarters to identify the most promising approaches to stopping the spread of HIV/AIDS around the globe. It had been more than ten years since the disease had presented itself to the world, and we still didn't have a clear strategy to combat it. Moralizing and judgment still reigned, as did fear.

HIV/AIDS was different in Africa than elsewhere; it was much more widespread and had multiple different syndromes. In many cities in Africa, the hospitals were overflowing, sometimes with two people to a bed and patients camped out on the floors. The streets were filled with people visibly sick from the "slim" disease (named for the way it emaciated bodies).

By 1991, our WHO team had grown from one person to four hundred, and we had started to build the foundation of countrywide epidemic-control programs in a hundred and twenty countries. But our strategy was still missing several pieces.

Out of the hundreds of initiatives to stop the spread of HIV/AIDS that my team and I reviewed in Geneva, only thirteen had produced data, and only four or five had been well proven to work. One of those successful projects was Wayne's.

For years, Wayne and his team had focused on reducing intravenous drug use in some of the hardest-hit communities in Chicago, work that involved getting to know people who used or sold heroin. A street-smart anthropologist and epidemiologist, Wayne was well-versed in both the science and the culture: He observed and empathized nonjudgmentally. And over time, he gained the trust of the community and its leaders. So in the 1980s, when HIV/AIDS ravaged the city's drug users, many of whom shared needles, Wayne was already positioned to help. He and his staff educated the community about the dangers of sharing needles, helped distribute clean injection supplies, and told as many people as possible about the new virus that was responsible for the deaths around them.

Two aspects of his approach stood out. The first was that he deliberately recruited, hired, and trained workers *from the community*, people fluent in the social codes, the slang, and the realities of their daily life. The second was that he and his team not only provided support to infected persons, *they also identified the close contacts* of those infected persons — those most likely to be exposed — so that they could seek services and support.

It was a lot like what we did to control TB in San Francisco and cholera in Somalia: public education, community outreach, active case finding, and contact tracing to interrupt transmission and reduce further exposure. And it worked, producing a 50 percent drop in new HIV infections among intravenous drug users.

This is a common epidemic-control approach now. But in the United States in the mid-1980s, it was novel — and not always popular.

In fact, there was tremendous pushback, even in the public health field. In the fight against AIDS, for example, many people (including public health workers) didn't understand why people sick with drug addiction were "worth their time". In their eyes, "those people" wouldn't follow up after initial contact, allow themselves to be contact-traced, or use the clean needles provided; they were already presumed to be a lost cause. But Wayne's detractors were wrong; in fact, a few years later, his work produced a 70 percent drop in high-risk behaviors (notably sharing and reusing needles) and an 86 percent drop in new HIV infections.*

We at WHO took note and adopted his approach in countries all over the world where transmission of HIV was occurring through IV drug use. Wayne led the team in this critical work on HIV/AIDS, and he and I were in close contact for the rest of my time at WHO.

"They were ready to draw chalk outlines around drug users," Wayne told me back in the 1990s. "But I knew it could work."

Five years later, when I reconnected with Wayne in Chicago, it quickly became clear what we should do next. Wayne suggested that colleagues of his at the University of Illinois Chicago would be eager to be part of what I was dreaming up, and with his help, I was able to establish a foothold at UIC, which gave us institutional credibility for fundraising as well as a home base in public health. It was time to get to work.

INAUSPICIOUS BEGINNINGS

My office at UIC was at the end of a seemingly abandoned hall in an old biology-lab building on Taylor Street. In my darker moments as I sat in the tiny, windowless room that smelled of industrial cleaner, I imagined that the residue of decades-old chemical waste had seeped through the floors and into the walls. One day, after returning from a Westside Health Authority meeting, I was sitting in my dismal office eating an equally dismal lunch (tuna straight from the can) when a cheerful-looking woman in her late twenties — a PhD student in public health, as I soon learned — walked in.

"I'm looking for Dr. Slutkin?"

I wiped my hands and pushed my lunch away. "Yes?"

"My name is Kathleen Monahan. I was told you're someone I should talk to. The truth is, I'm not really sure why I'm here," she said.

---

* One of the other few early success stories in reducing new HIV infections was Susan Allen's work in Rwanda, which used credible outreach workers and counseling and testing to reduce new HIV infections by 50 to 70 percent.

"But my friends went to your talk last week and said I should speak with you."

I'd been giving lots of talks on campus and around the city, many at the invitation of community groups who had grown curious about "the WHO guy" and were interested in hearing about the new approach.

"They said, 'This guy sees things differently.' They thought we'd get along."

Kathleen was employee number one of an enterprise that didn't yet have an official name. In 1995, we had begun by calling it the Chicago Project for Violence Prevention. We were a concept in search of a team, with an idea in search of a more complete strategy. We needed to learn everything we could about violence in Chicago and contact people who were currently doing, or attempting to do, the work of violence prevention and who might want to partner with us, join us, or contribute their thinking.

Kathleen started accompanying me to meetings across the city, and her straightforward and outgoing nature made her a magnet for other young activists willing to think outside the box. At a Westside Health Authority meeting, we met LaDonna Redmond, a friendly, confident, tall Black woman in her mid-twenties who lit up and immediately understood what we were hoping to accomplish. I don't remember my presentation or the conversations that day, but I do remember stressing the need for a strategy to fight this problem.

LaDonna approached me in the doughnut line after the meeting. "I like what you said back there," she told me. "About strategy. I want to know more about what you mean and what you do. And how to do it."

LaDonna's background was in fighting substance abuse, and she had worked at a halfway house for women. She understood disease and believed, as I did, that sometimes what looked like a choice was actually a symptom. A few days later, LaDonna stopped by my office at UIC; she wrinkled her nose, as everyone did, at the smell. It wasn't just the laboratory smells. The building housed an ancient smoking lounge, not yet abandoned, and the scent of untold quantities of Marlboros came down the hall.

"I thought this was supposed to be a school of public health," she commented.

LaDonna seemed less than impressed with my office that day, but she wasn't there for the scenery; she was there to learn. While she'd long been curious about the broader ideas involved in public health, her work had always, by necessity, been focused on the day-to-day. At the halfway house, that meant managing the new arrivals, helping the residents stay sober, and making sure everyone was fed, but she was now our liaison at Westside Health Authority.

"I want the bigger picture," she told me. She was hoping to learn more about public health and how it worked.

From then on, LaDonna and I met weekly for what I began to call "office hours." Sometimes Kathleen Monahan stopped by too, bringing fresh fruit and ideas with her. Our meetings covered the basic principles of epidemic control and how we might apply them. I also invited researchers from the scientific and public health communities, including Wayne, to our strategy sessions.

Sometimes, with the magnitude of the work ahead staring us in the face, Kathleen would call us grandiose for believing we could resolve a problem as massive as violence.

"But as a society, we have done it before — many times," I always told her, reminding her of all the diseases that people didn't even think about anymore because they were effectively gone, consigned to the history books. Plague and leprosy had almost disappeared. Cases of polio had decreased by over 95 percent since the 1980s. Smallpox had been eradicated about fifteen years earlier.

"Violence is no different," I said. "The only explanation for why it persists is that people have never treated it using the public health strategy of epidemic control. We have to try it."

EXPOSURE AND DOSE

From 1998 to 2002, the sociologists Richard Spano, Craig Rivera, and John Michael Bolland conducted in-depth studies of young people in the housing projects of Mobile, Alabama. They wanted to better understand the independent effects of exposure to violence in low-income neighborhoods.

At the time, there was already quite a bit of research tying early exposure to domestic violence to a whole host of health issues later in life — depression, PTSD, risky behavior. There was also quite a bit of research linking childhood and adolescent exposure to violence with violent actions in adulthood. Victims of violent assaults, for example, were more likely to exhibit violent behavior in the future, and there were strong indications that those who had suffered abuse as children were likely to be abusive toward their own children.

But Spano and his colleagues wanted to look deeper. How did exposure to violence predict future violence over time? And what qualified as exposure? Was it limited to direct experience — that is, being the victim of violence? Or was witnessing it enough?

To answer these questions, Spano and his colleagues interviewed 348 children and adolescents over four years (they promised them their responses would be kept confidential). First they asked the kids about violence they had *witnessed or experienced*:

- Have you ever been threatened with a knife or a gun?
- Have you ever been cut severely enough to see a doctor?
- Have you ever been shot at?
- Has a member of your family or a friend ever been shot at or stabbed?
- Have you ever witnessed someone cut, stabbed, or shot?
- Have any of these things happened in the past ninety days?

Spano and his colleagues asked the young people annually over the next five years about any violence they themselves had *been involved with*.

- How many times have you been in a fight in the past ninety days?
- How many times have you threatened to cut, stab, or shoot someone in the past year?
- How many times in the past year have you pulled a knife or a gun on someone?
- How many times have you stabbed or shot someone in the past year?

Often, correlations emerged instantly: A teenager who got beat up started carrying a knife; a young boy witnessed a gang shooting, then joined a gang. But what made the study so intriguing wasn't merely the correlations but the fact that they were what epidemiologists term *dose dependent*. Put simply, the more exposure a child had, the greater the risk of infection. Children who were exposed to intermediate or high levels of violence, especially those who experienced chronic exposure, were over 3,000 percent, or 31.5 times, more likely to engage in chronic violent behavior than those who were exposed to no or low amounts of violence. Those young people showed little or no violence in the years to follow.

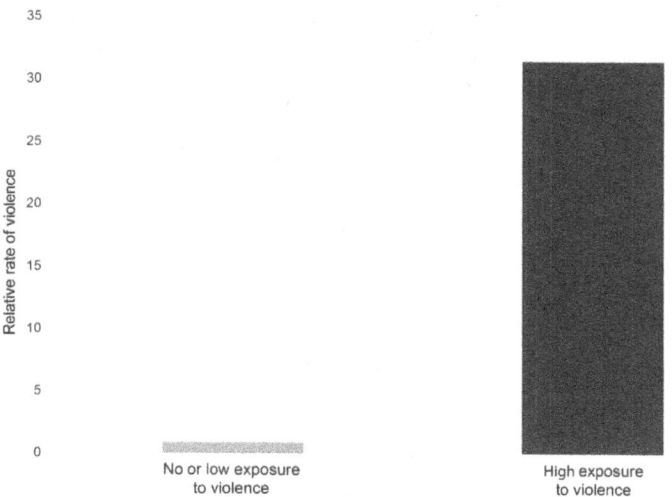

Higher exposure to violence results in higher rate of violent behavior.

A closer look at the relationship between low, intermediate, and high exposure over time can be seen here:

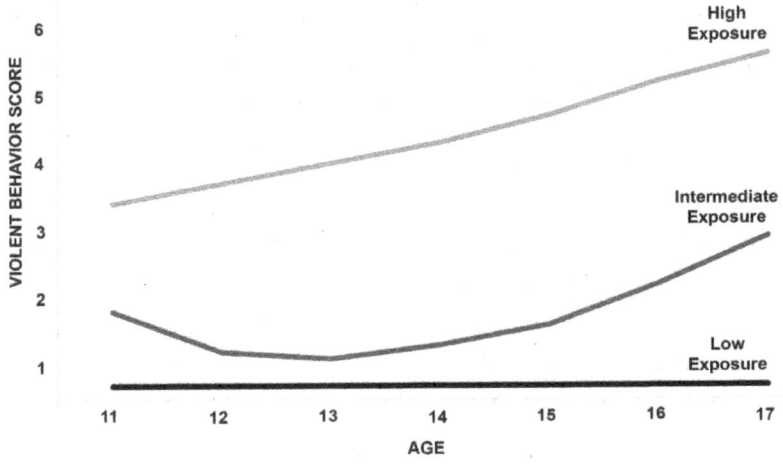

Higher exposure to violence results in higher rate of violent behavior over time.

Spano's study was a rebuttal of some stereotypical views about who experienced and engaged in violence for one important reason: Researchers controlled for poverty in their recruitment. All these kids lived in the same impoverished communities and belonged to families within a defined poverty level of between 57 percent and 91 percent. But they weren't all violent at the outset of the study, and how violent they became in the next several years was influenced overwhelmingly by one key factor: amount of exposure.

DEGREES OF EXPOSURE

For any infectious disease, the risk of infection depends on the degree of exposure, which can be estimated by considering *proximity* to a person or group, and the *dose* that person or group might be transmitting.

Dose is a measure of the actual amount of contagion your body experiences. Dose is the key factor in the infectivity of almost all contagious diseases. Some diseases can fully infect at very low doses; some require higher doses. But in general, the greater the dose, the greater the likelihood of an infection (putting aside individual variations in immunity, which we'll get to in the next chapter). Dose depends on your proximity to an infected person, the amount of time you spend close to that person, and the viral load (if the disease is viral).

For example, people who live in the same household as someone infected with TB have a higher risk of contracting the disease than relatives who visit only occasionally and a much higher risk of contracting it than next-door neighbors who rarely visit at all.

Viral load refers to the quantity of a viral agent present in a person's body. The concept of viral load helps us understand how much of the contagious agent your body comes into contact with when you are exposed. If the person standing in front of you in the Starbucks line is carrying an active — that is, symptomatic — COVID infection (meaning he has a lot of virus in his body), and he turns and sneezes directly on you, you could receive a high dose of the virus. If the Starbucks was crowded and not well ventilated and you spent twenty minutes just standing near the infected man, you would likely receive a sufficient dose to develop the disease.

Exposure means different things for different diseases. With airborne infections like TB, measles, and COVID, exposure can mean someone simply being in the same unventilated room as an infected person. But a disease like HIV/AIDS, which is transmitted through blood, semen, and other bodily fluids, requires a person to have direct contact with those fluids to constitute exposure.

With violence, exposure occurs *visually*. This can make infection even more likely in more circumstances than most other contagious processes, for a few reasons. First, you don't need to be physically close enough to it to breathe in air particles or share food, water, or sex; you just need to be close enough to *see* it. This means that several experiences in our environment have the potential to deliver a dose.

Further, proximity does not even need to be physical! Since the brain is the receptor, *proximity* may include social proximity, *perceived* social proximity, and even *desired* social proximity. You can be socially proximate in the real world to a gang, a fraternity, or any other peer network or you can be virtually proximate on social media through a group you belong to, feel kinship with, or simply *want* to belong to. That both physical and social proximity are relevant to exposure may explain why people can show symptoms of violence as a result of someone on social media promoting or normalizing violence. In fact, the *same brain pathway* that estimates closeness in *space* is used to assess closeness in *time* and closeness in *relationship*. In other words, a friend you talk to on the phone several times a week is still a close friend and influence even if he lives far away.* And he can still be a source of exposure — a social influence.†

A third difference is that dose can be *cumulative*. With contagious diseases like the flu, the exposure you had last winter has been cleared from your body by the time this year's exposure — which may be a new variant — occurs. But with violence, repeated past exposures and persistent ongoing exposures add up.

That additional dosage accumulates and changes your brain in a way that increases your risk of acute disease later. This was one of the findings from Spano's work as well.

Many things are so pervasive that they are hard to perceive as risks. Violence is one of them. It is ubiquitous or, more accurately, endemic in our communities and cities, in the news, and in our brains. But developing an awareness of the risks of exposure and learning how to reduce those risks can go a long way in diminishing your likelihood of contracting a disease. (There are ways to estimate and reduce risk that we will discuss later.) This is why it's essential for people to be educated on the disease of violence and *how it works*.

---

* This might mediate some of the combined effects of direct exposure and norms in anything from community violence to mass shootings to political polarization to war.

† In researching this book, I was amazed to learn that the brain uses the same neural pathways for social reward and physical reward, the same neural pathways for social pain and physical pain, and the same neural pathways for social proximity and physical proximity. And while this may be efficient in terms of evolution, all three of these brain pathways can get hijacked to produce the disease of violence. This may explain not only the effects of social media but that of felt or desired closeness with a political figure, or with an authoritarian leader.

TYPES OF EXPOSURE

Even though we know that the *amount* of exposure predicts the likelihood of infection and disease progression, there are, as with most things involving the human brain and body, a few variables. It is possible to have high proximity to violence but receive a low dose. Similarly, one can absorb a high dose without much proximity. To understand how these two key factors function, it might be helpful to examine a few situations and cases.

Scenario One

James has just started working as a prison warden. Though physically imposing, he has always been a gentle person and he has no history of violence. He applied to work in the prison only because he needed a job. He knew it would be challenging, but what he sees among the inmates — knifings, shankings, and beatings — shocks him. Not only that, but the other guards use excessive force on the prisoners. James does not. But he has already had to use his physical strength to defend himself, and he worries that soon he will be just like his colleagues, who hit inmates not only because they think they have to but also because they seem to enjoy doing it.* He recently found himself fighting the urge to push his wife around during arguments when he is frustrated and tired after his long overnight shifts.

Scenario Two

Stewart is a pilot in the US Air Force. All his life, he wanted to fly fighter jets. He fantasized about taking the helm of an F-22 Raptor and soaring through the clouds at nearly twice the speed of sound, flying in formation with his fellow airmen. His father and uncle had told him stories of navy fighters and the enemy planes they had shot down in the Korean War. He wanted to be just like them.

---

* This apparent "enjoyment" is sometimes seen in prisons, war, and other infections of the state in which belonging no longer produces a dopamine high, causing people to seek more of it in power and cruelty. (See Chapter 8.)

But his eyesight isn't perfect, so despite his stellar grades at the Air Force Academy and his promising performance in flight school, upon graduation he was assigned to a drone attack squadron and stationed at a base in Texas. Now his job is to pilot drones in several regions across the Middle East. Every day, he sits in front of a bank of computer monitors with a console of joysticks and levers in front of him. It's just like flying a small plane or helicopter — except Stewart is thousands of miles away from the terrain he glimpses through his virtual-reality goggles.

Most of the time, Stewart's job is surveillance. But occasionally, he is tasked with carrying out a strategic drone attack, dropping bombs or missiles on targets the US military has deemed a threat. He follows the target, often a truck convoy, and then, when he's given the order to attack, he points his joystick, locks on to the objective, and pulls the trigger, launching weapons that destroy the target on impact.

Most of the time, he can trick himself into thinking that he is just bombing a row of abandoned trucks or a cluster of empty buildings. But sometimes, he is zoomed in enough before he attacks to see a driver's arm hanging out of the window or a guard slowly walking a perimeter. That's when the guilt and remorse start to creep in. But even though he is fully aware that when he pulls that trigger, human beings generally die, the violence still feels to him more like a video game than real life.

Scenario Three

Julie has been a student at Grover Cleveland Middle School for about two weeks. She's new in town and is having trouble making friends in her seventh-grade class. One day after school, she sees a fight break out. Two girls from her class were taunting each other all afternoon. Slowly, the situation escalated from sarcastic remarks to threats and now to punching. It seems like the whole school has gathered to watch. Some kids from Julie's class cheer and egg the girls on, but Julie stands near the back of the crowd, feeling uneasy. These events are repeated over the next few weeks.

In all these scenarios, there is exposure to violence. But in each case, the exposure is different in amount and proximity.

James, the warden, is experiencing *a high, ever-increasing, and cumulative dose at close range*. Although he has no prior history of violence exposure and has just started his job in the prison, violence is all around him every day. Due to the cumulative effects of exposure, his risk will increase over time. Such persistent exposure has ripple effects within a prison and on the outside; it's already started, with James nearly bringing violence home with him to his wife, just as people carry other infections they get at work or school or anywhere else into their homes.

Stewart, the drone pilot, is getting *an indeterminate dose at low proximity*. This low proximity is both physical and social: Not only are his targets located halfway around the world, but he does not know their names, cannot see them clearly, knows nothing of their lives or families. They are nameless, faceless. Over the past decade, it has been found that drone operators like him are at high risk for PTSD. Even though they pilot their craft across the ocean from the actual field of combat, they often suffer from shame, guilt, and flashbacks. Still, they have not been shown to be at higher risk of future violence.

Julie, the student, is exposed to a *lower dose* of violence than James or Stewart, but her *proximity is quite high*, occurring right in front of her. Further, it involves members of her peer group, a peer group that Julie, as a new student, desperately wants to be accepted by. So while the schoolyard fight might seem like a nonevent — a story to tell her parents over dinner and then forget about — its effects on her could be pronounced. She might internalize the violence she witnesses and experiences, which can shape her understanding of what is normal, acceptable, and expected of her. She might one day join in the bullying.

So much of the initial research around adolescent exposure to violence focused on direct victimization — that is, a person who was the immediate recipient of a violent act. But Dr. Spano's studies and studies by several others have found that exposure to violence extends beyond being hit oneself. Young people with a history of chronic *vicarious*, or indirect, victimization were more than *ten times* more likely to be violent than kids with low exposure. This confirms that high proximity and high doses are highly predictive of future violent behavior, regardless of whether the violence was directed at the individual or at those around him. Like other infections, this disease doesn't care who the victim is or who is to blame. It will infect whoever is "close."

EXPOSURE DEPENDS ON WHO YOU KNOW

One of the original researchers assigned to assess Cure Violence's work in Chicago from 2000 to 2007 was a sociologist named Andrew Papachristos. He was the first to document the effectiveness of the epidemic-control approach and the ability of violence interrupters to significantly decrease retaliations in this initial seven-year period.*

A Chicago native, Dr. Papachristos had long studied social networks and how they functioned within gangs and other street organizations, specifically when it came to community violence. In a pioneering 2015 study in *Social Science and Medicine*, Papachristos and his colleagues analyzed six years of data from the city of Chicago, examining the cases of over ten thousand shooting victims. Prior studies had focused on transmission within smaller groups — a neighborhood, a gang — but their research took in the whole of the city. Using arrest data, Papachristos and his colleagues re-created social networks, establishing "degrees of separation" between shooting victims and the people who had shot them. This allowed the researchers to trace the movement of violence through these networks and see the varieties of exposure people experienced based on their proximity to violent events and to their peers.

What they found over the course of several papers was instructive. First, the vast majority of Chicago's gun violence was committed

---

* Papachristos was one of four researchers from four different universities using four different methods to examine the first seven years of work.

by a tiny minority of its citizens. About 6 percent of the city's population caused 70 percent of its nonfatal gunshot incidents. This was a major finding; it meant that the violence many described as being widespread in the city was in fact more limited.*

Second, the findings could not be ascribed to demographics alone. Models that attempted to track the violence based solely on factors like neighborhoods or race were not particularly accurate. But models that took into account both demographic data *and* social contagion — which Papachristos defined as spreading through social networks — matched up quite well and accounted for more than 60 percent of the over eleven thousand shootings. People often refer to "bad neighborhoods" when talking about violence in urban areas. Papachristos's findings revealed that the features of the neighborhoods mattered much less than the social dynamics — that is, the social connections — within them.

Third, Papachristos and his colleagues found that even *tiny increases in exposure* to gun violence increased the likelihood of someone becoming the victim of a shooting. Even a 1 percent increase in exposure tracked to a 1 percent higher chance of victimization, which meant that a person could be several degrees of separation from a shooting and yet be at significantly higher risk than someone who lived just down the street. This mirrors other infectious diseases, in which those who have less contact are less at risk.

These studies don't just posit a direct link between exposure and future violence; they show how proximity — in space and in relationship — relates to gradients of higher levels of exposure and hence to active disease.

In short, Papachristos's work shows that exposure to violence isn't just about where you live or where you are physically exposed; it's about *who you know*. It also shows that violence is transmitted in predictable ways. From the following image, one can see the cluster,

---

* This argues even more for employing the active-case-finding approach used for other diseases. Note that the percentage and specific people causing the incidents can change over time, hence the need to maintain case finding.

with the risk of disease increasing as you get closer in space and social relationship.*

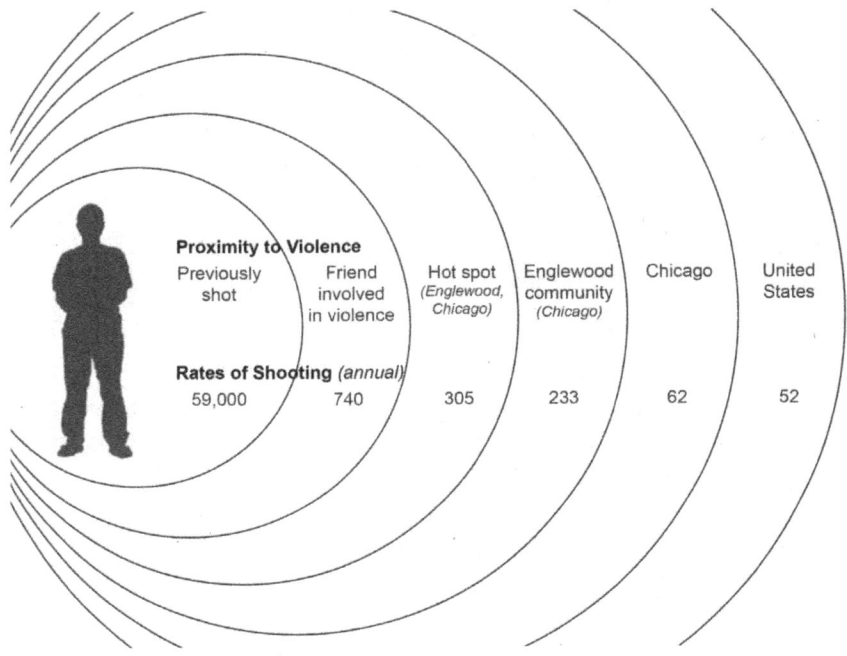

This is good news for several reasons.

For one, it shows that violence is not naturally endemic to a place or a people but the predictable product of proximity and dose.

These are things we can track. And these are things we can change.

It also means we can apply the standard public health strategy of contact tracing to find the highest-risk individuals and prevent future acts of violence. It means we can identify those in closest contact with known active cases (commonly referred to as perpetrators). We can figure out if children and teenagers are spending time with peers who expose them to violence and attempt to limit such contact. We can also better educate parents and grandparents and other caregivers about

---

* In chapter 8 we will discuss how the perception of social proximity (for example, interacting online with violent extremists or frequent exposure to an authoritarian leader who incites or normalizes violence) alters brain function in the same way.

how to work with those in the community to reduce exposure. Hospitals, health clinics, and schools can screen young people for risk by assessing past and current exposure and connect them to intervention services to keep them from progressing to active disease or relapsing.*

TRANSMISSION WITHIN AND BETWEEN DISEASE SYNDROMES

We must keep in mind that the different syndromes of violence are all part of the same disease. There are now over one hundred studies showing that exposure to violence makes people more likely to be violent; this is also how exposure works with other contagious diseases. Further, over thirty of these studies showed transmission *between* syndromes, meaning that a person exposed to one form of violence, such as bullying, might later display symptoms of another form, such as domestic violence, suicide, or even mass shooting. A victim of child abuse, for example, is more likely than others to commit child abuse decades later but also more

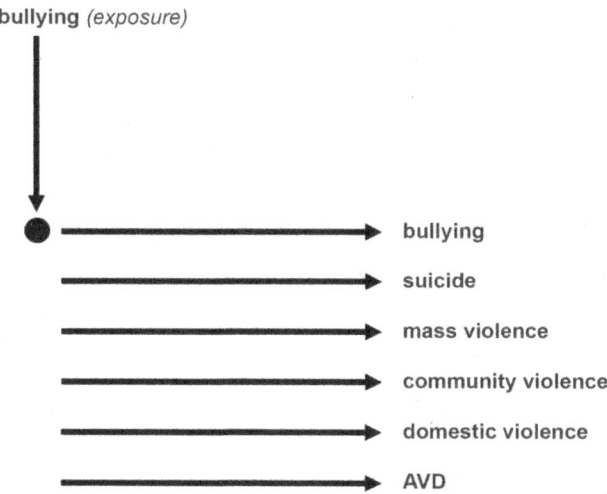

---

* Such hospital-based programs were set up across Chicago, and a national network in dozens of cities has grown. And there are many organizations and groups that can help with the behavior change and support needed. Screening for exposure in primary care and other settings is predictive as well.

likely to develop the syndrome of intimate-partner violence, community violence, or suicide. (Hence the importance of prevention and treatment of each syndrome to avoid the development of the others.)

Witnessing a shooting puts you at risk for more than being involved in a shooting. Having a friend commit suicide puts you at risk

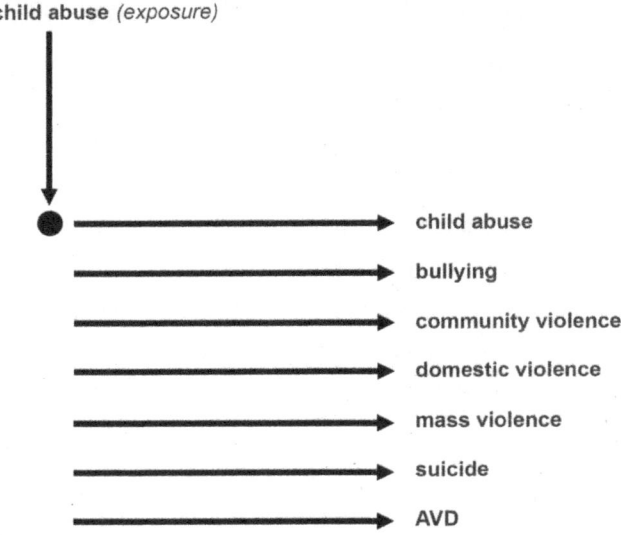

for more than committing suicide. Exposure to all forms of violence — including war — are risk factors for other forms of violence.

The fact that one type of violence can cause other types is why violence is categorized as one disease with multiple presentations or syndromes, just as TB, AIDS, and other bacterial and viral diseases can take many forms.

However, even with all we have learned and all the tools we have to reduce exposure, there will still be those who become infected, sometimes receiving high doses. And some of those infections will progress to full-blown disease. But others won't. Just as with any infectious disease, progression to an active case depends on the body's ability to fight off exposure and infection. When people begin to show symptoms of violence, it might mean that their internal immune-like defenses are insufficient or compromised. In other words, they have increased susceptibility.

CHAPTER FIVE

SUSCEPTIBILITY

The child who is not embraced by the village will burn it down to feel its warmth.

— African proverb

On the last day of his life, the seventeen-year-old boy with curly hair woke up early. He was in his mother's house, the same one he'd lived in his whole life, in the little room at the top of the stairs. It was like a cocoon, a place where he felt safe. Movie posters lined the walls; books were stacked neatly on the shelves. On his desk were his letters of acceptance to college and the rose he'd worn to his high school prom, pinned to the lapel of his tuxedo. Even three days later, it still looked alive.

The boy dressed quickly, kicking aside the dirty clothes on the floor in favor of a neatly pressed T-shirt, pants, and a coat hanging in his closet. His bags, two heavy black duffels, were waiting by the bedroom door. They were heavy on his shoulder.

It was 5:15 a.m., so early that the birds weren't awake yet, and the stairwell was still dark. He moved carefully, avoiding the creaky spot near the top of the landing, stepping gingerly on the outside of each stair. He stooped to avoid the low-hanging light fixture, then peered through the window at the Mercedes in front of the house. He and his father had bought it for $700 and spent months fixing it up.

But he had no thoughts of that now. No thoughts of all the happy times in this house — the birthday parties and Christmases and Friday nights he'd spent with his parents and his brother watching movies they'd rented at Blockbuster. The golden retrievers were sleeping next to the comfortable couch where he traded favorite lines from Monty Python with his dad; there was the spot at the breakfast bar where he ate pancakes with his mom, and behind the house was the lush suburban backyard where he and his brother had tossed a baseball around and played tag with kids from the neighborhood.

He wasn't thinking about any of that now. His thoughts were not of the love that he had been given, only the love that had been denied him. The times he wasn't invited. The times the phone on the wall in the kitchen didn't ring. All those late nights in his room with his diary open, writing poems that no one would ever read. Poems about love.

He was almost out of the house. All he had to do was take a step down, turn the dead bolt, ease the door open so it wouldn't squeak, and slip out. But then he looked back. And he must have made a noise.

"Dylan?" The boy couldn't see his mother, but he felt her presence; she was standing in the darkness in the doorway of her room. At that moment, he could have dropped the bags, walked upstairs, and hugged her. But he didn't. He couldn't turn back now. The plan — code-named NBK — was already in motion. Someone was waiting for him, and he couldn't be late.

"Bye," the boy said.

He walked out the door and shut it softly behind him.

NBK — short for "Natural Born Killers," after the 1994 Oliver Stone film — was the Columbine shooters' code name for the attack they carried out on April 20, 1999. The boy with the curly hair was Dylan Klebold. His friend and partner in the act was Eric Harris.

Together, the two teenagers shot hundreds of rounds of ammunition that day. They killed thirteen people — twelve students, and one teacher — and injured twenty-one more. And as tragic as this was, it could have been even worse. As law enforcement and investigators later discovered, NBK was supposed to be a *bombing*. In the months preceding the killing, the two teenagers had built dozens of pipe bombs, several of which they stationed in the school as well as in their cars on the morning of the attack. But these weapons failed to detonate, so the two boys had to improvise on-site. They began walking the halls of the school, automatic weapons and rifles in their hands, shooting indiscriminately. After less than an hour, their pace slowed. Together, they entered the library and never came out. Both boys turned their weapons on themselves.

Many readers of this book know most of the basic details of this story. The images of that day are burned into the brains of nearly everyone who lived in the United States at the time. The killings were discussed endlessly in the media, the killers' motives examined from every angle. Were they taking revenge on bullies? Did violent video games and music make them do it? Were they sociopaths?

I don't intend to consider these questions because they miss the point. They are attempts to find a reason, a rational explanation for what led these two young men to carry out this brutal, devastating act of violence.*

But as an epidemiologist, I prefer to focus on the underlying disease process of the violence itself — specifically, how did these two young men catch and develop such a severe case? How had they become so susceptible to infection, and how did this infection manage to progress to such full-blown disease?

How did violence work in them?

---

* Patients also come up with reasons other than exposure and susceptibility for why they get flu and other communicable diseases.

We have already learned that exposure is the essential variable, necessary for violence to infect the brain. And we have seen that the dose of exposure predicts the likelihood of the infection "taking."

But as we also know, not everyone who was exposed to COVID got sick, and not everyone who got sick died. The same is true for TB, flu, cholera, measles, and all contagious diseases. Many people are exposed to infection and never show symptoms. Others do. Who does and who doesn't get sick has to do with exposure but also with one's ability or inability to fend off the progression to symptomatic disease.

This is the variable called *susceptibility*. Exposure is what happens from the outside — what is going on in the community, in the environment you are in, who you know. Susceptibility is how you handle the infection on the inside. Susceptibility is what is going on within you.

It's what we call a *host factor*, an existing internal state.

HOW INFECTION BECOMES DISEASE

When an agent of infection encounters a human body, there are many possible obstacles to infection, replication, and progression to full-blown disease.

There are, of course, external defenses to prevent infectious agents from entering the body — distance, barriers (like masks or condoms; these are partial protections that can stop some infections and decrease the effects of others), and the physiological defenses at the body's entry points, like moist mucous membranes in the nose and mouth and acid in the stomach. The body is better at blocking or deterring external influences that might be toxic or infectious than most people are aware. The skin, the largest organ in the body, acts as a barrier against many potential infections, as do the respiratory and gastrointestinal systems.

If a potential contagion does manage to breach the body's first line of defense — the physical barrier — the immune system is the next line of defense. It begins working to identify, repel, immobilize, and even digest potentially harmful pathogens. The human immune system is so efficient that healthy people often repel threats without even knowing they've been exposed to them. The B and T lymphocytes and other white blood cells detect, swarm, and disable or destroy invading entities; they make antibodies when some aspect of the body is in contact with infectious agents. That is why we don't experience symptomatic infections every flu and cold season and throughout the year.

Most of the time, bodies are quite efficient at blocking harmful outside influences. But when people are worn down and tired, malnourished, taking medications that suppress the immune system, or simply get older, they become more susceptible to disease. That means they are not only more likely to catch illnesses that their bodies would normally repel but also more likely to experience severe symptoms.

The susceptibility factors for many infectious diseases are usually related to age, sex, metabolic factors, and immunity. For example, very young and very old people are more likely to become severely ill with flu, tuberculosis, measles, and cholera, among other diseases. Similarly, malnutrition and immune deficiencies make people more susceptible to these and many other infectious diseases. We became aware during the COVID pandemic that certain people — the elderly, people with metabolic conditions such as diabetes and obesity, and those with immune deficiencies — were more susceptible to getting severe cases. (Though not being vaccinated was the largest susceptibility factor for severe disease and death once vaccines became available.) In all these cases, the underlying condition of the person (that is, the *host*) leads to a lesser or greater ability to contain infection in a more benign form.

With violence, too, there are known factors that make people more at risk of severe and acute disease. They are related to brain processes but operate in the same way as factors like malnourishment and advanced age do in bacterial and viral diseases: They weaken the system that is supposed to contain infection.

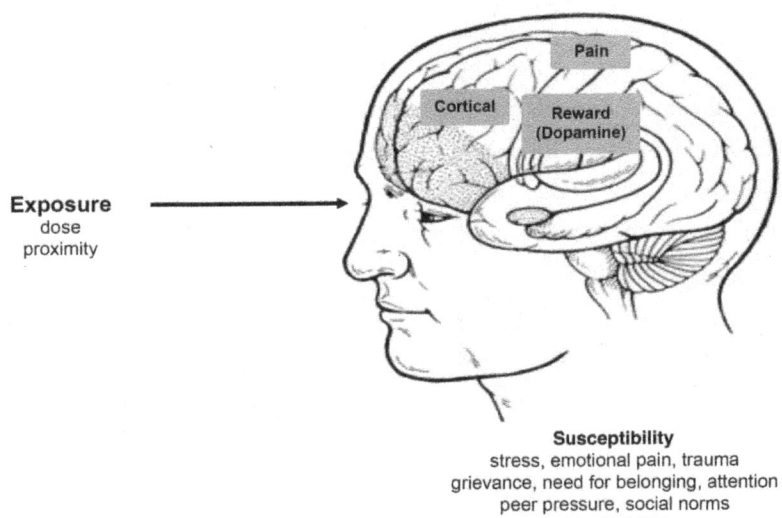

There are four broad factors that can diminish immune defenses and cause the *progression* from infection to disease:

Stress, emotional pain, and past trauma
Grievances and the need for belonging, attention, and status
Peer pressure and social norms
Age and gender

When you are stressed or triggered, certain physiological processes kick in — your heart and respiratory rate increase, your muscles tense, and your body releases stress hormones. Anxiety, nervousness, volatility — these are names we give to the bodily processes accompanying stress.

The brain is designed to process stress, but it does not always do so appropriately. Stress registers in the amygdala, causing the fight-flee-or-freeze response. The hypothalamus activates the pituitary gland, prompting it to release a precortisol hormone, ACTH, which stimulates the production of cortisol in the adrenal glands. The prefrontal cortex, which manages decision-making and control, is a potential regulator of some of these processes, but when you are experiencing extreme stress, the processes mentioned above often overwhelm your rational attempts to control your behavior. And function is changed.

And it's hard *to turn that system off*, especially when memories or past experiences are activated by life circumstances or events. This is what being *triggered* means neurologically, and it can occur months, years, or even decades after a stressful or traumatic incident or period.

However, if you have already contracted violence, high stress can be the trigger that pushes you further into fight territory, especially if you believe you have a legitimate grievance and if the social norms in the community, at home, or both are such that violence is accepted or even expected.

If you feel that an insult has been directed at you or if someone says something demeaning about a friend or romantic partner and your brain is already primed for violence via prior exposure and infection, the signs and symptoms of violence can be activated.

Consider the example of a man who as a child witnessed his father's repeated physical abuse of his mother, swore never to do it himself, and yet decades later did exactly that? When he saw his father hitting his mother years ago, the image imprinted in his brain. This imprint lived, dormant, for decades. Then one day, when he was insulted and fired from his job, he went home to his wife, who called him a failure; to his children, who were screaming; and to a pile of bills.

Pain and grievance present.

Stress high.

And the social norm that he learned as a child, that violence against women was acceptable within the home, was also present.

And so, without doing what we might consider *thinking*, he raised his fist and did what his father had done and what he'd sworn he never would. A script of violence that lay dormant in the brain for decades was activated.

None of this was the product of a reasoned decision, nor was it mere impulse. It was the progression in the brain's networks from exposure to infection to latency to activation of disease.

The brain's frontal lobe helps control these pathways, but only to a point. This limitation is especially relevant for young people, as the frontal lobe is not fully developed before age twenty-five. And alcohol shuts the frontal lobe down even more, which is why alcohol is often found to be a factor in the acute activation of violence.

Preexisting or newly acquired belief systems also influence susceptibility, particularly *obedience to authority* and, in some cases, *religiosity*,* both of which have been linked to certain types of violence, including hate crimes, violent extremism, and wars.

Social norms are enormous influences that can tip the scales toward violence. If the norms around you accept, expect, or praise violence, *you* are more susceptible. You have less immunity. But the opposite is also true: If violence is taboo in your social circles, you don't want to risk the disapproval of the people around you.

One day, a staff member named Tio came by my office. "Hey, Doc!" he said excitedly. "I finally got what you've been saying all these years about norms." He went on to tell me that he'd been at a bar the previous evening, and around two in the morning, someone pulled out a gun. Tio feared that all hell would break loose. But instead, several other patrons in the bar approached the armed man and said, "What are you doing? What's wrong with you?" The man put the gun away and the whole place quieted down.†

---

* This is a controversial area because of the lack of clarity about these terms; however, there is literature related to strictness and context. See chapter 8 for further information.

† Once, when I was called down to the ER at three in the morning, a particularly rowdy young man started punching the walls. He even turned a gurney upside down. We had just moved to a new building at SF General, so I said, "You don't understand — this is the new hospital. We don't do this anymore." He stopped. I still laugh at this story — at the fact that I thought to say this and at how well abruptly changing expectations worked.

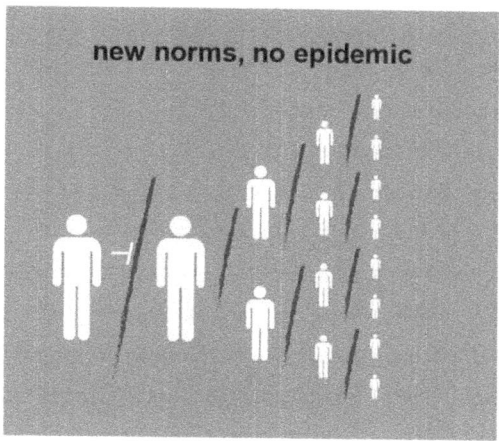

The opposite of susceptibility is resistance, or *immunity*. Immunity prevents an infection from progressing to disease. In the human immune system, antibodies and T cells are sophisticated and complex defenses that keep a dormant disease in check. However, the systems within the brain do not behave like an on/off switch, and in some cases, circumstances, emotions, and latent, deeply ingrained scripts overwhelm the brain's ability to hold a sickness at bay.

That's exactly what happened to Chris.

SAVING FACE

At nineteen years old, Chris was quiet and reserved — not the kind of kid who got into trouble. He had never been arrested but was sadly familiar with the criminal justice system. His older brother had been in prison for ten years, and having seen those narrow cell cots, the cold steel toilet, and drab cinder-block walls many times when visiting his brother, Chris had sworn to himself that he would never view them from the other side of the bars. He stayed out of fights, never experimented with drugs. When other kids joined gangs, he hit the books. He wanted to be an engineer or maybe a doctor.

But on this Monday morning, he woke up in a jail cell. He knew that from now on, things would be different. All his plans — the late-night study sessions, the hours of after-school tutoring, the community college brochures folded neatly in his desk drawer at home — were out the window. He had been charged with murder.

It had all started Saturday night. Two of his friends, Tony and Del, came by his parents' house with a girl he knew. They were on their way to a party, and they wanted Chris to go. He didn't want to. It was already late, and he knew they were going to cause trouble.

Tony and Del were brothers. They were new to the neighborhood, and in their old community, they had been involved with violence. They were friendly but volatile, and they took things personally.

"Are you guys invited to the party?" Chris asked.

"Nah," said Del. "But there's a problem we need to take care of."

Chris looked from one brother to the other. They were smiling. The girl, who was still in the car, was not.

"Come on, man," Tony said, leaning on the porch railing.

Reluctantly, Chris climbed into the Suburban with Tony, Del, and the girl. On the way to the party, he learned the real reason behind this expedition — they wanted to get even with someone there who had slept with Tony's girlfriend.

This was not Chris's fight. Nor did he want it to be. But once he was in the car, there was no way for him to extricate himself from the situation without losing face. He was in it. For the sake of his reputation, he had to go along.

At the party, Tony and Del quickly found the man they were looking for, and the three men exchanged words. Their voices kept rising until they were audible even over the thumping bass of the sound system and the chatter of other guests. Then the man cocked a fist and swung. Del pulled a gun and fired three shots in quick succession. And Chris was behind him, part of the scrum and then part of the fight that ensued.

When the police caught them in the car as they tried to peel away from the house, one person inside was already dead. By the time Chris arrived at the city jail that night, another two had been admitted to the hospital with major injuries.

At the jail, cops kept talking to Chris about his choices. The choice he'd made to get in the car that night. The choice he'd made to accompany his friends to the party. The choice he'd made to stand with them while things got worse.

But it hadn't felt like a choice to him at all.

"It just happened," he said.

A strong sense of belonging and acceptance, especially in a supportive culture, along with a balanced mental state free of undue stress and anxiety can strengthen immunity to violence. So can the ability to resist peer influence, although it is not always easy.

It's hard to resist peer pressure, especially at an age when the frontal lobe — the internal guardrail of rational action and planning — is not yet fully developed. But peer pressure is not a problem only for teenagers. The need for social acceptance is a biological and neurological reality for all of us. When you anticipate that some action will earn you respect, belonging, recognition, acknowledgment, credit, or status, it can be extremely hard to resist.

We often think of physical needs and psychological needs as different — physical needs are seen as real, while psychological needs are just nice-to-haves. But that's not the way it works.

If your reputation is very important to you or if your position within a social group is threatened, social reward can seem like a crucial necessity. The dopamine that you get from social acceptance and approval is so powerful, it can drive you to do whatever it takes to be accepted, liked, and approved of — even if that means going along with violence.

In Somalia, reputation is highly valued. It is a matter of mostly social custom or what might be considered informal law in Somali society to resolve conflicts in ways that allow people to maintain their social status in the eyes of their peers.

For example, someone who caused an injury to a neighbor might be told by one of the wise elders who mediated conflicts to compensate the neighbor with two goats or a chicken or a few months of free labor. This compensation allowed the victims of these crimes to save face — to protect their honor without having to use violence.*

This custom reflects a vital truth: Humans don't just *want* social acceptance and status. We seem to *need* it.

A HURT AND A NEED

In her memoir *A Mother's Reckoning*, Susan Klebold attempted to reconcile what her son did with who she believed he was. Her son and his friend had planned the attack in her own basement, loading guns and filming each other ranting furiously about the pain they would inflict, and she'd had no idea. She had suspected nothing.

She wrote that, in the immediate aftermath of the attack, "the idea that Dylan could have been centrally involved in this monstrous event" was beyond her ability to accept or even grasp. "Instead," she wrote, "I conjured a million alternative explanations.... Was he duped into participating, thinking the ammunition was fake? Had it been a prank gone terribly wrong? Had he been forced to participate, under some kind of duress?"

Both she and her husband, Tom, Dylan's father, "believed with all of our hearts that Dylan could not have killed anyone, and we clung, not just for hours and days, but for months, to that belief."

And even after it became clear that he *had* done that — after the FBI visited, and after she toured the school, and after she saw the videos that Dylan and Eric Harris had made in her own basement — she still could not square the sweet, goofy, and sometimes sad child she'd known with the menacing, leering, *angry* man she saw on the tapes.

Many of the narratives that emerged in the aftermath of the tragedy construed Dylan's actions as retributive and vengeful, yet they

---

* In Somalia, I saw this firsthand; my colleague Qassim Aden Egal, the nephew of the president, brokered such arrangements. And Abdikamal Ali Salaad, the head of the RHU (and son of the great sheikh Ali Salaad), also spent some of his days in these mediations.

were curiously untargeted. He did not go after a specific bully or a group of classmates who had tormented him. Dylan had grievances. But mainly, he was lonely. He *felt* alone, even when he wasn't. He felt unloved, even though his family loved him.

"I feel so lonely, w/o a friend," he wrote in his journal. And then, as though the universe had been listening, Eric Harris came along.

Unlike Dylan Klebold, Eric Harris was outgoing, sociable, and charismatic. Active in team sports, he was extroverted; he prided himself on the ability to get people to believe things that were patently untrue. His default response to pain was not depression but anger edging toward rage. Aggressive and vindictive, he fantasized about beating, killing, and raping, plotting vengeance for small slights.

The two met in seventh grade, and Dylan Klebold and Eric Harris formed a strong friendship, playing video games, building sets for school drama productions, and sharing summer jobs. Each gave the other something he lacked: Harris found a quiet acceptance in Klebold, while Klebold saw in Eric Harris a model for how to direct his depressive, self-destructive tendencies outward instead of keeping them bottled inside. Unlike Harris, who drew swastikas and guns and violent scenes of death, Klebold plastered the pages of his journals with hearts. Page after page cried out for love and cursed existence for keeping it from him. "A dark time, infinite sadness," he wrote. "I want to find love."

It wasn't exposure to violent video games* or films or music alone that led Dylan Klebold to violence. It was that the acute, constant, irrepressible feelings of loneliness and pain weakened his immunity, similar to the way a preexisting immunodeficiency weakens the immune system of someone exposed to COVID.

---

* In 1995, at a global meeting on adolescent health held by WHO and UNICEF in Chiang Mai, Thailand, I was cornered by colleagues from many nations concerned about violent US media infecting their countries. One participant talked about the Arnold Schwarzenegger movie *Terminator* and other movies that had come to Paris, and a colleague from Thailand asked if I and other Americans could please come help them work on reducing violence, since the problem was new to them but they assumed the US had expertise.

The extensive media coverage of such high-profile events combined with the high susceptibility of young men like Dylan help explain why mass shootings are a particularly contagious form of violence, according to an in-depth mathematical study of this phenomenon by researcher Sherry Towers. When viewed through the lens of susceptibility and exposure, the fact that the number of school and other mass shootings rose greatly after the Columbine event should not surprise us. Many mass shooters have said they were inspired by this event.

Many infectious diseases increase in infectivity in the presence of open wounds or sores. With HIV, for example, studies show that for people who have genital sores — a break in the barrier of skin or mucosa — exposure to HIV is anywhere from twenty-five to fifty to, in some studies, over one hundred times more likely to result in infection. And that infection, if left untreated, is likely to result in disease.

For young men like Dylan Klebold, hurt and need is like that sore. They carry their need for love, acceptance, and connection like gaping wounds on their bodies, an open access point for disease. Research also shows that nearly all the mass murderers of the twentieth century were beaten, bullied, humiliated, or neglected during childhood.[*]

The disease already existed latently in young men like Dylan. And in the face of pain and need, their natural defenses aren't enough to resist, counteract, or fight off the contagion. Maybe they've endured a lot of loss, are being abused, bullied, disrespected, or ridiculed, or feel as though they've been wronged. Perhaps they've been rejected romantically, fired from a job, kicked out of school, or cast out of a group, and now they feel desperately alone and unloved. And maybe they feel they have no place to turn, no one to talk to, nowhere to put their rage, their despair, or their hurt. They know hurting others is wrong. But they are also desperate for anything that will soothe their pain. This is likely why, according to Violence Project data, 43 percent of

---

[*] See Chapter 8: Infections of the State.

mass shooters intended to die during the shooting, and an additional 33 percent had a history of suicidality prior to the event.

The good news is that sores can be treated. They can heal. And the same is true for the needs and grievances that make people more susceptible to violence.

WHO IS AT RISK?

During an epidemic, one of the first things field epidemiologists do after determining what the disease is and how it is being transmitted is locate where the majority of new infections are occurring. They ask: How fast is it moving? Who is it infecting most? And who is getting sickest and dying? This final question often leads us to the most susceptible populations. This is where we need to direct more of our resources and attention.

For TB, the most susceptible are the youngest, the oldest, and the most malnourished. TB also shows up in young adults and anyone with underlying respiratory issues like chronic lung disease. But the very young, the very old, and those who are malnourished are most likely to die from it. Being in a poor nutritional condition is a susceptibility for many infections, lowering immunity.

For COVID, we learned quite quickly that the disease posed a much higher risk of death for older persons; people over sixty-five died at almost one hundred times the rate of people between the ages of eighteen and thirty, and more than 80 percent of the deaths overall were in people over sixty-five.

With COVID, exposure carried much more risk for the older population than for others, but both the very old and the very young are more susceptible to severe disease and death from influenza and several other respiratory infections. That's because children's immune systems are still developing and don't protect as well as they do later on, and older people's immune systems lose their power to fight off disease.

For violence, a similar developmental effect comes into play, only in this case, the immune defenses are functions of the developing brain. This is why children and teenagers, with their less fully developed frontal lobes, are so susceptible to it.

Gender also factors into one's risk level for many contagious diseases. Female hormones seem to protect against certain diseases and increase susceptibility to others. Male gender correlates with higher rates and severity of disease for HIV, TB, influenza, hepatitis B, and, indeed, for violence. The highest risk factor for violence is being male and between fifteen and twenty-five years old. I don't think we pay enough attention to this.

According to data collected by the Violence Project as of May 2025, one hundred and ninety-two of two hundred mass shooters were male, and 84 percent were between eighteen and forty-nine years old. And FBI data shows that 88 percent of murders are committed by men. According to the CDC, 96 to 98 percent of mass shootings and 80 percent of all suicides are committed by men.

The reasons for this are likely due to a combination of biological and cultural factors. Regardless of age, males have a less robustly developed frontal cortex (the part of the brain that correlates broadly with executive control and decision-making) and a more active amygdala (the part of the brain that correlates with impulsivity and large emotional swings).

Further, according to the Violence Project, of the men who were mass shooters, 69 percent intended to die by suicide in the mass shooting or had a prior history of suicidality, demonstrating their pain or hurt. According to news reports, 25 percent were veterans, showing the crossover between the syndromes of war and mass shootings. And though these findings might be controversial, recent research suggests that violent trauma leads to real and lasting physiological changes in the brain that accentuate innate differences and may make the male brain more susceptible to violence.

But biology is not the whole story. If it were, some countries wouldn't have much lower rates of violence than others do.* The reasons that the United States ranks 128th among 163 countries in peace indices, for example, are largely cultural. They include individualism; a culture of aggressive posturing in government, in business, and on the streets; inadequate government and community responses to shootings; society's acceptance of violence as inevitable; and parenting styles that emphasize obedience and control. Europe and dozens of countries around the world have moved toward more nurturing parenting approaches, but the United States has been slow to change.

There are different norms for men and women across countries and cultures. Unfortunately, many men have been socialized in societies, communities, and families to feel that using violence is a normal, even expected, response to an insult or grievance. The more threats and violence people see on display, the more they internalize them. We all internalize norms and behaviors, even those that make us more susceptible to disease (such as smoking). These norms inform how we handle exposure, and our scripts guide the specific behavior.†

Another social accelerant to disease progression in violence is exposure to racist or sexist ideologies, harmful beliefs, and distorted stories. Norms that hinge on the idea that some people are better than others, more deserving than others, or more to blame than others give the brain its pathway from pain and grievance to anticipated relief, which increases the likelihood of progression from exposure to infection and from infection to disease. If exposure is reduced and the pain is treated with a different story, a different perspective, and a place to belong, the risk of progression decreases.

People who are taught their entire lives that members of another group are inferior or inhuman are primed, years in advance, to attack

---

* In other words, there are differences not only between men and women but also between men in one place and men in another.

† The US norms regarding acceptance of violence are higher than most other countries. A related variable is inner feelings of self-worth, which varies among nations. Teachers from Tibet and other Asian countries were surprised to find that their students in the US and Europe did not feel good about themselves.

and harm others. But even if they are *not* taught that directly, indirect exposure to such ideology can accelerate people's path toward the disease of violence. Think of Dylann Roof, the teenager who shot and killed nine people at Emanuel African Methodist Episcopal Church in Charleston, South Carolina. He was not raised by white supremacist parents, but his exposure to that ideology online in his teens normalized it and pushed him further and further into a worldview that encouraged violence against anyone who was not white. Impoverished, abused, and aggrieved by his perceived lack of opportunity, he became more and more susceptible to violence with each violent post he saw; his brain became a tinderbox awaiting the first spark.

Identifying specific risk factors for violence, however, is more difficult than identifying susceptibility to TB or COVID. After all, pain, grievance, and the need to belong are much less visible than, say, a person's age or degree of malnourishment. The risk factors of violence are also harder to quantify. How does one assess, with any degree of accuracy, the level of grievance in a nineteen-year-old boy whose girlfriend has just left him for a guy in a rival gang? How can you assess the anguish of a teenage girl who has been bullied since the first grade? What algorithm can put a number on that kind of pain?

While we do have several tools already in use to identify people most susceptible to contracting violence, none of them are good enough. Adverse childhood event (ACE) scores, for example, account for childhood abuse, neglect, trauma, and other forms of exposure to violence, but they don't capture the pain and need a person is experiencing now, in the present. We need better tools to aid parents, teachers, and public health officials in early detection.

A group from the University of Michigan and the CDC worked on developing a clinical screening score for predicting future risk of violence based on prior victimization, community exposure, peer influence, and fighting. However, with so many people in the United States relying almost entirely on emergency departments and urgent care centers for medical treatment, and in the absence of community health workers, there is little consistency of care or opportunity for active case finding and early detection or follow-up. And by the time violence hits the ER, it's usually in the late stages — gunshot wounds, broken bones, stabbing injuries.

Therefore, in some settings, including mass shootings or political violence prevention, the most effective way to identify those at risk for violence in the acute epidemic setting is by being in the community or in touch with the community — by tuning into what friends, neighbors, and family members see and hear and using public health strategies of active case finding and contact tracing. Active case finding requires two things: *manpower* and *social connection*.

In the mostly private and fragmented US health-care system, this kind of public health approach has not been the norm, even for conventionally understood epidemic diseases.

It doesn't have to be this way.

For other diseases and in other places, it isn't.

Even when I worked with the Refugee Health Unit of the Somali Ministry of Health (Wasaaradda Caafimaadka), for example, there were approximately one million refugees spread out in forty tented camps across the desert. (The tents, called aqals, were made of sticks and cloth; the refugees brought the sticks with them from Ethiopia.) We knew this population was highly susceptible to infectious diseases, including diarrheal diseases, measles, pneumonia, malaria, and TB, based on their young age and visible malnutrition. In fact, the whole population was likely highly susceptible due to malnutrition — in same cases extreme malnutrition — alone. We had only about six doctors and a dozen nurses and a paucity of resources. But *we had a system* — a network of approximately fifteen thousand community health workers (CHWs) and traditional birth attendants (TBAs) who had been recruited and hired from the refugee population itself. These CHWs and TBAs were in constant contact with the refugee population, doing active case finding for disease. TBAs knew and visited every pregnant woman and helped with every delivery, and they stayed in continuous and active contact with the moms and babies. The CHWs were actively looking to identify people with acute or chronic coughs or diarrhea or fevers in the refugee camp and throughout the entire population.

A public health approach to violence requires similar systems of outreach, detection, and care. We *cannot wait* for people to become sick and infect others; we must *look for* the people who are most susceptible to infection as well as for people with active cases who are most at risk of imminent injury or death.

That's what we did in Chicago.

TALKING TO PEOPLE

It took five years to solidify a strategy, acquire funding, and win support from communities throughout the city. But by 1999, we had several strategy papers and enough funding* to begin forming a coalition within a community. We chose West Garfield Park because it had the highest number of killings of any district in the city (and, we were told, in the whole country) at the time and because we had the support of Bethel New Life, a local community group led by Mary Nelson and Mildred Wiley, both of whom were eager for the outreach.

In time, I was able to get start-up funds from the DOJ, the CDC, and two leading and forward-looking Chicago foundations. This allowed me to hire a few more frontline public health workers to bring the message and the intervention to their communities.

These people needed to be credible, connected, and committed. They needed to have access to and trust within the community so they could find out where transmission was occurring, interrupt it, and help people begin to consider changing their behaviors and lifestyle.

Linda Toles was one of our first hires. She had lost her son to a shooting just a year prior, and the trauma of walking into a cold, tiled

---

* Including a grant from the Robert Wood Johnson Foundation, which enabled us to guide an epidemic-control pilot at small scale.

morgue and seeing "my baby boy's" big toe sticking out of the white sheet atop a metal tray had driven her into a very deep despair.

Through her grief, she made it her mission to do everything she could to ensure that what had happened to her son would never happen to anyone else's child.

Marilyn Pickford came to us after leaving her customer-service job with a telehealth company. She had grown up on the east side of Garfield Park and had heard about what we were doing and planning.

"What do you know about public health outreach?" Norm, a new hire who would go on to become one of our key leaders, asked her in her interview.

"Nothing," Marilyn admitted. "But I know how to talk to people. I know how to keep them on the line." Self-assured and openhearted, Marilyn did more than keep people on the line — she heard them, understood them, empathized with them. And never judged them.

Marilyn became the first outreach worker for Cure Violence (then called CeaseFire), and Linda followed soon after.

People like Marilyn and Linda were our eyes and ears in the community — and they were also the community's eyes and ears. They would walk the blocks for hours, talking to the guys on the corner and the grandmothers on their stoops, trying to find out what was going on so they could help stop the violence disease from spreading. They tried to reach those who were most susceptible so they could provide support and help them heal from their prior and ongoing exposure to daily violence. And they let people know what CeaseFire was doing and helped them see how that work benefited them and everyone in their community.

In a highly affected community with so many shootings, this approach had its dangers. One of the first times Marilyn walked a block, she approached two young men hanging out on the corner, said hello, held out a flyer, and explained who she was and what she and the project were doing. The men were wary but receptive, and they seemed to warm up when she mentioned where she had gone to high school. They knew some of the same people.

"Anyway, nice to meet you," Marilyn said. She was feeling accomplished and relieved that one of her first outreach interactions had gone so smoothly when out of the corner of her eye she saw something flying toward her. Then came the crash of shattering glass — a bottle hitting concrete.

Across the street, a tall man was riding by on a little BMX bike.

"Don't talk to her! She ain't y'all's people!" he yelled.

The words were out of Marilyn's mouth before she even thought about them: "Shit, if I was your people, I woulda shot your ass!"

This was definitely *not* the sort of thing that she had been trained to say. Her immediate reaction was to apologize, but before she could say anything, the two men next to her began to laugh.

"You're all right," one said. "That's the hood comin' out."

"We got you," said the other, looking with renewed interest at the flyer Marilyn had given him.

Marilyn already knew that the best way to earn trust was to be completely honest and completely herself. When she walked neighborhoods, she knew she was entering other people's space. She had to give something in return — not just a flyer, but her attention, her understanding. She had to give a bit of herself.

And it wasn't lost on her that, as one of the only women on the outreach team, she could get people to open up when others couldn't. Men would tell her personal things because they did not feel threatened by her. They could be vulnerable with her in a way they couldn't be with Tony, Reggie, or Rick, outreach workers on the team she was now leading. While talking to men about future shootings and killings, she often got the feeling that they wanted to tell someone what they were going to do so they could be talked out of it.

They sought her out, these men. They lived in a hypermasculine world in which most relationships with women were complicated, caught up in status and feuds. Marilyn was uninvolved, safe. She did not take sides. She listened.

CARING EYES OPEN

Our outreach workers were jacks-of-all-trades. They were community liaisons, helping us keep tabs on potential hot spots and volatile situations. They were part of a support network, helping victims and their families access resources. They were like contact tracers in a TB epidemic, following an incident of violence back to its source. Keeping track of the susceptible.

They were what I thought of as a cadre of paraprofessional public health workers, people who hadn't been to medical school or nursing school or maybe any other degree-granting educational institution but who knew what it was like to be exposed constantly to violence. These people had a kind of knowledge and feeling no school could teach. They knew the neighborhoods. They knew the people. They knew the language, the customs, the scripts. And they could see in a few seconds who was infected, who was *affected*, and whose prior and current exposure was likely to result in active disease.

But to control the spread of violence, we can't rely on the efforts of these public health workers alone. People in the community need to be educated and trained to recognize the signs a highly exposed and acutely susceptible person might exhibit in their speech, online posts, and behavior. And they have to do it before that person progresses — sometimes rapidly — from an early stage of violence to a severe and lethal one.

Imagine groups of trained public health outreach workers employed by the city or by nonprofits walking around their own neighborhoods where violence has been prevalent, greeting people by name, keeping tabs on who's been in conflict, who's been erratic, who's been making threats. Imagine teams of high school or college students trained in identifying violence and potential violence looking for early symptoms, making daily rounds of their classrooms and lockers or dorms, checking in with people to see how they were doing and offering help to those who needed it. And in the workplace, imagine an arm of the HR department focused not on documenting and punishing infractions but on keeping tabs on feuds or grievances with the potential to escalate to violence. Once they recognize these high-risk cases, these teams need to have somewhere confidential, trusted, and helpful to turn to with that information. As it currently stands, law enforcement and the medical establishment (hospitals and mental-health professionals) are where people commonly go to report an at-risk individual. The former is punitive, which prevents many from reporting. Who wants to get their son or daughter, their friend or family member, arrested? And with the privatization of health care and the hollowing out of the social service infrastructure, the current medical establishment is ill-equipped to deal with violence.

These teams need to be able to work confidentially and watch for changes over time, because susceptibility is not a static state. People can become more susceptible in response to a triggering event like an insult or less susceptible when something happens to make them feel respected or accepted, like getting a compliment. Thus the disease can accelerate acutely or gradually due to these and other outside factors.

We see this again and again in our work and in the field more broadly. We know that violence causes violence, which causes more violence, and so on. This is especially true for people who have experienced a high and cumulative dose of exposure and whose brain defenses are compromised. The good news is that your body's ability to fight off contagion is, to some degree, within your control. Smoking a pack a day makes someone more susceptible to respiratory infections like COVID, and quitting smoking does the opposite. For violence, if the experiences and norms people are exposed to weaken their immunity to it, then exposure to new and better ones can bolster immunity. In this, peers can help.

There is in fact a lot you can do to interrupt this physiological progression so you can keep yourself free of disease and avoid spreading it. When you protect yourself, you're also helping others.

Understanding how exposure works in the brain (whether you're aware of it or not) allows you to make different choices to limit your exposure. It also helps you see people who engage in violence differently — you can be more sympathetic about the exposure they've experienced. All of us have pain and grievance and a need to belong, at least to some degree. And we need to help one another with those things.

We can develop systems to treat this epidemic of violence by actively interrupting exposure among people, by interrupting worsening or progression of the disease, and by interrupting retaliation and further spread.

PART THREE

INTERRUPTION AND ELIMINATION

CHAPTER SIX

INTERRUPTING SPREAD

There is a crack, a crack in everything, that's how the light gets in.
— Leonard Cohen, "Anthem"

Camilo remembers the moment he realized his life had to change. He was in his childhood bedroom with a gun. A gun he was pointing at his mother.

"What are you doing?" she screamed over and over. "What are you doing?"

Camilo's hand was shaking; the steel barrel of the pistol wobbled in the air between them. Tears streamed down his face. *I don't know,* he wanted to say. *I have no idea.*

EVERYTHING I TOUCHED TURNED TO PAIN

Camilo grew up in Cali, Colombia, in the late nineties and early two thousands. Technically, it was a time of increasing peace in the country, which for decades had been racked by political violence.

The bloody days of leftist guerrilla groups battling right-wing paramilitaries were slowly receding into the past. But the neighborhood where Camilo grew up was as dangerous as ever; the violence had just morphed into another form.

Highly organized *grupos* with ties to drug cartels ran roughshod through the hillside barrios, spreading violence as part of daily life. So did smaller, younger *grupitos* without any ties to the larger gangs. These smaller groups, which were frequently composed of young men living under tough circumstances and in constant danger, vied for control, jockeying for status and notoriety, and were eventually incorporated into one of the larger citywide organizations. These mergers were not peaceful, and they were often coercive. Shootings were constant, and although most killings were targeted, many people were caught in the cross fire.

Camilo lived in a small six-room house with thirty other people. The family was desperately poor. He and his eleven brothers and sisters would play in the street during the day but rushed indoors whenever they heard gunshots or saw the approach of a motorcycle or groups of men they didn't know. Each of the siblings had dropped out of school by age ten or eleven to make money in the streets. At twelve, Camilo and some of his friends decided to "take over the barrio" — to form their own *grupito*. He got a gun. He and his friends began robbing people on the street and holding up small shops.

Camilo committed his first killing at thirteen.

And then, just as his *grupito* was gaining power and clout, one of the larger gangs swooped in. Every day, its members waited by the school, leaning nonchalantly on the fence near the entrance. They waited by Camilo's house and held court on the corner of a street they didn't live on. They pulled up their shirts to show guns, started fights for no reason. They seemed casual and at ease, but also menacing. It was a performance designed to intimidate the younger guys — boys, really. The gang wanted them to see what they were up against so they would allow themselves to be subsumed.

Camilo and his friends weren't being recruited by this rival gang; the gang wanted to *acquire* them, swallow them up. And the larger group's tactics became brutal.

One day, five of Camilo's friends were killed in front of him. The gang was sending a message: *Join us or die.*

So he did. He ran drugs. He robbed people. He kidnapped people.

"From the age of twelve," he told me, "*mi vida fue una desastre —* my life was a disaster."

To survive, he had to *normalize* his actions in his mind. He had to think of what he did as his job. Camilo had to see violence as a normal part of his daily life, because the alternative was death. It was, literally, kill or be killed.

Camilo didn't believe all the gang's talk about brotherhood. He had real brothers. His *grupito* had been something else entirely.

He came to accept the utility of violence; he believed it was the only way for him to protect himself. Over time, however, he also began to *enjoy* it.

He had felt powerless; violence gave him power. He had felt weak; violence made him feel strong. It made him feel *good*. Even a little high.

He wouldn't be the one to hurt. He would be a person who could hurt others.

He would be in control.

"Everything I touched turned to pain," he later told me. I wasn't sure if he meant the pain he caused, the pain he was in, or both.

In his childhood bedroom, Camilo was hyperventilating, his chest heaving, sweat pouring down his face. His hand was shaking, and it never shook. At the end of the barrel, he could see his mother's terrified face, her eyes wide with fear.

His mother, who had always provided for him. His mother, who had given him his life, was now facing the end of hers at his hand.

"Who are you?" she asked, fear in her voice. "Who have you become?"

This was the moment, Camilo told me, that his life changed course.

Every day, he had pushed down the pain and the constant fear. He hadn't allowed himself to picture the faces of the people he'd killed or kidnapped, or to remember the desperate cries of people begging for their lives. He'd sleepwalked through his days, numb and cold. And now he couldn't anymore.

Camilo lowered the gun.

He wept in his mother's arms.

TRANSFORMATION

When I spoke to Camilo, I felt as if I were speaking to two people. The first was a polite, kind man with a soft voice. He was thin and angular with high cheekbones, wide-set eyes, and a mouth that often flashed a brilliant smile.

When he talked about his current life, he was expressive and eager; he proudly listed the soccer tournaments he'd helped sponsor, the food drives he'd organized, the young men he'd mentored.

But when I pressed him to describe his old life, his face shifted. Everything in his manner became withdrawn. His brow furrowed; he rubbed his eyes and mumbled his answers to my questions in Spanish.

At times when we spoke, he cried quiet tears, remembering things he'd done, the person he'd been. It was clear to me he was still healing from the events of his earlier days, that his mind was still working to fight off the infection of violence inside.

The day after Camilo pulled a gun on his mother, he called Angelica, a woman from his neighborhood who had been like another mother to himself and his friends; she had known them since they were toddlers. He told her he was in trouble. She helped him get off the streets and into a mental-health facility, and when he emerged a month later, he felt like a different person — clean, sober, calm, and more in control of himself.

Ten years older than Camilo, Angelica understood his and his friends' struggles because some of those struggles had been hers too. She'd never judged their lifestyle, although she'd urged them sometimes to be safer. She took them to see live music and let them watch TV shows on her phone until the battery died. She asked them about their lives and teased them about girls.

She also encouraged them.

"*Tienes carismo*," she always told Camilo. "You have charisma. People follow you."

And people had — in the *grupito*, in the larger gang. Now he wanted to use that power to do something different. He wanted to pull people from the life he'd once had, to intervene before they found themselves pointing guns at their own families.

He wanted to lead young men like himself somewhere new, somewhere beyond the street violence and the drugs, the *grupitos* and the gangs. But as he contemplated changing his life, a nagging thought persisted in the back of his mind:

Would they follow him there?

A SECOND LIFE

Camilo is like a lot of the men and women who have worked in violence intervention using the model our organization developed and adapted over the past twenty-five years. Men and boys like Camilo are too often spoken of as a lost cause, people to fear and blame. They're not seen as individuals who got infected and then ill with violence, much less people who might be part of the solution rather than part of the problem.

Yet one of the most powerful insights in the field of public health and epidemic control is that it is precisely people like Camilo who are the most effective at helping to curb the violence epidemic in their own communities.

But curbing an epidemic isn't always straightforward. Treatment is not always available. And the existing public health infrastructure is not always sufficient to support outreach work.

To interrupt the transmission of these diseases, we need to follow a new playbook, one grounded in the world of public health.

PUBLIC EDUCATION AND BEHAVIOR CHANGE

Even when vaccines and treatments exist, our most formidable tool to stop an epidemic from spreading is helping a population adopt safer behaviors that both protect them from the disease and keep them from spreading it to others. In addition to providing medication (when it is available) and care, we must help people understand the disease that threatens them. There can be no behavior change without public education.

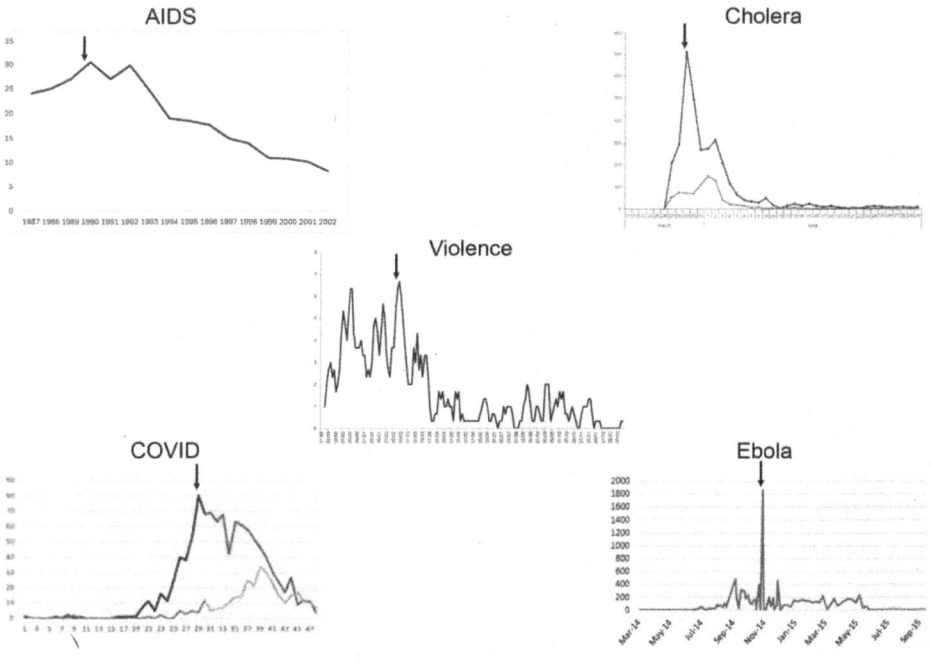

Effects of Behavior Change on Epidemic Diseases[*]

---

[*] Behavior change groups represent epidemics of AIDS in Uganda; Cholera in Somalia; Violence in Logan Square, Chicago, United States; COVID in New Zealand; and Ebola in Sierra Leone.

For a cholera outbreak, this means showing mothers how to hydrate their children fast, even when it doesn't seem like the children can keep any fluids in their bodies, and seek help quickly. For an HIV/AIDS epidemic, it means encouraging people to limit the number of partners and use condoms — and providing those condoms for free. For a TB epidemic, it means urging people to take their daily meds, and for a respiratory epidemic like COVID, it means educating people on the efficacy of getting vaccinated, wearing masks, avoiding crowds, and practicing social distancing.

These are all behaviors aimed at reducing or interrupting transmission. And whether officials succeed in improving the health of individuals and the whole community depends on whether those behaviors are adopted. *There is no epidemic control without changes in behavior.*

At the outset of an epidemic, in its hottest zones, behavior change is frequently all we have to fight it. But public health officials cannot *force* behavior change. It requires collaboration and involves a great deal of trust and understanding. Because in truth, the community does most of the work. The role of field epidemiologists is to explain the situation, if needed, help a community understand the threat of the disease they face, and let them know what tools and approaches are available. We are there to guide, train, and support. Supporting communities is an art and a science — and requires continuous learning.

I remember the moment it clicked for me. I was in Somalia for the first time, helping with the tuberculosis epidemic. TB patients must complete a four- to six-month course of therapy to cure the disease and prevent relapses months or years later, and the problem was that TB patients would not stay on their meds. This led to relapses and more people infected. The fact that the population in the refugee camps had a tendency to nomadically wander made it that much harder to stop the spread.

I met with about fifteen village elders and sheikhs to discuss a plan for managing the TB crisis at the Bo'o camp. I asked for their help in educating the community about the disease and in convincing people to accept our care.

I spoke with the men for over four hours. I explained about the bug that was so tiny, it was invisible; I told them the bugs were released into the air from someone's cough and inhaled by someone else, and the bugs multiplied in the next person. I told them about the drugs that could cure people of the disease forever when they were taken as instructed but that if people started taking the drugs and then stopped, they could get very sick again, and this time the disease might be much harder to treat. By stopping the drugs, people would endanger the community while putting their own lives at risk. I answered questions for hours.

When I was done, a deep and deafening silence descended.

Eventually, the great sheikh with the red-hennaed beard said softly:

"Why didn't anyone ever tell us this?"

That's when I more fully realized that trying to get people to change their behavior without first helping them more deeply understand the disease was a losing battle. A lot of people don't understand diseases and don't know what to do to avoid catching them. This is what public education is about.

The elders and sheikhs went to work. And pretty soon, the Bo'o camp went from 65 percent completion of therapy to 85 percent, and that included the seminomadic patients. That percentage is almost the point where research shows TB transmission no longer occurs. It's what epidemiologists call a marker, the metric by which we measure success in controlling an infectious disease. For TB, the marker is the percentage of a population that completes treatment. For measles or COVID, it's the percentage of the population that gets vaccinated. And with violence, one important marker of success is the number of successful interruptions.

ACTIVE CASE FINDING AND OUTREACH

We know that to stop a disease from infecting a community, we need to identify and reach the people and populations most at risk of developing active cases. But it's not enough to seek out the most susceptible; we also need to find those who are already very sick.

Active case finding is what the TB outreach workers did in San Francisco, what the sheikhs and community health workers and TBAs did in Somalia, and what outreach workers and violence interrupters do in many US and Latin American cities.

Active case finding goes hand in hand with public education; you can't educate people at risk if you don't know who they are, and you can't find people with active cases without public education. These elements are the bread and butter of epidemic control.

Uganda had a countrywide public education strategy* for HIV/AIDS led by the president. But they also had local health workers doing active case finding to reach people and communities with high levels of transmission.

When I was working to combat TB in San Francisco in the early 1980s, we sent outreach workers not only to the communities but also to the emergency department and the wards at SF General to look for patients who showed signs of the disease. Sometimes I went myself. I'd talk to the nurses and the residents on their rounds, check in on any ER patients who were showing symptoms — the hacking cough, the severe weight loss — or who had already been diagnosed† with TB.

Patients who were found to have active TB were treated with TB-specific antibiotics. This would not only eventually cure them of the disease but quickly reduce their infectivity to others. We also did meticulous contact tracing. Outreach workers interviewed close contacts — family, coworkers, friends — tested them for TB, asked if they were experiencing any symptoms. Those who were infected but

---
* This included trainings through every one of twenty-six sectors as well as community meetings throughout the country to change norms.
† The diagnosis of TB is suspected by symptoms and X-ray findings and confirmed by sputum smear or culture.

not symptomatic were given preventive treatment; those had active disease were treated. We then did the same with *their* networks, following the potential trajectory of transmission. We kept records and made house calls to the newly infected to ensure they were being cared for.*

Within four years, with the continued support of the city, San Francisco's robust public health department, and the CDC, we reduced the number of TB cases by nearly 50 percent, from five hundred to just under two hundred sixty. This number fell[†] to sixty cases in 2023 and it is still on its way down.

For the violence epidemics in Chicago, Baltimore, and New York and in Mexico, Colombia, Honduras, and dozens of other sites where we seeded activity, the public education campaign was paired with the active case finding and violence interruption.

Active case finding was what Angelica did for Camilo: She identified a person with disease who was in acute distress. And it's what Camilo went on to do for others. He was no longer an active case himself.

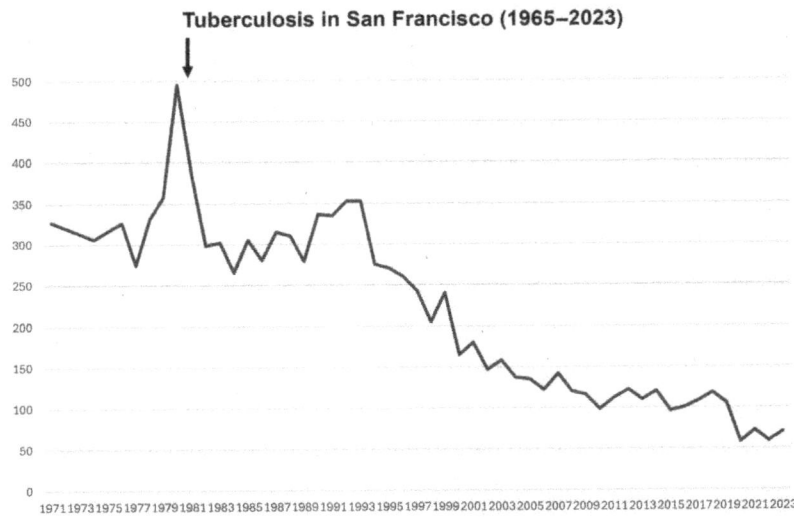

Tuberculosis in San Francisco (1965–2023)

---

* The follow-up is so important that the global strategy now calls for daily check-ins and even, to ensure patients are taking their medications, directly observed therapy (known as DOTS). For violence, follow-up on the most active cases similarly requires continued check-ins after a violence interruption.

† There were a few years where it fluctuated, largely due to HIV causing increased TB disease as previously mentioned.

Without realizing it, Camilo had spent most of his life preparing for that job, amassing street education and street cred, developing connections and relationships, and, most important, getting to know the population from within.* Moreover, all the exposure to violence and the susceptibility of the peer group and culture he grew up in allowed him to understand the disease very well.

So when he became a violence interrupter in 2015, the highest-risk people and communities knew him. They trusted him. And they listened to him.

COMMUNITY RESPONSES

We discovered the power of public education to shape community responses back in the early days of our first pilot in Chicago. Probably the only request I ever made of the University of Illinois in those days — beyond an office and a phone — was for a larger-than-usual heavy-duty photocopier. It was a beautiful machine, fit for a newspaper or a publishing company. It could print three hundred pages a minute, in full color, and produce pamphlets, posters, photographs — it was a veritable Kinko's in the bare solitude of our offices. As soon as the copier was delivered, Kathleen and I began testing its capabilities, pushing it to the limit. I'm not sure the machine was ever given a chance to cool down. We made thousands of flyers and leaflets. We'd flood the streets with them after a killing, handing them out to whoever would take them — kids on the street, men sitting on their front steps, moms behind barred doors.

This was a strategy we'd used in Uganda during the AIDS crisis. We printed tens of thousands of posters with the slogan the Ugandans came up with: "Zero Grazing" (it meant don't stray beyond your current partners). The Ugandan team blanketed the cities, towns, and countrysides with them. I knew the initiative was working when, years

---

* Not all can do it; some are not ready (or not ready to be supervised). Recruitment and hiring is an intensive process, and we don't always get it right.

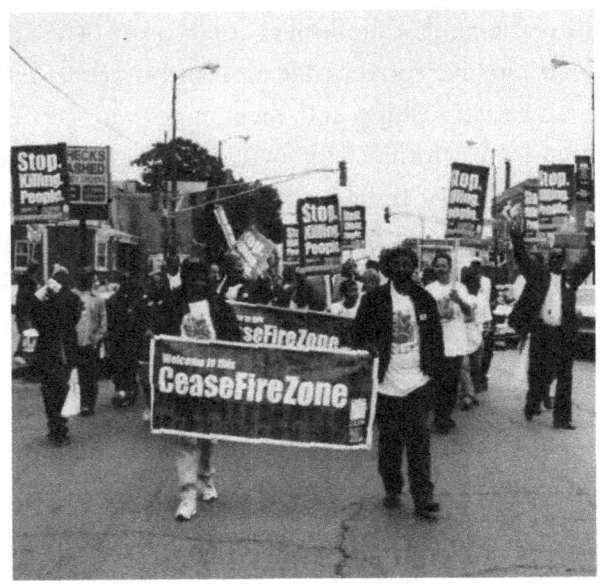

later, UNICEF complained about the mess of condoms found on the shores of Lake Victoria.*

Some of our first posters in Chicago read STOP KILLING PEOPLE. Beneath this message was all the necessary information for a planned march or event at the site of the shooting. Other posters were more involved. One featured a full-color photograph of a young boy's face. DON'T SHOOT, it said. I WANT TO GROW UP.

Outreach workers — at first, there were eight — handed these flyers out and put posters up inviting people to prayer vigils we planned along with the local clergy. Cardinal Francis George joined us on some of these neighborhood marches. With Cardinal George's help, I had previously put together a network of seventy churches, synagogues, and mosques with the goal of getting the clergy involved in our mission.† This later grew to one hundred forty places of worship.

---

* Likewise, in Chicago I knew our public education effort has sufficient intensity when the city's sanitation department complained of too many bumper stickers attached to lampposts and elsewhere.
† Years later, Cardinal George mediated a high-intensity conflict between two Latino groups after first praying with them.

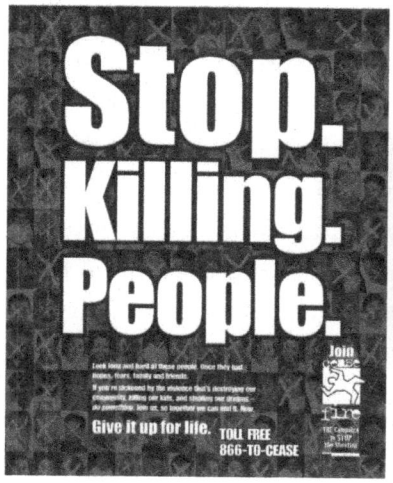
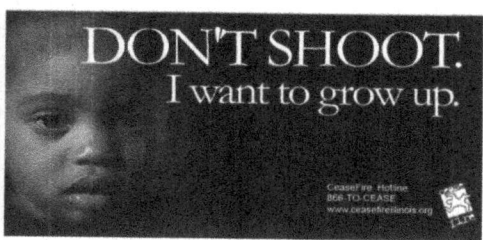

We knew that many shootings happened late at night, so with the assistance of local organizers, the outreach team arranged midnight barbecues and invited everyone in the community to come out for free hot dogs and burgers. In partnership with local music promoters, including Tony Braggs, a music promoter himself who wrote a Cease-Fire song, put together hip-hop concerts and handed out T-shirts with CeaseFire and STOP THE KILLING printed on the front and back.

The community was very receptive. No one wanted their streets to be unsafe. Even the drug dealers didn't want the violence; it brought heat from the police. And gangs didn't especially want violence in their neighborhoods — it was bad for business. At one of the first community responses I attended, I handed a small pamphlet about what we were doing and why to a young man, who said to me as he opened it, "Good idea to stop the violence. None of us want this. But don't talk to us about the drugs."*

Also, by framing things in terms of disease, we made fighting violence a *nonjudgmental* act. Our marches, protests, and speeches weren't designed to cast blame or point fingers. As we were always

---

* The focus on violence was an essential step, although we also helped people with substance issues.

telling people who asked us about what we were doing: "Our job is to help people not cross the line. And stop the shootings."

We kept a heightened community presence in high-risk areas, and we handed out flyers and gathered at the site of a shooting within twenty-four hours. Our goal was to prevent people from forgetting about the violence in their community and to encourage them to be part of the solution. We were aiming to change the social norm that violence was expected and routine. Violence could not be ordinary. It could not be something that was usual and normal and that happened because of grievances or arguments or a fight over a woman or money or what they were selling or where they were hanging out.

Violence had to become unacceptable. And that meant treating *every act* of violence as an incident to be objected to, an event that merited marching in the street and making our voices heard.

Within a few weeks, we noticed something disheartening. If a child was killed, our protests were well attended. Hundreds of people packed the block where the killing had occurred and chanted "Stop the killing" along with Norm and the team, all hoisting their signs high overhead. Reverends and pastors showed up to offer words of comfort to the family and the crowd. But when the victims were older teenagers, it was different; people asked me why they should bother showing up when a gang member had been shot. "They're just shooting each other!" I would hear. Clearly, another round of education was needed, and soon the community changed its tune. *Anyone killed became a concern to everyone. And all shootings resulted in a community-wide response.*

The work started in February 2000. That summer, there was a ninety-day period with zero shootings and zero killings.

There were two or three shootings in midsummer, and after that, another ninety-day stretch without shootings or killings.

At the end of the year, there had been a 67 percent reduction in shootings.

I recall visiting the community during the first of these zero-killing streaks and talking with moms and grandmas who were sitting out in their front yards and telling us that they had not felt safe sitting out in the open like that for years, if ever. They were also now using the park across the street, they told me, a very small park with a playground that they said had never been used for playing.

The following year, the *Chicago Sun-Times* published an article with the headline "Treating Crime as a Disease Works." Around that time, I saw Terry Hillard, the chief of police of the Chicago Police Department, at a large community meeting. We were both hanging back in the balcony. "We all know what happened in West Garfield Park was due to you and your team," he said graciously. And then he added, "But you'll never do this on Chicago Avenue" (in West Humbolt Park). And yet we did.

Over the next three years, from 2001 to 2003, we replicated our pilot program in several more neighborhoods. The result was a 45 percent drop, on average, in violent events compared to control communities, neighboring communities, and the city as a whole.

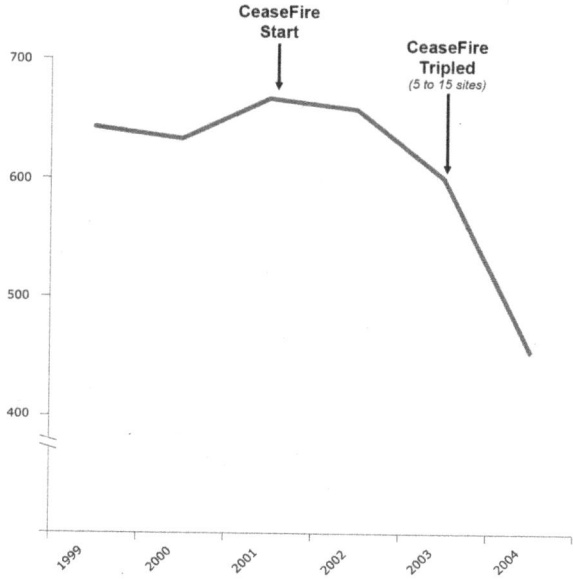

INTERRUPTING SPREAD

One day, I was at Bethel New Life discussing the need for more focused outreach and more active case finding when I was approached by Tio Hardiman, a community organizer. I had seen Tio at prior meetings and been impressed with how authoritatively he spoke about life on the streets.

"I grew up on the streets," he told me. "I've seen violence firsthand. I've seen people get killed, okay? And you're right. When it happens once, it happens again. When you see it, it does something to you. This thing spreads. It's not just a bunch of isolated incidents. You can catch it." Then he told me he could see the wisdom in what we were doing and wanted to be part of it.

Tio had grown up on the west and south sides of Chicago, raised by his uncle and grandparents. When he was a child, his uncle had fallen into alcoholism and addiction, and his house became a gathering place for people struggling with substances. He described eating "salt sandwiches" when there was nothing else in the house and dodging "ghetto rats" the size of raccoons. He survived beatings and navigated the gang warfare of the 1980s and 1990s by befriending everyone he could. He had the gift of gab — he could talk his way out of almost any fix — and he had so many friends in so many places that the gangs largely left him alone. Tio knew all the gang members but somehow avoided becoming one of them.

"God blessed me with a vivid imagination," he said. "I've been able to see through my circumstances and see something better. And I think what you're saying makes sense. It might sound crazy to some people. It sounds kind of out there to me. But I think it can really work."

Tio told me about something that had happened when he was twenty and living with his grandparents in the Henry Horner housing complex. On his way up to the ninth floor, he saw a kid surrounded by teenagers in the hallway. One of the teens had a baseball bat that he was slapping against his hand. "Join up," he kept saying. "Join up."

The message was clear: If the boy didn't pledge loyalty to the gang, he'd be beaten to within an inch of his life. The boy knew it too; he had lost control of his bladder, and his eyes, wide with terror, darted from one tormentor to the next.

"Whoa," Tio said. "Y'all step off. This kid's too young."

Ten pairs of eyes turned to Tio. When the teens recognized him — a friend of their leader and a lot of the other gang leaders in the area — they backed off, mumbling.

Tio had been doing that kind of thing his whole life, he said. Then he gave me his pitch. He could help CeaseFire do more, he said. He knew the major players. And he could find outreach workers who carried even more respect in the community to help stop more shootings before they happened.

For a few months, Tio worked for us as a consultant. But after winning another grant, we had the money to bring him on full time.

Tio recommended we hire two men, Chip Edwards and Tony Picket. We already had outreach teams at that point, but Chip and Tony (known locally as Batman and Robin) alerted me to the fact that the outreach workers were doing both too much and not enough.

A NEW CATEGORY OF WORKER

Outreach workers could not do the day job *and* the night job. And violence didn't keep regular hours. Shootings happened at midnight or two in the morning. But work needed to happen during the day as well. Sometimes a young person needed* help going back to school or applying for a job to keep from getting swept up in some gang dispute

---

* Working in TB control, I learned that an outreach staffer for any epidemic has two functions: One, stop the disease by ensuring people are treated, and two, help people with whatever else they need. Nurses Sally and Pat at the TB program in San Francisco taught me this well — they provided bus tokens for patients, always had food around for them to take home, and occasionally helped with housing. When people have acute needs, the disease is not usually the main thing on their minds. The same is true for violence — our workers are there to stop the disease and help people with their other basic needs.

on the streets, but by the time our outreach workers were available, the damage was done.

It was clear that we needed a new type of worker. Our outreach workers were playing the long game, attempting to educate people about violence contagion and helping to change behaviors and get more support over days, weeks, and months. Chip and Tony pioneered a *more immediate, more active* style of intervention: the direct interruption of violence. This approach required access to and credibility with some of the major players, people who were tough to get to. But Chip and Tony had long histories and tight relationships with the gang leaders who ran the various blocks. Their names brought respect.

Chip and Tony advocated for what we then came to see as a new category of public health workers: violence interrupters.*

For some diseases, interruption might mean getting people vaccinated. If administered on a large enough scale, effective vaccines, like those for polio, measles, and smallpox, drastically reduce transmission, effectively eliminating diseases from many populations. But there is no vaccine for most communicable diseases. We still don't have one for AIDS, even though it has killed over forty million people worldwide.†

For other diseases, stopping the spread might mean treating people with medications so that they are less likely to transmit the disease to others. This is how epidemic control works for tuberculosis. Because TB is spread through the air, every person with active disease who coughs is a major risk to everyone in the vicinity, so interrupting transmission means case finding and treating as many active cases as

---

* New categories of professional and paraprofessional workers often emerge during epidemics. For AIDS, there are several new categories of workers, including counselors, drug-treatment providers, and public educators. For violence, too, we have developed new violence-specific categories, such as trauma specialists and patient advocates. But violence interrupters marked the *first new category for the field.*

† There are now a number of highly effective therapies for HIV infection, medications that have improved and saved millions of lives. But it took fifteen years for those medications to be developed, and at the start of the AIDS epidemic, all we had to stop transmission was behavior change.

possible. But as we will see, treatment involves not just medications but also changing people's thinking.

For violence, interruption might, on rare occasions, mean one person using his high level of street cred to mediate a conflict, putting his body on the line and using himself as a shield until a better solution can be reached. More commonly, interruption means heading off conflicts before they go too far and preventing retaliations before they become ongoing contagions. It means speaking to people individually and in a safe space to cool things down, shift their thinking, and help them arrive at better solutions. In some cases it means following the chain of transmission through families and communities, patiently intervening in dozens of microconflicts, and handling them the same way.

Chip and Tony began by focusing on the hottest zones, places where shootings were common, and quickly showed they could head off violence before it happened. They would get information on what was being planned and intervene swiftly and reliably. It became clear that if we could build a network of interrupters who were as intimately connected as Chip and Tony, our efforts could have a broader and deeper impact. We would be able to identify brewing conflicts and arrive in time to stop outbreaks. This constituted a big advance in how the organization operated and how the field developed.

In 2004, with the support of the state, CeaseFire expanded from five to fifteen communities in the city and five cities outside of Chicago. Aware that managing such a team would be time-consuming and labor-intensive, I asked Tio to coordinate the interrupters working with community groups across our rapidly expanding territory. I held monthly meetings of the sites to review the data and progress and discuss strategies for strengthening the efforts further.

Within weeks, CeaseFire's employee ranks included interrupters like China Joe, Fonzo, and Monster, affectionate nicknames that came from street life. Many came from difficult backgrounds, and some had spent time in prison, but they were clearly "out of the game" or "on this side of the line." A big advantage was that we now had access to multiple rival groups, as people were selected for their prior contacts with whom they still had personal relationships and respect. Critically, they knew they had been part of the problem in the past and were committed to righting those wrongs.

They were on board with our mission. And although their résumés alarmed some of our supporters, others saw their value.

CeaseFire's tenth-floor offices at UIC were soon filled with dozens of interrupters — one to three for each community group, which also included a violence prevention coordinator and six to eight outreach workers. I was proud that we had been able to find the right staff, and I loved seeing them all come out of the elevators and convene in the conference room for weekly strategy meetings. And I loved hearing their tales of successful interruptions, their intel on trending hot spots, and their strategies for defusing conflicts. Each meeting was a partially open forum, steered by Tio, who sat at the front of the room like some combination of teacher, drill sergeant, and motivational speaker.

Many of the interrupters and their work stick in my mind. James, nicknamed Monster, had spent years in prison and had been a high-level player in a major gang. He was widely respected but also feared for his unpredictability and his physical strength.

Others might have considered Monster a liability, but we saw a person looking to get back on his feet, a changed man who wanted to avoid going back to prison and who wanted to use his "juice" on the street for good. He impressed me, as they all did, with his dedication to doing something positive.

One of Monster's first interruptions was particularly legendary (although I probably wouldn't have approved of it if I'd known about it before it happened). Two rival crews were fighting over territory, not in adjacent blocks or corners but on opposite sides of the street. Gunmen stationed in the second-story windows of row houses fired day and night across the avenue. Children were scared to walk to school for fear of being hit by a stray bullet. Parents were terrified to walk to the corner for milk or food. Older people couldn't get to the pharmacy to pick up prescriptions. The block was eerily quiet and empty during the day.

Monster had taken part in occasional turf wars like this in his time. The standard approach to that kind of conflict was to shut down the street. But that would mean that kids couldn't even play tag on the sidewalk or shoot hoops in the alley. Monster believed that was going too far.

So on a Wednesday afternoon, Monster drove his van down the center of the street, parked in the middle of the block, got out of his van, and addressed the crews involved.

"Shoot me if you want!" he said, throwing his arms in the air. "But I'm not leaving until y'all stop shooting up the damn neighborhood!"

Silence on the avenue. He could see faces and gun barrels at the windows, but not a single shot was fired. He climbed into his van and shut the door. And stayed there.

Not a single shot was fired that night either. Or the next day.

Or the day after that.

For two days, Monster stayed in his van, talking on his cell phone to Tio. Other interrupters brought him food so that he'd need to leave the van only to use the bathroom. And after two days, the leader of one of the warring groups approached the driver's-side window.

"This gotta stop."

"You're telling me," Monster answered.

Monster made some calls, and within a few minutes an emissary from the other rival group was at the passenger window.

"No weapons," Monster said, opening the back door.

He worked out an agreement with them. One group would confine its activities to the north side of the street, the other to the south. There would be no shootings when children were present. The street would be a safe zone until midnight. That was the start.

If anything happened, Monster would come back and park his van in the street again.

This was not the way it was usually done. I was not thrilled about the level of confrontation and risk involved, but interrupters like

Monster were serious about stopping the shooting and had the street smarts to understand how to go about it.

In another situation, two gangs were planning a retaliation against a much stronger one. They kept egging each other on. Then a few of our interrupters arrived with a bucket of chicken wings and a three-liter bottle of Sprite and asked if they could come into the apartment where the gang members were making their plans to watch *Scarface*. It defused the tension, opening the door to a conversation about why the retaliation was not a good idea.

Some of the stories I heard from our interrupters sounded like something you might see in a movie. Some, like the one with Monster and his van, were built on codes of masculinity and bravado.

But far more often, interruptions were subtle. Intimate. Quiet. And many times, they involved mothers and grandmothers.

One interrupter went all the way to Milwaukee, picked up someone's grandmother, and brought her back to the city so she could help talk her grandson down. Even when young men listen to no one else, many of them (and many older men) will listen to the women who raised them. It is a rare dressing down that can both shame its recipient into unloading his weapons and also shower him with unconditional love.

"Young men — they do respect a mother," Linda Toles, the mom who had lost her son to violence, told me. She could cajole them, she could yell at them, she could tell them to change, and they'd listen to her because of what she had been through and because of her obvious love for her own lost son.*

Even if the mother isn't involved, merely invoking her is often enough to change someone's behavior. Questions like "What would

---

* My theory is that when a woman yells at a man, he hears his own mother. And it is believed that there is nobody more important to a boy than his mother. (A surprising finding of the later Department of Justice study of our work was that the outreach workers were seen as the most important people in clients' lives — next to their mothers.)

your mother think about this?" and "Is this what your grandmother would want you to do?" can carry great weight.

This was certainly true for one of our interrupters, Max. While serving a twenty-year sentence for killing the man who'd murdered his brother, Max came to a startling realization: His mother had now lost both of her sons to violence. One was dead, and the other was locked up. His mom died at home during his sentence with no son at her bedside. Upon his release, Max became an interrupter, and in one particularly powerful incident, he was tasked with convincing a young man not to avenge his brother's death. "Don't rob your mother of both her sons," he advised him.

Early on in our work in Chicago, a third of our interrupters were women, and this is true today as well. Over and over, we've seen that many women have the ability to reach people in a different way than men do. They are seen as less threatening even when scolding and they're often more trusted. Men can many times let their guard down with women more easily than they do with other men, and other women may feel more comfortable with women as well.

This is important, given that nearly a third of the world's women have been subjected to physical or sexual violence or both from a partner or another person, according to UN estimates. And our experience is that in many situations the most trusted people intervening in familiar, domestic, and sexual violence can be other women as well.

Every week, I heard stories from interrupters and outreach workers about domestic disputes defused; a man dissuaded from hitting his child's mother; two sisters taken someplace safe after sexual abuse by their mother's boyfriend. In instances like this, interrupters checked back in with the women frequently, helping them access the services they needed to heal and giving them both informal counseling and referrals to organizations that could help.

Reports like these made me think about how we could do more in this area. Alma, one of our interrupters, once told me, "It's the men who are making the mess. We're just cleaning it up."

THE PRINCIPLES OF INTERRUPTION

There is no one "right" way to interrupt violence. But there are principles that guide the work. We train our staff on them, and they have trained thousands; these methods have gone national and international.

The violence interrupter's goal is to ensure there is no further violence. How to go about it depends on the who, what, where, and why of the situation and on the actions and reactions of the multiple people involved.

Interruptions don't happen by chance; they involve much more than simply walking up to a heated situation and magically resolving it. A typical interruption takes days, weeks, even months of careful observation and decision-making. You need eyes and ears on the street, people who know the major players and who understand the history of the conflict. You need *information*. That information might come from an interrupter. It might come from an outreach worker. It might come from concerned neighbors, friends, or family.

As with all forms of public health outreach, everything is done with confidentiality and trust. That's one of the core principles of the public health lens.

Many of the potentially violent events we interrupted early on in Chicago and, later, in other cities and countries were the result of years of violent conflict. Some of the communities we work in have been functionally at war for thirty years. Stepping into such a conflict without knowing the background and context is a recipe for failure.

For each planned interruption, a team spends time developing a strategy. What do we know? Who has the best contacts? What do we need to find out? What might be said, and to whom? By whom? Who is best positioned to make contact and attempt to head things off? What might be some of the better approaches to try? Who else do we need to call on to help?

So much depends on selecting the right interrupters, people with preexisting relationships, access, credibility, and trust. Entrusting this work to an expert who the people and groups don't know personally is a mistake made throughout the field of community violence and for other syndromes of violence as well.

As Tio once put it, to reach people, to defuse situations, "you can't send in a bunch of social workers." Violence, particularly violence within communities, is not a problem that can be solved from the outside. The only reason we got anywhere in West Garfield Park and other communities was that we hired interrupters who had grown up there, who had family there, who knew the streets and corners and could connect authentically with the people who lived there.

We didn't just need locals. We needed locals who had firsthand experience with violence. People who had credibility and trust not only within communities and neighborhoods but within the street organizations whose conflicts they would now mediate. People who also had personal relationships with the current shot callers and leaders of these groups.

This was equally true in the epidemic-control work I did before I focused on violence. If we wanted to reach Somali refugees, we needed to hire other Somali refugees. If Wayne wanted to help change behaviors among intravenous drug users, he needed to hire former intravenous drug users. People trust people they recognize themselves in and, ideally, already know.

In the early 2000s, our organization was sometimes condemned for hiring "gang members" and "criminals." But we were praised for giving ex-cons a second chance just as often. My response was the same to both groups: I wasn't doing this as a favor or as charity; this was how public health worked!

We had chosen our interrupters the same way we'd selected people for other disease outreach. But this field was different in that it was surrounded with a cloud of moralism that threatened to get in the way of interrupting the disease's spread.

We hired people who had personal experience with violence because they were the ones best equipped to stop it. They knew the disease's characteristic signs and symptoms and knew what to say to help change the behaviors of infected people.

I didn't care about their past as much as I did about who they were now. Their past mattered only insofar as it had introduced them to the disease. It should not be lost how dedicated these men and women were, and are, to using their social currency to help people and for the greater good.

Before we hired Tio, reaching even these potential interrupters was difficult; we didn't have enough of the right connections. But with Tio on board, our web of influence grew. We were able to attract dozens of workers, and the more who joined us, the more credibility we earned. Pretty soon, it became fashionable for the elder statesmen of the streets to take on this new role of interrupter and healer, and many of our best interrupters embraced the chance to get out of the game without losing credibility in their world while also redirecting that credibility toward a new purpose.

One of our most respected interrupters in those days is a guy called China Joe. Everyone loved to listen to Joe. His voice was hard, raspy, and Southern, with a curious lilt. He once told a story at an interrupter meeting that caused even the most seasoned people in that experienced group to shake their heads in disbelief and admiration.

Here's the story China Joe told: Through his sources, he had heard that a group of young men were planning to shoot all the members of an entire household, including a grandma and five kids. It was a retaliatory murder — one of their brothers had been killed, and to avenge his death, they were going to kill the person who had done it along with his whole family.

It was a horrible tragedy in the making, one that Joe worked for days to prevent. As he drove to the house hoping to avert a massacre, he stayed on the phone with one of the men, trying to convince him to wait or reconsider. Then he received a call from one of his contacts letting him know about another act of violence being planned on the other side of the neighborhood. Since he couldn't be in two places at once, China Joe called someone he knew who was involved in the second conflict, told him what was going to happen to the family in the first dispute, and said that he needed their help to stop it.

At this point in the story, he paused, clearly having a good time telling it.

"And?" one of his listeners asked.

"And they dropped it, man. They loaded up into their car and drove over. Instead of staying with their own dispute, they came to help me cool down the first scene and save a family they didn't even know."

"Damn," someone said.

"Crazy."

"Two birds, one stone."

"Nah." Joe smiled. "No stone, all birds alive."

Interruption is, by definition, a context-dependent act. Sometimes we'd have a good run without shootings for months and then there'd be an outbreak, forcing us to regroup. Our tactics changed as new cases arose, new leaders appeared on the scene, or new factions developed out of the blue.

But there were a few guiding principles that we always kept in mind regardless of what specific methods we chose.

1. **Nonjudgmental listening**

   Interruption is health care. Like other health-care workers, interrupters are trained to be calm, cooperative, and nonjudgmental. To interrupt an act of violence, they have to understand who is at risk of acting and why. Any time spent talking is time people are not reaching for weapons.

2. **Validation**

   Listening not only ensures that interrupters know what is going on, it also allows the people involved to vent, to *get it all out*, which can help them calm down. Interrupters do not judge, criticize, minimize, or tell people what they're feeling. Instead, they support people in the effort to do the nonviolent thing. They use short, reassuring phrases; "Okay, it's okay" and "You're fine" work best. "I get it," an interrupter might say. "I see how you're feeling. Sounds terrible. Sorry this is happening." They speak positively, concisely, and they do not argue. Their goal is not to be right but to prevent violence.

3. **Cooling down**
   You can't interrupt anything if tempers are high. As we've seen, violence is salient to the brain, and under conditions of stress, anger, and other heightened emotions, the amygdala may be fired up. When the amygdala is "on," the frontal lobe is turned off. When in this state, the brain relies on its familiar script. So the first thing an interrupter must do is lower the temperature — give the person another outlet for his anger, get him to a different location, or give him something else to focus on. Anything to calm the nervous system down.

4. **Buying time**
   Often, rational appeals aren't enough to convince someone not to behave violently in that moment. So interrupters take a different approach — they put it off. "Come on, let's go have a slice of pizza, and then we'll talk about it," they'll say. "I hear you, let's just go have lunch first." This is a calculated strategy. It gives the person time and space to cool down, but it also shows the person that the interrupter cares, that they are listening, that they are both on the same side.

5. **Ensuring safety, both physical and social**
   Once the temperature has been lowered and interrupters have bought time, they have to be able to bring all the parties into some kind of agreement, however tentative. The agreement

might be a more involved resolution. It might be simply an agreement to walk away. Or it might involve more.*

The goal of the agreement has to be safety — physical safety, of course, but also social safety. All parties have to feel that they will remain safe as a result of the mediation. They must not fear physical violence or other social consequences.

Typically, the biggest hurdle is ensuring that everyone saves face. All parties have to exit the situation feeling that they have maintained their reputation and gotten a win. When negotiations get complex, the interrupters have to be able to see the conflict from both sides and engineer a solution that allows each side to avoid social and reputational costs.

6. **Catalyzing a perspective shift**

    Interruptions prevent violence in the short term, but they also tend to have long-term effects, changing the way infected people view violence and altering how they might respond in the future if they are triggered. For example, an interrupter might do some or all of the following:

    - Convince people that refraining from violence will help them avoid future threats to their safety: "If you do something here, it's likely more guys will come after you."
    - Help people see that the time has come to go on the *defensive* rather than on the offensive and that, strategically, violence isn't the smart move.
    - Assure people that the situation has already been resolved or that the other person made a mistake and is sorry: "He's more afraid of you than you are of him.

---

* It is not always necessary for the sides to meet and agree. Sometimes it is enough for each side to meet with their respective interrupters and agree to stop if the other side will.

You don't have to do anything" or "He wants to give you the money he owes you."
- Reframe letting it go as an act of magnanimity: "You're letting them off easy because you're bigger than them. You're bigger than this."
- Encourage people to consider their children or what their mothers might think: "What type of example do you want to set?"

These techniques encourage acutely symptomatic people to see violence as a considered *choice*, an option that they can take or not, and help them navigate this choice without pressure. For so many, violence has always been an inevitability, something that just happens, like vomiting or the hiccups happen. But the fact that the disease of violence primarily affects the brain rather than autonomic processes in the body means that people can exert conscious control, especially if they are given help or shown a physically and socially safe way out. This requires interrupters to be *guides and partners* in this cooling-down *and shifting* process.

In Chicago and many other cities, our interrupters and outreach workers stay in frequent contact with people for months to years after an interruption. In fact, there is a robust *protocol* for the follow-up that includes gathering information from the people involved in the conflict, their neighbors, family members, social media, and more, all aimed at ensuring that they *remain well* and *don't relapse*. This is what physicians and health-care workers call *longitudinal care* — continued and focused attention on patients' needs. It includes providing referrals and care for other issues they might have, such as mental-health problems, lack of education, or trouble finding jobs. This *sustained contact* encourages long-term behavior change, and over time, the new behaviors become the norm.

THE POWER OF INTERRUPTION

Guadalupe Cruz was one of our earliest and most effective interrupters in Chicago and one of our most important staffers when we took the organization's work to other countries.

Whenever Lupe (as she was known) walked into a room — whether it was in Honduras, Culiacán, or Juarez, and whether its occupants were members of drug cartels, Salvadoran gangsters, or teenage girls trying to survive — people listened to her. Soft-spoken but firm, she radiated a sweet but powerful confidence. She connected with people who were hurting as well as those whom others feared with endless empathy beyond what most of us have seen in action.

In her work coordinating Cure Violence's efforts across Latin America, Lupe often faced suspicion. People who have experienced violence or have committed violence are usually distrustful of outsiders. "You don't know what it's like," they said to Lupe. "You have no idea."

"Yes, I do," Lupe always said. "I know exactly what it's like. The streets raised me."

Lupe was from Back of the Yards, a historically Mexican American neighborhood in Chicago that has more recently become home to tens of thousands of Venezuelan migrants. The daughter of Mexican immigrants, Lupe never knew her father. After her mother succumbed to addiction, she and her two brothers, Frankie and Sergio, were put into foster care with an abusive family. Sergio ran away first, then Frankie, and when Lupe was twelve, she ran away too. The three of them slept in abandoned cars, in alleyways, and occasionally on friends' kitchen floors. Lupe and her brothers were wards of the state, but the inattention of incompetent caseworkers allowed them to run scams: Lupe would get friends' parents to sign papers saying they were her aunts or uncles so that support checks would arrive. She never saw this money, but it helped keep her in good graces with adults who could occasionally help her.

Their childhood was extremely dangerous, but she recalled parts of it with fondness. There was a freedom to it, and a strong bond.

When her brother Frankie was in a group home, Lupe would call and pretend to be his aunt, then break him free for a weekend. She and her brothers were wild. They would do anything for one another. Once, Lupe hid Frankie in an alley dumpster so he could avoid a truant officer; she knocked on the side when it was safe for him to come out.

They were always hustling. Lupe's brothers quickly became involved with various Latino street gangs, in particular the Two-Six. This was in the late 1970s and early 1980s, and the groups were still nascent. Drugs were a factor, but they were not, at least at first, the stated raison d'être of the gangs. Solidarity was. The street organizations were forging an identity based on their ethnicity in opposition to the Black gangs that held sway elsewhere in the city. For someone like Lupe and for young men like her brothers, the gang was a stand-in for the family they had never had and a connection to the country they had never visited. It gave them a sense of belonging and a story they shared.

It also gave them scars. Violence back then was usually in the form of rumbles, essentially street fights between rival groups. Although there were weapons — knives, razor blades, baseball bats — there were far fewer guns on the streets in the early 1980s than there are now. No one could afford them.

But that didn't mean that the violence Lupe saw was minor or that it couldn't completely derail a life. She saw people beaten beyond recognition. People hospitalized. She'd seen her brothers incarcerated, her friends injured, some of them killed. She'd even had a hit put on her. She knew what it was like to be scared for your life. What it was like to hurt someone. What it was like to feel like you *had* to hurt someone just to survive.

Perhaps that's why, even as she rose through the ranks of the Two-Six and eventually became the first woman on the "board" of the gang, Lupe was looking for other ways to live. She graduated from high school and used her education and connections to open a series of businesses in Little Village. She ran Candie's and Junior's, arcades that catered to teenagers and young men, as well as a clothing shop that specialized in Western wear.

Lupe got married, had three kids, ran her businesses. But she didn't forget the streets. One evening, three young gang members, all of them girls, broke into her arcade and demanded protection money. Lupe laughed in their faces.

"You think I'm scared of you?" she asked. "I've *been* you. Get out of my store."

Lupe was clearheaded enough to get out of the game before it was too late. And she was proud — proud of what she'd accomplished, yes, but also *proud* in the sense that her head was always held high. She'd scrapped for everything she had, and no one was going to take it from her. When her husband told her after years of marriage that she was worthless, that no one would ever love her like he did, that she wouldn't be able to live without him, she left him immediately. Kicked him out of her apartment and then bought a house with her own money. She and her kids slept on the floor for months before Lupe could save enough for a couch and some beds. But no one, not even the father of her children, was going to tell her she couldn't make it on her own.

When Lupe first heard of CeaseFire, the program was in its early days. At that time, she was a successful businesswoman. She didn't seek the organization out; it was her brother Frankie who introduced her to us.

Frankie had just gotten out of prison. One of his friends from inside had been released and was working with CeaseFire. He knew that Frankie would need a job and that, as an early member of the Two-Six, he had incredible knowledge of and credibility within the Latino gang world of Chicago. He invited Frankie to a meeting, and Frankie asked Lupe to go with him.

She wasn't impressed. At the time, CeaseFire did not have much traction in the Latino community. We didn't know the major players, we didn't know whom to hire, and, Lupe saw, we didn't understand the culture.

But something resonated with Lupe. The idea that violence was a disease, that it was passed from person to person — it made intuitive sense to her. She'd seen the way that violence and loss spread through generations. She was desperate to raise her children differently, to break the chain of violence in her family. She wanted it to stop with her. And she could see the logic in taking that energy to the community around her.

Lupe began as an interrupter in Chicago in 2002. At first, she worked mostly with Latino gang members. It was a world she knew well, a world by which she was not intimidated.

For much of her life, Lupe had been like a second mother to many kids in the neighborhood. She recognized herself in them. She could tell when a teenager wasn't getting enough to eat, when a boy didn't have a safe place to stay, when a sixteen-year-old girl was pregnant and scared of her boyfriend. Her own kids often got frustrated with her for emptying the family fridge to host impromptu barbecues in the yard. "Mom, you're going to bankrupt us," they'd say. But Lupe ignored them; she just pulled the cover off the grill and poured in charcoal so she could grill for whoever needed a plate.

Becoming an interrupter was a new way to help those kids. She could not only give them a safe place to stay but also change the *conditions* of their lives. What CeaseFire was doing in Chicago was what she and her brothers had been doing for years. But now they'd have a larger organization as a resource, funding to ease the financial strain, and, crucially, a new framework to use: public health.

Lupe quickly established a reputation for fairness, directness, and tough love. And the more she worked, the more she gravitated toward women and girls. She could see the pain in their eyes, the danger they were often in. So many of them were seeking to escape abuse from their parents or boyfriends. They longed for protection and often found it in the arms of other men or in gangs. They adopted a tough pose, but they were angry, distrustful, hurt — and often terrified.

Lupe had found a way out of the game by going to school and

building the skills to become an entrepreneur, and she helped the girls plot a similar course. What were some skills that they had and that they could monetize? What were they good at, and could it help them in school? Who were their friends, and how could they support one another?

She thought often of those three girls who had broken into her store. Where were they now? Lupe asked around, and within a week, she had gotten calls from all of them. She listened to their problems. Gave them advice. Gave them a place to stay when they needed it. Something to eat. Reassurance.

A month later, they were back in school. A year later, they graduated. Two of them went on to start businesses as cosmetologists and beauticians.

This was proof to Lupe of the power that nurturing intervention had over young lives. But it was also proof something else: the power of breaking the chain of transmission.

Because two years after breaking into Lupe's shop, these young women became interrupters themselves.

This was just the start.

CHANGING THE NARRATIVE

In 2004, after CeaseFire had expanded from five communities to fifteen, Chicago moved from the sixteenth most violent city in the country to the forty-second. And we saw a 50 percent drop, on average, in killings across the CeaseFire sites and a 25 percent drop in killings across the city. This made sense because the CeaseFire sites were strategically located in the neighborhoods that were previously determined to be the main hot spots.

Local press began to report and sometimes celebrate the fact that 2004 had seen the lowest number of homicides in Chicago in thirty-eight years. They ran articles with headlines like "Treating Gun Crime Like Disease Shows Results: CeaseFire Program May Cut Shootings by as Much as 67%" (*Chicago Sun-Times*) and "Homicide

Capital Becomes Role Model" (*Philadelphia Inquirer*). The DOJ secured federal funds for us, which allowed further expansion. We got a major award from the US Attorney General's Office and an official endorsement from the US Conference of Mayors; our organization was featured in a cover story in *New York Times Magazine* ("Is Urban Violence a Virus? Blocking the Transmission of Violence") and in a piece in the *Economist* (which referred to our work as "the approach that will come to prominence").

We were featured on major networks like PBS and CNN, and an award-winning documentary on our organization, *The Interrupters*, played around the country and around the world.

The first independent evaluation of our work was funded and supported by the Department of Justice and assessed our first seven years, from 2000 to 2007. The study employed four different universities using four different methods: hot-spot mapping, time-series analysis, confidential interviews, and, perhaps most interesting, gang-network analysis. The results showed a 41 to 73 percent decrease in shootings over the seven neighborhoods. In two of these neighborhoods, the number of retaliation killings fell by 50 percent, and in five of these neighborhoods, *retaliations dropped 100 percent — to zero!*

We had shown that the epidemic-control approach to violence — identifying the susceptible in highly exposed populations, public education and community responses, active case finding, and using interrupters with access, credibility, and trust to interrupt the transmission — worked.

It worked in West Garfield, where in one year, the community team was able to reduce shootings by 67 percent.

It worked in Logan Square, the most violent area in the city at the time, where killings eventually went to zero.

It worked in Auburn Gresham and Englewood and East Rogers Park — some of the most entrenched violence hot spots in the Chicago area — where retaliations *ceased to occur*. And the public narrative about violence was changing too, not just in those neighborhoods but in health departments and even in the media.

"The science is clear: violence is undeniably a public health issue," said Dr. Leana Wen, Baltimore's health commissioner. "Like other public health crises, we can prevent violence by identifying risk factors, treating it as a disease, and preventing violence before it starts. That's powerful, and it's cause for hope."

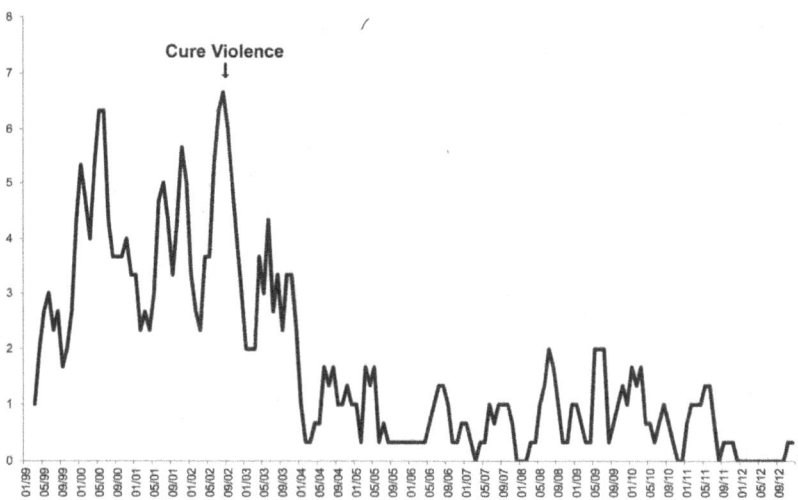

Even the mayors were beginning to speak up publicly. In July 2025, for example, Baltimore mayor Brandon Scott announced that the city was seeing its lowest number of homicides in fifty years, and he attributed this success to the strategy of approaching gun violence "as a public health threat instead of simply a crime issue" and addressing that threat at the source by "investing in violence interrupters, community organizations and trauma-informed support systems in impacted neighborhoods."

In August 2025, Chicago saw fewer shootings than it had at any time since the mid-1960s, with a 37 percent drop in shootings from the previous year and a nearly 60 percent drop since 2021.

As I write this, we are seeing record lows in homicides not just in Chicago but in cities across the country, and it's impossible for me not to attribute this in large part to a national anti-violence movement led by Black and Brown leaders, community activists, and billions in funding from the Biden administration that allowed for the hiring of more outreach workers and violence interrupters, far more than the eighty to one hundred we were able to hire from 2000 to 2004 when we expanded our efforts in Chicago to fifteen other cities and beyond. (This movement is now better known as community violence intervention, or CVI, among dozens as well as hundreds of local names.)

It was well known that health interventions that stopped epidemics in one city, country, or region also worked in other areas, although they always required adaptations to culture and circumstances. We manage TB the same basic way in Seattle and Tanzania, just as we manage cholera with the same principles in Sudan and Bangladesh. Although the local cultures differ, the fundamental approach doesn't. But in the early days of the organization, we knew we would need support soon from the international community if we wanted to make the approach work in cities and countries with the highest homicide rates in the world.

But we also knew we would need systems and support to scale up the approach anywhere. And we would need to either find these systems or design them. To best adapt the approach, we would need to learn some of the details of local norms as well.

CHAPTER SEVEN

NORMS AND SYSTEMS

The organization that would become CeaseFire (and eventually Cure Violence) started with no name, no money, and no home, in part because we had no proof of concept, just an idea. But we had no opportunity to provide proof of concept because we had no funds.

Raising money was a full-time job, and for a while we were barely scraping by. It would take money to hire and train people* in outreach, persuasion, behavior change, de-escalation, and carrying out a coherent long-term strategy.

And in the mid-1990s in Chicago, that's exactly what we needed to do. Chicago was having a huge epidemic of violence, and the disease was spreading unabated.

There were over twenty hot spots throughout the city, so it didn't make sense to limit our efforts to just the Austin community or West Garfield. A major problem that I saw then was the lack of any existing system at all, much less one we could scale to many different neighborhoods across the city. This was a new problem for me. I had worked in less developed countries that had better public health systems than this. We would have to work with communities to create a system and

---

* Community health workers of every type need to be paid. It was a big mistake we made years ago, thinking serious problems could be solved by volunteers alone.

we would have to study and likely have to help change some attitudes and norms.

I understood early on that if we were going to make any headway, we needed to listen and talk to the people so many others reviled — the gang leaders, the drug dealers, the people society feared and called *criminals*, a word I disliked. Health care and epidemic control has no use for morally charged words and labels. If we were to succeed, we also had to help people drop their deeply felt preconceived notions about who violence affected. We would have to train a lot of people to understand the disease without letting biases, fears, and judgments get in the way.

FACE, FUNDS, AND FEMALES

One of the first members of the Cure Violence team was Jamaican-born Norman Livingston Kerr, then in his twenties. He came to us from Bloomington, Illinois, where he'd run a program that helped rehabilitate gang-affiliated youth. A former high school basketball player, Norm had gotten to know a lot of the young men in the community when he began hosting impromptu three-on-three games in the rec center. On the court, the conversation was mostly bragging and trash talk, but off it, Norm found a new openness in the young men, a willingness to talk about their lives. He became someone they could trust. He connected in a way that I, a white doctor new to these communities, was not always able to do.

When working to stop epidemics in the past, I had learned that to get a grip on what was happening, we needed to understand both the disease and *the way people perceived the disease*. We needed to listen to those affected by it and those working to stop it. I needed them to tell us how they understood the violence in their neighborhoods.

In the fall of our first year, LaDonna worked with Bennie Lee, a leader in Chicago's Vice Lords gang, to convene a summit with young men from the community. All were affiliated with various gangs (or *groups*, as my organization called them). They ranged in age from fourteen to twenty-six. All of them had experienced high levels of exposure to violence.

Most had spent time in prison, where shootings, beatings, and retaliations were common. In short, they were not only highly susceptible, but also highly exposed, and they were certainly infected at some level. And in need of some help. When I asked LaDonna why the oldest was only twenty-six, she shook her head ruefully.

"Many of these kids don't live much longer than that, Doc."

The point of this summit was twofold: First, to listen to these young people's experiences with violence and learn what was normal for them. And second, to demonstrate these young people's *humanity* to members of a community that feared them, to show them that these men were not fundamentally bad or evil; they were fellow human beings suffering from a disease.

This second point was especially important. So many times in those early years, we came up against preconceived notions and fear. People in the community were scared of the violence and of the "sort of person" who enacted the violence. In fact, they were afraid of young people.

I saw this in white, Black, and later Hispanic spaces and at the most grassroots-level community meetings and the highest tiers of political power. And people who were deeply fearful of violence often dehumanized those whom they associated with it, similar to the way that people with certain physical illnesses, such as HIV, have historically been dehumanized. Society blames the people infected.

This is what happens with epidemics. People fear things they can't control and don't fully understand. They fear for their safety and the safety of their families. That fear distorts thinking and changes norms.

If my organization was going to have any success in treating this disease, we had to get the public to see those who had it as fully human.

I'll never forget the looks I saw on some of the faces during the "gang summit" with Bennie Lee. The audience filled the back room of the Westside Health Authority, and the usual attendees seemed nervous. These were mostly activists who spent a lot of time discussing the problem of drugs but who were seldom in the presence of the young men who sold them. Some of the expressions I saw were disapproving — brows furrowed, heads cocked. Some were more stoic. Other people looked friendly but uncomfortable. Some of the loudest voices I'd heard in earlier meetings were noticeably quiet that day.

"Okay, everyone," LaDonna said. "Let's get started."

The room was silent except for a cough at the back of the room and the sound of shuffling papers. Bennie sat near the front, a regal man with a goatee wearing a black beanie. After years of incarceration, he had recently completed his master's degree at Northeastern and was now working as a nonviolence coordinator and consultant for organizations helping previously incarcerated people reintegrate into society. He called them "returning citizens."

After talking a bit about his own life — the pressures of his upbringing, his leadership role in the Vice Lords, and his subsequent time in prison — Bennie turned to the teenagers beside him.

"So," he said. "Tell us. What is life like for you?"

The young men were shy at first, smoothing out oversize T-shirts, fiddling with their braids, but in time, they grew more talkative. They opened up. They were being listened to, taken seriously. They neither evaded nor bragged. Violence was an inescapable fact of their lives, a facet of their ecosystem, or, as one man I'll call Jerron said, "It's just part of the game."

I asked them, "What do you fight over? What do people shoot or even kill over?" The answers boiled down to four main items: turf, money, saving face, and women (or, as they said, "females").

"Face, funds, and females," one of the young men said, smiling.

Much of the violence they reported between rival groups was over money, reputation, or territory, the exact same things warring countries fight over. Several young men wanted to narrate the long and difficult histories of their gangs. These stories and traditions were important to them, a part of who they were. But we tried to limit the amount of gang lore discussed; we were more interested in the relationships, the mechanics, and what they considered the reasons for killing. (Later, we instituted a policy of calling the various gangs "Group A" and "Group B" and so forth; it helped neutralize some of the emotions that came up when speaking of rival gangs. The practice is still used by our organization and widely in the field today.)

One young man named Anthony told us that people got shot over extremely small debts — ten dollars that you never repaid could get you killed. Another man, DeAndre, detailed several fights, shootings, and deaths over women, often because someone was with someone else's "girl."

We learned that it didn't matter if the police were around or what kind of prison sentence they might get because they knew a lot of guys who had "gotten away with" killing. And the consequences were the farthest thing from their minds when they felt they "had to do it."

All of this was normal. These were the norms of the community as the young men experienced it.

Underlying many of the stories was a need to save face. As Chris, the most voluble of the bunch, told us, "On the street, your reputation is everything. Sometimes you do things not because you want to do them but 'cause you have to."

"Why?"

"To keep your name."

I could think of a few world leaders who had the same problem.

About halfway through the meeting, I could see empathy on the faces of the men and women in the audience. The thought of young people dying over ten dollars or to protect their reputations pained them.

"Babies," one of the women remarked after the meeting as we lingered over the terrible doughnuts and worse coffee. "Those poor babies."

The more these men spoke, the more we could see their pain and hurt. There were a lot of aha moments for people, including one law enforcement officer in the audience who later told me he now understood why these kids were still in gangs and why the streets were still dangerous despite all their efforts to curb the violence.

This called to mind what I'd seen for many epidemics. I'd witnessed the afflicted being dehumanized and blamed,* but I'd also seen how much empathy and understanding emerged once certain perceptions were reversed.

Going forward, I knew we would have to understand the unwritten rules and norms within the communities we were trying to serve. And in order to do so, we needed to design a system that people within these communities could trust the way they trusted the workers.

A DIFFERENT KIND OF EFFORT

In CeaseFire's early days, we conceived of violence interruption as something that had to happen in person and in real time. If you wanted to stop others from shooting, you had to be there with them. After all, these were very heated arguments, sometimes steps away from where the shooting that the interrupters were trying to prevent might occur. They were dealing with disease transmission day to day, minute to minute, second to second with people who had been hurting. This wasn't the kind of work we could do from a distance.

Direct contact in the community was also important for less confrontational modes of violence prevention — the pamphlets outreach workers handed out, the T-shirts they wore, the rallies they organized and attended carrying signs that read STOP KILLING PEOPLE. The outreach workers were in contact with the people who were most affected, and their work was visceral and personal; public education by definition involves dealing with the public, meeting them where they are.

After several successful years in Chicago, CeaseFire began to expand. In doing so, we were forced to confront a central reality: The efforts in the different areas could not exist in their own separate

---

* We see this dehumanizing today in the United States. It is an urgent national issue; violence is being done to people intentionally on a large scale to create more violence. We'll discuss this more in chapter 8.

silos. We needed some way to coordinate them. We had to ensure that workers were where they were most needed and that we provided them with the necessary resources and support while also keeping them from getting hurt, just as we would for public health workers in a hot zone of any dangerous epidemic. We needed government officials to be on board. We needed funding to pay our teams and ways of monitoring and measuring our results. And we needed to be able to do all this within communities, between communities, and across a city.

The work of stopping any epidemic requires systems, ones that exist within the overall public health framework. It can't be just a series of individual projects or programs. It has to be built into the infrastructure of a community, city, state, and country. This is how we lowered tuberculosis rates in San Francisco from the highest in the country to near elimination levels; it's how we eliminated cholera from Somalia and how we dramatically dropped HIV/AIDS rates in the most affected countries in the world. This is how these and many other diseases are continually managed globally, resulting in large reductions trending toward elimination.

In my years in San Francisco, in Somalia, in Uganda, and at WHO, I worked hard with my colleagues to build and strengthen systems. You can't have an epidemic-control effort without a community-based health system. There are too many moving parts — too many people to coordinate, too many variables to measure, too many ways to innovate and adapt to changing situations.

In Somalia, for example, the Refugee Health Unit had already built a network of over ten thousand community health workers and traditional birth attendants spread out across forty camps to help with issues ranging from diarrheal disease, pneumonia, and measles to malnutrition and complications related to pregnancy. Because of this amazing system already in place when I got there, we were able to immediately deploy forces to successfully combat TB and cholera.

By striking contrast, at one point, the United States was *the only country in the world* that did not have a national system and plan to stop the spread of HIV/AIDS. The United States has excellent clinical-care systems (if you can pay for it), but it lacks the community health system that other countries have. Luckily, we were able to tap into a global system that WHO had in place.

Time and again, I've found that the work of systematizing public health requires convincing people with power, influence, and funds to invest those resources in getting rid of a problem that they have been complaining about but not attempting to fix. For example, during the HIV/AIDS epidemic, my supervisor and mentor Dr. Daniel Tarantola and I spent many hours trying to get the US government to develop a national plan for dealing with the crisis. This work happened in conference rooms, in politicians' offices, at foundation galas held in opulent dining rooms. In the case of violence, we were able to garner support from people like Ada Mary Gugenheim of the Chicago Community Trust, Susan Lloyd at the MacArthur Foundation, and Marjorie Craig Benton and Gigi Pritzker and Michael Pucker. The City of Chicago didn't understand our mission and in fact fought it.

As a default, we used the university as the backbone of our system. But the community organizations that were credible in the affected neighborhoods were the real system and did the work.

In the absence of a functioning community-based health system, we built our networks from the ground up, seeding neighborhoods through activists and community centers. We got funding from the CDC, the DOJ, more private foundations (in particular, the Robert Wood Johnson Foundation), and then the state. We cultivated relationships with community leaders and clergy and attempted — usually unsuccessfully — to court key city officials. Despite our best efforts to win the police over, they distrusted us. The mayor's office disliked us, not because our approach didn't work but because (or so I was told) they couldn't take credit for it.

I recall so many meetings with Chicago city officials — council people, police chiefs, even the mayor — in which I was politely granted the floor, only to stare at the faces of an audience betraying not even a flicker of urgency. Law enforcement was not interested in a nonpolicing intervention, and the health department director at the time said it was not his problem.

So we built our own infrastructure that worked in parallel with the city, just as many NGOs and the CDC built the refugee health system in Somalia when the Somali government did not have such a system.* There were some advantages in both cases as we could do the work with less interference from government. But this was suboptimal compared to having actual support from the government.

I wasn't used to the lack of interest being displayed by Chicago's city officials, especially when the people themselves had so much interest in stopping the violence. When I dealt with epidemics abroad, most governmental officials *wanted* new solutions. They might fight over credit, but in the end they trusted the recommendations and suggestions we at WHO provided. If our input could help them solve the problems they had to fix, they listened. But I wasn't representing WHO anymore.

SYSTEMS AND SUPPORT

When we began to expand outside of Chicago, we were pleasantly surprised to find much more consistent support from some local governments, even in cities where we had few if any connections.

The first city outside of Illinois where we attempted to replicate the model was Baltimore. We were operating without any of our normal points of contact. In Maywood, Aurora, Rockford, East St. Louis, and other pockets of Illinois, we'd been able to rely on the systems and local networks we'd built up or helped strengthen† and on the trust and goodwill we had gained through our success in Chicago.

---

* There wasn't even a system for the nonrefugee population. Years later, when it was found that the mortality figures for the refugees were better than those for the nonrefugees, I was asked to help build the primary care system with the Somali director Dr. Qasim Aden Egal.
† Some of the groups we partnered with had only one or a few paid employees, often without a lot of experience with data or financial reporting, much less with epidemic system variables, of which there were more than a few.

Baltimore was brand-new territory, a smaller, East Coast city with a longer history of extreme poverty than Chicago due to de-industrialization and the decline in the volume of goods being shipped to and from the port. We didn't know the west side from the waterfront. And so much seemed to be going wrong there — drugs were ubiquitous, and in 2006, the year before we started our work, Baltimore had recorded three hundred killings, more murders per capita than almost any other city in the country.

Widespread poverty, skimpy social services, a high murder rate, a thriving drug trade, and declining industries. Baltimore, according to one early visitor from Cure Violence, felt like a failed state.

In a place like that, where do you start?

BALTIMORE

Our entry into what had once been called (rather optimistically) "Charm City" came largely by happenstance. I was giving a speech attended by many of Chicago's policymakers, public health workers, and politicians. This was something I did from time to time to raise awareness of our work locally and, increasingly, nationally and to attract funding.

After the talk, I felt a tap on my shoulder.

"Dr. Slutkin?"

The woman was serious and brisk, in her late twenties, with a firm handshake.

"I'm Catherine Fine," she said. "I've been told to talk to you about Baltimore."

Catherine had heard of our approach and thought it might work in her city. Could I tell her more?

A few days later, we met in my office, and I outlined the approach we'd taken in Chicago. She understood the idea that violence was a disease, that it was infectious, and that it was necessary to first interrupt the spread before beginning to change norms. I told Catherine about our challenges and our failures as well as our successes. I said, "We know this can work."

She nodded, took a few notes. Then she glanced around the messy office. It was more lived in now, as I had been there for ten years and acquired a few shelves of books, but it was still an unimpressive space, littered with old pamphlets and posters. It seemed a funny place to ask my next question:

"Do you think you can raise a million dollars for this?"

In Baltimore, Catherine was our connector and interpreter. She was a young, brilliant, and highly proactive member of the city's health department, and she knew the city's government and public health apparatus as well as anyone. But she wasn't one to be bound by bureaucracy if she felt something needed to be done right. She saw the city's violence epidemic through a different lens than the government, law enforcement, and even the health department did. She believed the epidemic-control approach could work in Baltimore and had fought hard for our partnership.

So much of the discourse around violence in Baltimore was about gangs and drugs. But Catherine saw it as another public health problem. With our help, she and her colleagues were able to secure about a million dollars in funding from the federal government that was earmarked for violence prevention. They put out a call for proposals and met with assorted community groups, looking for the most effective partners. As one after another filed into the health department's offices in downtown Baltimore, Catherine came to a realization:

"We aren't the ones who are going to do this work," she said. "These are the real public health workers in our city. These are the credible messengers."

One of the first groups we decided to work with was led by Leon Faruq, a respected community activist on the east side of Baltimore. Tall, slender, with a neatly trimmed beard and a studious manner,

Faruq had been out of prison for about six years after having served twenty-seven years for a murder he did not commit. Now he was determined to help others avoid incarceration. In prison, he'd been widely respected for the way he helped many on the inside fight their sentences just as he had his own. On the outside, he was connecting many of the men he'd known in the Maryland House of Correction with jobs as community-outreach workers. While in prison, some of them had experienced a profound spiritual rebirth, inspiring them to change not only their own lives but also the communities where they'd grown up.

Faruq had charisma, trust, and connections. And his mission dovetailed with Catherine's and with ours. Before we even had the support of local government at the higher levels, Faruq began putting the CeaseFire epidemic playbook into action through his organization, Living Classrooms.

As had happened in Chicago, the results drove support. It took months — months during which Faruq's outreach workers didn't have offices or even a logo — but once the program started to show quantifiable positive results, city officials began to take notice. Daniel Webster, a researcher at the Johns Hopkins Center for Gun Violence Solutions, quantified the data in four Baltimore neighborhoods over the first four years, and found significant reductions in shootings, homicides, or both in three of the four of the most violent neighborhoods in Baltimore, including Cherry Hill, which saw a 56 percent decline in homicides and a 34 percent decline in nonfatal shootings, and McElderry Park, which did not experience a homicide in the first twenty-three months the program was running.

Once the results were in, everyone wanted to help.

THE GRANDMOTHER TEST

Within a few months, Baltimore began to show clear and obvious results. With the support of the mayor's office and the health department, the initiative — now called Safe Streets — attracted more funding, enabling it to hire more outreach workers and interrupters and open offices in more neighborhoods.

Baltimore had a lot of problems. But by collaborating across multiple spheres of influence — local government, the health department, community organizations, and the police — Safe Streets was making real progress. Many of the communities were beginning to pass what I would call "the grandmother test" — older women were once again sitting on their porches in the evening rather than hiding inside for fear of gunshots. And children could play safely outside.

Communities like McElderry Park and Cherry Hill registered multiple streaks of several months to over a year without a shooting. The longer the streak, the more the community was invested in keeping it up. This led to a change in norms — violence became unacceptable, at least within certain sections of neighborhoods. And when violence was unacceptable, so too were the activities that led to it.

MooMoo — born David Fitzgerald — was one of the many interrupters Safe Streets hired after those initial successes in Cherry Hill and McElderry Park. He liked making an honest living doing something that served his community, and the interventions themselves kept his days interesting. But the work didn't become what he now describes as a real calling for him until one cold day in February three years into his work with Safe Streets.

It was a frigid, rainy afternoon with that icy rain so particular to Baltimore winters. Monument Street was mostly empty, its residents huddled under the housing-project awnings. Shivering in his black parka, MooMoo stepped out of a corner store, a rapidly cooling coffee in his hand. Another quiet day — day 302, in fact — without a single shooting or killing in his neighborhood.

As he sipped his coffee, MooMoo saw two men shuffling toward him. One was walking with his head down, his hood up, white earbud cords trailing from his ear to his pocket, bobbing his head to music. The other was half a block behind, dressed in all black, his hand positioned somewhat awkwardly near his hip.

When the first man stopped, the second man stopped. When the first man started walking again, the second did too.

MooMoo had been around the block a few times — literally. In fact, he'd grown up in this very section of Monument Street, on the fourth floor of the housing project just down the block. He'd seen enough shootings to know what one looked like in the minutes before it happened: the target walking obliviously down the street, his would-be assailant trailing him for a block or two, working up the nerve to shoot. So when the first man — the potential victim — got within shouting distance, MooMoo called out and waved him over. MooMoo knew that the second man would never fire a shot right in front of him and that his orange Safe Streets shirt would assure the first man that he had his safety in mind.

"Go inside the store," he said, handing the man a five. "Buy a Coke or something."

Although confused, the man took the money and sauntered through the door. He didn't even take his earbuds out.

That's when the second man approached. He was taller and more intimidating than he'd looked from far away. More muscular too, with broad shoulders and an intimidating expression.

"I know what you're doing," MooMoo told him. "And you can't do it here."

"I can do whatever I want," said the other man quietly.

"Not here!" said MooMoo.

And then he began to follow the interrupter playbook, trying to distract, to redirect, to keep the man talking. As long as he was talking, he wasn't shooting.

But the man was having none of it.

"You can't stop me," he said. "That orange shirt you're wearing doesn't mean anything to me. Y'all think you're doing things, but you aren't doing *shit*."

Now another man walked up. He dapped the potential shooter and joined in. "Bum-ass orange jackets don't mean anything," he said.

This made MooMoo mad. Here he was, spending his days and most of his nights trying to keep a streak of peace alive, trying to keep people from shooting each other, and these corner boys were clowning him.

"You think I give a shit if you shoot him?" he said. "Shoot, don't shoot; kill, don't kill — my check still comes in the mail."

As soon as he said it, he regretted it. Then the two men in front of him started to laugh.

"You stupid?" said the man MooMoo assumed had a gun. "They ain't had a killing here in a year. I'm not trying to ruin that!"

MooMoo poked his head in the corner store. The man with the earbuds was gone. He'd probably slipped out the back. When Moo-Moo turned around, the corner was empty. There was no trace of the two men he'd just been speaking to.

But the street was quiet. There was no shooting.

But, that night, MooMoo couldn't sleep. He kept thinking about the intervention he'd attempted that afternoon, the interruption that wasn't. MooMoo's pride was hurt. And he felt regret, too, for bringing up his paycheck. He knew that he had done it in anger because he'd wanted to show them up.

He also thought those corner boys had been right — he couldn't have stopped the shooting. The would-be shooter hadn't gone through with it because he knew about the streak* and didn't want to screw it up.

The norms had changed. There were new expectations. The community to which the shooter belonged had collectively decided that on this block in McElderry Park, shooting wasn't okay anymore.

Before this incident, MooMoo had seen himself as a kind of bouncer for the neighborhood, a type of security guard squashing beefs so everybody could get through one more day. But now he saw that the job wasn't about him.

---

* This became the second streak of over a year of zero killings from McElderry Park; Cherry Hill has had four streaks of over a year.

It was about changing the norms of the community, one interruption at a time.*

INTEGRATING SYSTEMS

Baltimore taught us a number of valuable lessons.

First, it taught us that the Cure Violence approach could work outside of the state of Illinois and far from the networks of influence we'd built. That was significant, because it meant that this was a replicable strategy that didn't depend solely on the strong links we had developed over the years in the communities. Others could take the idea and run with it using *the same basic epidemic playbook.*

We also learned that it could work *quickly*. From 2007 to 2010 in Cherry Hill, one of the first Baltimore neighborhoods Safe Streets targeted, there were sixty-five interruptions — forty-six involving gang members and forty-one with weapons on scene — resulting in the 56 percent reduction in killings mentioned earlier. And even later, from 2011 to 2021, Cherry Hill had four streaks of *over a year* without a single killing.†

In 2023 and 2024, the city achieved historic safety milestones, including 23 percent further drops in homicides and a 34 percent reduction in nonfatal shootings citywide. In 2024, several sites, including Belvedere, Park Heights, Woodbourne-McCabe, and Franklin Square, went more than a year without a single homicide. In prior years there had been *nine* streaks of one to three years across five communities.

Although Baltimore's struggles were immense, our success there showed that the epidemic approach could be adapted to even the most challenging situations. And it showed that when this system was plugged into an *existing structure* — as I had seen for other epidemics,

---

* Studies by Daniel Webster in Baltimore correlated homicide reductions with number of interruptions and found changes in norms in the target community had spread to the neighboring community.

† In 2014 when I brought board members to Cherry Hill, they asked the workers what they did every day and what the police thought of the success. At that time, there had been four hundred fifty days without a killing. The workers said some of the police officers didn't like it so much because they weren't getting paid overtime.

in other countries — rather than our building a new system in parallel, it could be implemented quickly so it could start saving lives and bringing communities back to life in a short time period, and even begin to show progress toward local disease elimination.

Baltimore also taught us how much easier the work of violence epidemic control, including interruption, was when there was commitment and support at multiple levels — the communities, the city, the public health department, and the police. In Chicago, people in the mayor's office resented the fact that when the approach showed positive results, they couldn't take credit. Some in the police department saw us as getting too much credit at best and "aiding criminals" at worst.* And the health department at the time saw our work as unconnected to theirs — violence, in their view, was a police issue (although this has since changed).†

But in Baltimore, we had a mayor who not only accepted but welcomed our help, a police department that supported the efforts, and a public health department that actively led the approach. There was more buy-in, not just in the communities where outreach workers and interrupters were but at the highest levels of government. This ensured a sense of stability and a long-term commitment to the mission. The program has weathered some lean years in the almost two decades since, but it has become an essential part of the city's approach to violence.

As of this writing, the Safe Streets program, which has had the support of every single Baltimore mayor since 2007, is managed by the Mayor's Office of Neighborhood Safety and Engagement (MONSE) and is supported by Mayor Brandon Scott's Comprehensive Violence Prevention Plan along with hospital-based programs, reentry services, youth programs, and victim-support initiatives. Baltimore has standardized and professionalized its outreach workforce, integrating

---

* In Chicago, the local commanders commonly asked for more workers: "How come there's no interrupters on the other side of the highway?" But chiefs didn't want to give us credit when speaking to the press.

† During my first conversation with a health commissioner in Chicago, the official told me that the issue was "None of our business, we don't know what to do, and we have no money." That attitude shifted with later commissioners.

trauma-informed practices and ensuring coverage in even more of the city's most affected neighborhoods.

That's how it should be. All cities should invest in violence prevention the same way they invest in other public services. And they are now beginning to do this. Cities fund their schools, fire departments, and water-treatment facilities. Sometimes they even pay for public stadiums for sports teams. With community involvement and local government support, together we had successfully built an infrastructure and implemented a system to treat violence as the public health crisis it is and always was, and it has been replicated, adapted, and improved upon even more.

Today, Chicago, Baltimore, New York, Los Angeles, and dozens of other cities have adopted the epidemic-control approach. All have systems operating in or alongside central government, reaching epicenters in their respective cities. Further, there are now over sixty cities with an office of violence prevention. Over sixty additional cities have been seeded with the approach and most of these have begun to develop systems within this framework. More than fifty major trauma centers, emergency departments, and hospitals have connections to this system, and thousands of community groups are doing epidemic control. Their results contribute to a growing dataset documenting the effectiveness of the approach and add new information.

Any system of epidemic control must do more than just interrupt acute events. There also must be continuity of care and sustained management of the epidemic over time. To achieve this, the interrupters, outreach workers, and other staffers need to be integrated with the city government, health department, law enforcement, and health-care system.

Each of these actors and institutions have an important role to play. The interrupters stop transmission in the acute phase. Outreach workers help with active case finding, contact tracing, and follow-up care, as well as with educating the public about the danger of the disease. The public health department, too, works in public education, spreading the message of how violence is transmitted and what can be done to stop it. This is a very simplified diagram of what a citywide epidemic-control system looks like in the United States. (For ease of reading, this diagram is missing several elements, including multiple social service agencies for individuals, families, and communities.)

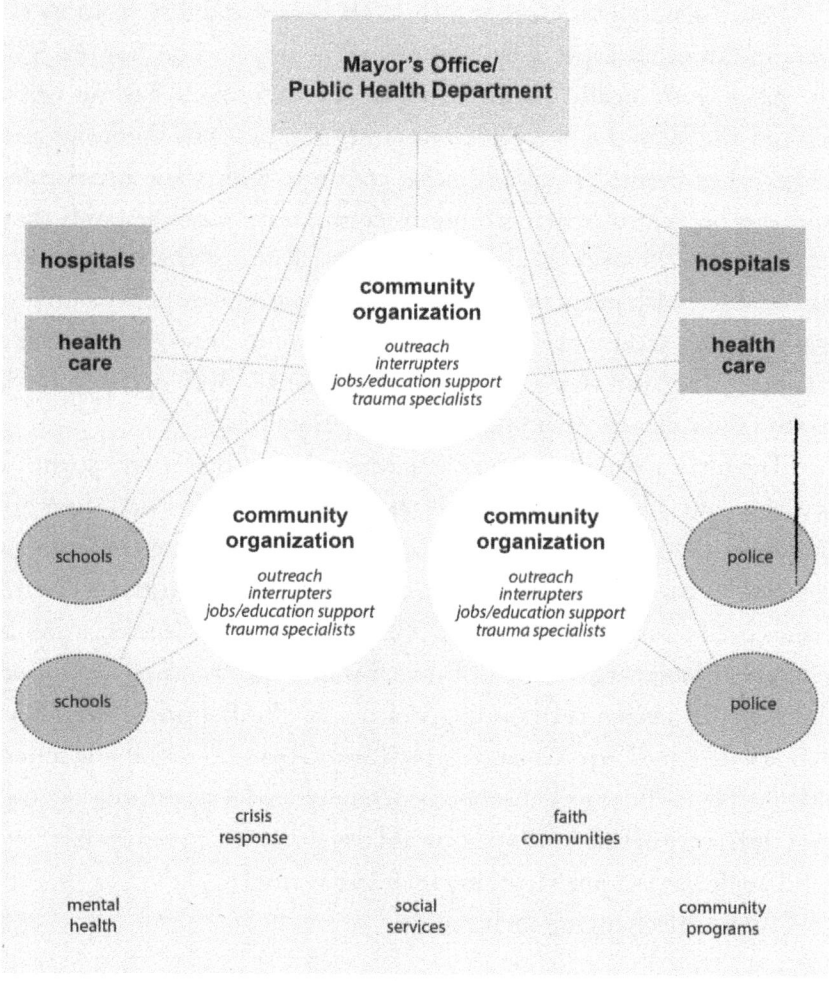

Police departments remain a critical part of the public health and public safety infrastructure, and they have taken on some new roles as well. Police officers now routinely contact interrupters prior to an anticipated act of violence in the community and commonly ask the core violence-intervention team to handle it. The team manager might then advise local police groups that a situation is under control. Although there might be sharing of information as to whether a situation is going to get hot or remain cool, Cure Violence teams do not provide confidential or identifying information to police, as this would limit the trust needed.

Police generally understand this. There is variability in cooperation and in other aspects depending on the city and on how each of the parts work locally. In the best case, police provide backup when needed and keep the peace at community responses to shootings and some other events. They of course continue with their usual roles and can be helpful when talking to community residents, and they do intervene themselves, although it's always best if the intervention can be done with persuasion rather than violence. The police's understanding and acceptance of the role of community intervention teams has been a big and very important norm change. Both agencies work to stop the violence, each in their own separate role.

The final, and perhaps most important, lesson Baltimore taught us is that norms can change in *quantifiable* ways. Stories like MooMoo's are quite common. Over time, countless outreach workers, interrupters, and community members have reported changes in people's attitudes toward violence. But it isn't just anecdotal. A study by Daniel Webster, at Johns Hopkins Bloomberg School of Public Health, quantitatively measured the shifts in norms surrounding violence in the Baltimore neighborhoods where the Cure Violence approach was put into action. He found that people in those neighborhoods demonstrated a statistically significant difference in their attitudes toward using violence to resolve conflict.

People weren't just changing their behaviors.

They were changing their minds.

THE FIRST PILLAR: COMMUNITY

The first pillar in any system is the community itself. This is where the people are; this is where the suffering is. But it's also where we take care of each other and where behavior change happens. The community is where behaviors are formed and where the safest practices and habits are normalized and shared.

The community is where we see whether we are expected to wear masks or not, whether to cover our mouths when we sneeze or cough or not, and whether to discourage violence or not.

It's where someone goes to the barber and tells him he "taught his wife a lesson," and the response is "You did what?" It's where someone who is thinking about shooting someone else tells his friend and the response is "No way! You're not thinking right, let's cool down" or "What's wrong with you?"

The community is where there is trust and where local expertise, services, interrupters, outreach workers, and trauma care specialists are available when people are in a crisis; where they can alert one another to potential violent events; where the schools, the churches, the synagogues, and the mosques can put up posters, leaflets, and flyers to help educate the public and discourage hate and violence; and where people celebrate their first yearlong streaks without shootings.

The community is where epidemics are stopped, and the stop is celebrated.

THE SECOND PILLAR: GOVERNMENT

By the mid-2010s, we were scaling the violence outreach and interruption approach we'd developed in Chicago to fifteen cities across the United States, including Baltimore, New York City, Kansas City, New Orleans, and Philadelphia, with the support of mayors and governors.

Although we had our struggles with some police departments and city leaders, most mayors and governors tended to appreciate that the epidemic-control approach — it made sense to them, was data-driven and efficient, and it produced results. Not all the time and not immediately, but when done right, it worked much more often than it didn't.

Our expansion into New York came totally out of the blue. One day in 2009 we were informed that the local city governments had received funding from the State of New York to implement our approach in nine highly violent communities in New York City and five other cities in the state.

Community activists had been lobbying the state legislature for something — anything! — that would work, it was explained to me years later. They didn't have a specific approach in mind; all they knew was that the violence had rendered their communities "unlivable" and that nothing seemed to be working.

I myself was in a bit of a panic, as there were no specific directions as to how these considerable funds were to be used. So I called the New York City health department — known as one of the best city health departments in the world — and they ultimately agreed to be the coordinating center for these efforts. A process was put in place at the community level that mirrored the one in Chicago, except that this time, there was a very interested and supportive mayor and health commissioner. New York City benefited from that support then and continues to benefit from it to this day.*

At multiple points during this period, one or more New York communities where Save Our Streets operated went one year or longer — up to three years in some cases — without a shooting, a killing, or both. Most notably, this occurred in Brooklyn twice, the Morrisania neighborhood of the Bronx three times, and in Yonkers four times. As I was writing this chapter, New York City reported five days without a single shooting *across the whole city* — unheard of in that city — and overall, killings declined by more than 25 percent in 2025. Multiple evaluations by the John Jay Center, the Department of Criminal Justice, and other organizations have shown not only strong and statistically significant reductions in shootings and killings, including a 63 percent reduction in shootings and a 37 percent reduction in gun injuries in the South Bronx and a 50 percent reduction in

---

* The central coordinating center in New York City has shifted back and forth between the mayor's office and the health department, which is fine.

gun injuries in East New York, but also shifts in norms and increased trust in government.

An initiative that started with nine communities expanded over the years to over forty throughout the boroughs, with an annual investment that grew from about thirty-five million dollars in 2015 to nearly one hundred million a decade later. This was partly due to funding from Mayor Bloomberg and then Mayor de Blasio, who, years later, spoke about how the system and infrastructure helped communities deal with COVID at the same time.* Thanks to significant investment from the city and the work of impressive leaders and community groups, New York City has managed to build one of the largest and most robust violence-reduction and crisis-management infrastructures in the country.

THE THIRD PILLAR: HOSPITALS AND HEALTH SYSTEMS

In 2002, Elena Quintana, our evaluation director, attended a presentation at the Cook County Hospital by a trauma surgeon named Rocky. Elena heard that when a person was seen in the emergency department for a gunshot wound and later discharged, the average time before that person returned with another gunshot wound was nine months, and nine months after that, on average, the person would be shot again and this time wouldn't survive.

She thought our organization should reach out to these people on their first hospital visit, and together with a public health student named Kristen Donaldson, she had written up a plan for how to do it.

The plan called for *new norms* in the hospital *and* in the community. The chaplain would be trained to talk with the patient, then alert Elena. She would send interrupters from the neighborhood to talk to the patient's friends, who were usually in the hospital's waiting room, preparing the retaliation, a response that was then normative and automatic; "like a reflex," as Elena put it. The outreach workers would give the friends other things to do — praying, donating blood,

---

* It is common that cities and countries with well-established public health systems with community health worker–based outreach be used for multiple epidemics as needed.

helping the patient's wife or mom buy groceries, helping get the children to school. At the same time, the community would be swarmed with interrupters working to lower the temperature so that one person with a gunshot wound did not turn into five or ten or twenty more flooding the emergency department that weekend.

This plan soon grew to include every hospital in the city that had a connection with CeaseFire and has now become the third pillar of the system in Chicago. Similar projects were developed around the same time in Philadelphia, Oakland, and Baltimore. Since then, this model of hospital-based intervention has grown into a national movement, implemented in at least fifty hospitals (and as of this writing, it is expanding to Uruguay, the first pilot program of its kind in Latin America).

THE FOURTH PILLAR: POLICE SUPPORT

In 2004, Bill Bratton, then the chief of police in Los Angeles, came to meet with me. He said he had been struck by CeaseFire's contribution in Chicago and hoped that the same method we'd used to reduce shootings and murders in some of that city's most violent neighborhoods could curb murder in his city. He told me that while big-city police departments had made headway in cutting violence in recent years, they were beginning to look for strategies beyond more aggressive policing. "They all believe there's something to be done in the realm of intervention," Bratton told me.

Over the next few months, I was invited to meet with a variety of government officials and community groups. Pretty soon, our chief operating officer, Candice Kane, was working with the city's Advancement Project* on a proposal for a citywide program for training interrupters (in LA, they called them "interveners"). Together with community safety expert Guillermo Cespedes, they developed the LA Gang Reduction and Youth Development program, which is still

---

* Led by Connie Rice, a prominent civil rights attorney who had made her name and career suing the LA police department.

in place today, thanks in part to political and financial support of multiple mayors, Chief Bratton, and, later, Chief Charlie Beck.

On August 28, 2014, the most notorious neighborhood in LA marked three years without a homicide, a success attributable to a combination of efforts by community activists, gang interventionists, and the LAPD. "It's really incredible to think there are kids who have been in Jordan Downs for the last three years and can say, 'I've never seen a homicide,'" Captain Phil Tingirides said at a public-housing meeting.* "We knew we had to change and help change the community," said Donny Joubert, a gang-intervention worker. "Gang banging just isn't as interesting or important," Kathy Wooten, a longtime Watts resident, said.† Norms were beginning to change here as well.

Years later, LA chief of police Charlie Beck and I were invited to present together at an International Association of Chiefs of Police meeting attended by the police chiefs from the fifty largest cities in the United States. They sat around a square table with Chief Beck and myself at the podium. I spoke first, describing how epidemic control worked and how it had worked in over fifteen cities. But the real star of the show was Chief Beck, who described all the different gang-related interventions that they had used prior to adopting the approach. He cited interventions with military-sounding names like Operation Hammer and Operation Gangs Busted and CRASH, and displayed a graph showing that none had resulted in any meaningful change. Then he pointed to where the graph took a quick and steady dive after the approach and system had been put in place.

A lot of people came up to Chief Beck afterward, but the most notable one was the very same Chicago police chief who had actively opposed our work. "Charlie," he said, "you've been talking about this

---

* Between 2001 to 2011, seventy-eight people were killed in the housing developments of Nickerson Gardens, Imperial Courts, and Jordan Downs.
† Connie Rice told me that "Jordan Downs with no killings was like having a brothel with no sex."

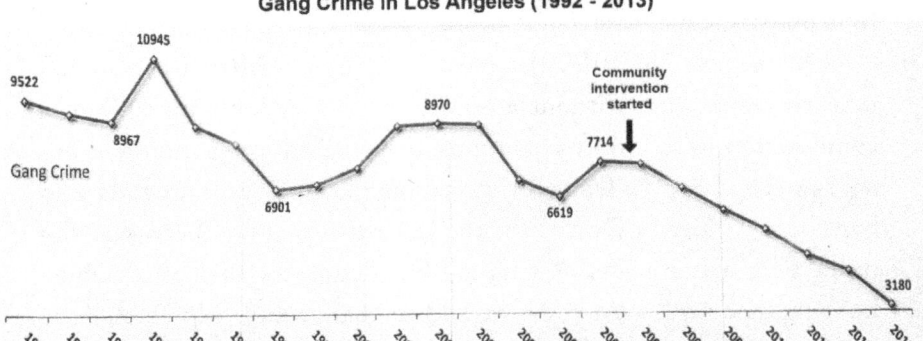

for a long time, haven't you?" Charlie replied in the affirmative. And then the Chicago chief conceded, "Well, maybe there's something to it." Even the most reluctant police departments were starting to recognize that there was a different way of approaching the problem of violence, something other than "punishing bad people." Public health was getting its hearing. This was one of several turning points that led to a better relationship between the fields of violence prevention and public health in the shared goal of eliminating this epidemic.

LOOKING ABROAD IN HOT ZONES

As the successes mounted, I and the rest of the organization's leadership saw our work as part of an international effort. We had been visited by representatives from over thirty countries, and we were getting inquiries from organizations such as UNICEF and USAID and, later, the Inter-American Development Bank (IDB). After all, disease has no respect for national boundaries or borders. We felt an obligation to spread these ideas that were working, and we were told the approaches did not exist in other parts of the world. And the new understanding of violence as a disease was resonating widely.

In our planning sessions, we drew circles on a world map to mark the epicenters of the violence pandemic at the time: the United States, Latin America, and the Middle East. In the mid-2010s we were contacted by USAID to support their efforts south of the US border. We knew the scope of the problem. In the preceding decade, the United States and Latin America had the highest rates of homicide in the world and accounted for roughly 36 percent of global homicides, with an estimated 165,617 killings in 2012 and a homicide rate more than ten times the global average. In 2022 Latin America and the Caribbean had 8 percent of the world's population and accounted for 29 percent of all homicides.

Thanks to Lupe Cruz and her team, we were able to seed communities throughout Latin America with capable, trusted interrupters; we partnered with existing programs to introduce our approach just like we had in Baltimore. Lupe was tireless in her efforts to train and guide teams in locales as disparate as Cali, Colombia, and Juarez, Mexico, effortlessly navigating the sociopolitical terrain of almost a dozen countries over the next ten years. She now supervises Cure Violence's activities in Latin America, working with former cartel members in Culiacán, drug dealers in Honduras, and at-risk women and girls in Colombia. In each country, Lupe and her team spend significant time and energy learning the local power structures of violence. In some places, one cartel might have near total control, which makes things easier because there is only one set of alliances to learn and gain access to. In another, several competing groups might be fighting for territory or power, significantly heightening the complexity of the system for interrupters and other staff.

Early on, the going was tough, in some countries more than others. The types of violence varied as well. The past century of Latin America's history is rife with several overlapping violence syndromes (which we will discuss more in chapter 8) — civil wars, insurrections, genocides, state violence against marginalized groups (in this case, Indigenous peoples), guerrilla and paramilitary violence, military violence against civilians and even the church, and drug cartels and their bloody wars for authority or control. In several of the countries, the populace has become numb to violence. And when there is no infrastructure for anti-violence work — no infrastructure or system for community work, period — it can be immensely challenging to establish a foothold.

This was the case in San Pedro Sula, Honduras, which in 2014 was the most dangerous city in the world, with a murder rate of 187 murders per 100,000 people — more than ten times the rate in Chicago and twenty times the rate of most US cities. Rival gangs — chief among them MS-13 and Barrio 18 — ran the streets, recruiting new members from an impoverished population with little hope and few other options. Every morning, bodies could be seen floating in the river, the latest victims in a bloody and seemingly endless violence outbreak.

When Brent Decker, our chief program officer, responsible for oversight of all US and international work, and Frank Perez from Cure Violence Global's first team visited San Pedro Sula, they found no organizations or people to partner with. Local community organizations had been overrun by the gangs and cartels or their members had fled. There was no government system or community infrastructure to work with, no strategy for curbing violence at the local level. The people lived in constant fear surrounded by loss. The epidemic had taken over life.

After her first visit, Lupe told me that she had never seen anything like it. It was heartbreaking, even for our most experienced team. As Lupe later recalled, the amount and the brutality of the violence in Honduras made the lethal violence we saw in Chicago "seem like child's play."

Five years earlier, the Honduran military had staged a coup, deposing President Manuel Zelaya and sending him into exile in Costa Rica. The ensuing instability was dramatic: The military began to systematically persecute anyone suspected of loyalty to the previous regime; the police arrested and beat civilians; and violence skyrocketed. Gangs ruled the neighborhoods, extorting businesses, facilitating the trans-American drug trade, and staging public executions. Civic institutions crumbled as people fled from the country by the thousands.

In the eyes of many, Honduras was a lost cause. Things were so chaotic that one US government staff member said that there was nothing left to do but call in the US Army, a view shared by many foreign officials. Like General Gani in Somalia, who suggested killing everyone infected with cholera, US officials believed that the only solution to the problem of violence was more violence.

Implementing our usual playbook of enlisting the help of community members who had access, credibility, and trust didn't seem possible. Such messengers simply could not be found. There weren't any former gang members with whom to make connections; they were all dead, in exile, in prison, in draconian "rehabilitation programs," or hiding out in churches, sanctuaries where wanted men could be protected for a time, although they were eventually returned to the streets and often killed within days.

Once, Brent Decker was approached by an American pastor, a white evangelical in his fifties. The pastor showed Brent a photo of some of the biggest cartel leaders in the country, tapping each one with his finger.

"We want these guys gone," he said.

The implication was clear: The pastor wanted these men dealt with. Disappeared. Perhaps even killed.

"I think you have us mixed up with someone else," Brent said. "We want to *work* with these guys!"

When even the churches had thrown up their hands, what could we do? When there no longer existed any civic life to speak of that wasn't touched by the cartels, how could we make connections? We would have to keep looking.

When there was no will within the communities, no systems in place to embed our people in, where could we start? We would again have to create our own system.

Brent and his team spent the days riding around in a black Suburban supplied by a local host, its lights on, the windows down, and everyone's hands visible so that anyone affiliated with MS-13 or Barrio 18, the two most powerful gangs, would know they were not members of a rival group and would not shoot at them by mistake. Nights were spent in the International Hotel, the front entrance of which was guarded by five soldiers with automatic weapons. No one went out after dark.

"I don't know why you're sending us here, Gary," Brent told me. "There's nothing to build on here. It's impossible right now."

YO SOY PASTORA

On the third week of their trip to Honduras, the advance team held a talk in a church in San Pedro Sula. They weren't expecting much. They had organized similar events there before, and both attendance and trust had been low. When people spoke, they spoke quietly, as though they were afraid of being overheard. And nobody knew how to get to the people who were doing the killing.

But then, halfway through that session, a woman near the back of the room stood up. She was barely taller than the church pew in front of her, but there was gravity in her voice when she introduced herself.

"My name is Lourdes," she said. "I know the people. I know their families. And I can help."

She was a *pastora*, she told them, a minister. Her church, where she served alongside her husband, a local school administrator and pastor, was called Cristo es la Roca (Christ Is the Rock). Lourdes knew the community deeply. People came to her with their problems. And she knew just how much everyone was suffering from the relentless violence.

The next day, she brought Brent and Frank with her into the community, visiting homes, churches, and other meeting places. Quite quickly, they saw that spiritual dedication was a big part of what made Lourdes and her team so effective in earning the public's trust. It was not uncommon to see someone take up the spirit at one of their services, dancing in the aisles or speaking in tongues. In the midst of the devastation, religion gave people the strength to live and work another day.

Lourdes Henriquez was born in Santa Barbara, one of the eighteen regions (known as departments) of Honduras. The granddaughter of Chinese immigrants, she, like many Hondurans, grew up in a mixed-race household. Her father was a businessman who bought and resold electronic goods out of their home. Her mother was busy raising Lourdes and her eight siblings. Money was tight, but they were happy.

In the late 1970s, Lourdes and her family moved to San Pedro Sula, where she attended school during the day and helped her father sell batteries and other electronics at night. Back then, the city was peaceful and relatively affluent. It had long been a textile hub and a center for industry and trade.

Foreign companies were pumping money into Honduran factories, where labor was cheap and regulation minimal. The explosion in textile growth attracted new workers — Hondurans from other parts of the country first, then migrants from elsewhere in Central and South America. All these groups arrived quickly and were crammed into increasingly crowded neighborhoods, which caused conflict. So, too, did the arrival of some of the larger gangs from the United States: MS-13 and Barrio 18, which had been formed in Los Angeles by first-generation Salvadorans and Guatemalans who were being deported back to Central America under the United States' increasingly draconian immigration policies.

To make matters worse, many immigrants, desperate for money, worked twelve-hour shifts in the factories, seven days a week. That left children largely unsupervised and often unsupported. Many turned to the family structure of the gangs for protection, connection, and a sense of belonging.

At least at first. Over time, as the gangs gained power, they became more ruthless, and strove to control every facet of daily life across vast swaths of the city. The children of San Pedro Sula didn't choose to join these gangs; they were conscripted into them. The gangs extorted local businesses, kidnapping owners' children and murdering them if their parents refused to pay the *impuesto de guerra*, or "war tax." They sold drugs with impunity, siphoning product from the drug routes the South American and Mexican cartels used to ferry drugs through the Caribbean to the United States. They competed viciously for territory, conducting shoot-outs in broad daylight, commandeering private homes, and coming and going as they pleased. They killed with abandon, utilizing increasingly powerful weapons: high-capacity pistols, automatic weapons, even grenades.

It was not unusual to see a body riddled with bullet holes lying in the middle of the street. Nor was it unheard of to witness a kidnapping in the middle of the day, passersby standing helpless and silent.

Living with this relentless fear day after day had led tens of thousands of Hondurans to pick up and move — west through El Salvador and Guatemala, north through Mexico, then across the border to the United States. By 2019, hundreds of thousands of Hondurans had emigrated, and more were fleeing the country every day. But even when so many others had abandoned the neighborhoods to the gangs, Lourdes and her congregation remained. This gave them enormous moral credibility. It also earned them access to and the trust of some of the most notorious gangs in the city.

It didn't take Brent and Frank long to decide to work with Lourdes. At first, they had to conduct separate trainings for their new outreach workers — people Lourdes knew well and had recommended — dividing them into small teams based on the neighborhoods they called home. Each neighborhood was ruled by a different gang, and while the new workers weren't affiliated with any themselves, they had lived their entire lives in fear of crossing the borders of gang territory, lest they be accused of being an informant for a gang. Why risk that when the mere rumor of someone spending time in a neighborhood ruled by another group could be a death sentence?

Together with Lourdes, the new outreach team came up with a list of things that could get you killed in San Pedro Sula, a strategy Cure Violence workers used in cities where they didn't yet understand the cultural patterns. They needed to know what the local norms were before they could help people shift away from them.

In communities in the United States, the lists of what could get you killed usually consisted of ten or fifteen familiar items, variations on what we'd learned at that Westside Health Authority gang summit: owing someone money, insulting someone's manhood, crossing into someone else's turf, dating someone else's girlfriend. As always, face, funds, turf, and females.

But in Honduras, the list stretched on and on. Twenty items became thirty. Thirty became forty. In the end, the group counted fifty-three things that could end in a person's death, everything from having the wrong gang tattoo to expressing frustration over prices at a fruit stand.

The citizens of San Pedro Sula were a perpetually exposed group in a highly susceptible population. This was not because the gangs and cartels were always at war; it was because over the years, violence had become so widespread that it was *seen as normal*, a part of everyday life.

If a teacher said something to a girl at school that the girl's father didn't like, he didn't write a letter to the school or ask to meet with the teacher; he called people in one of the gangs and told them that the teacher was spying on them, essentially signing that teacher's death warrant. If someone had a problem with where a neighbor placed her trash cans, he didn't ask the neighbor to move them; he called friends in MS-13 and asked them to take care of the situation.

In a city where almost nothing functioned — where the politicians were openly corrupt, the civic infrastructure nonexistent — the gangs were the only place to turn. In other words, violence had become the norm because it was one of the only systems that still worked.

In time, Brent realized that for the Cure Violence approach to be successful in Honduras, they would have to convince people that there were other ways of resolving conflicts. And to do this, the organization needed to partner with Lourdes so they could reach the people doing the majority of the violence.

Lourdes, Brent, and a team that included Lupe and her brother Frankie established five main categories into which most violence fell:

1. Community violence that used the gang infrastructure
2. Gang violence against the community
3. Gang-on-gang violence
4. Gang violence against the state
5. Gang violence against international drug cartels

They realized that they would not be able to stop the violence in categories three through five at that time. They didn't have the access, the manpower, or the resources to effect broad changes in international gang culture. But they *could* make a difference when it came to community violence that used the gang infrastructure and gang violence against the community if they could find a way to reach the populace — including gang members — on a neighborhood level.

Lourdes's church knew the local gang hierarchies, and Lourdes and her colleagues knew the players, which meant that they frequently knew about brewing disputes before they erupted into violence. Brent and the Cure Violence team realized that if they could train the church's workers to provide community members with basic conflict-resolution methods, aggrieved parties wouldn't feel that they had to reach out to the gangs for help.

This was a quiet, subtle form of intervention involving a shift in norms at the local level.

"The interrupter model," Brent told me, "with the orange shirts and the up-front confrontation? That wouldn't work in Honduras. No one would listen to that. It was much more like a domestic-violence interruption. We didn't say things like *Don't go to MS-13 with your problems* or *This is wrong*. We just showed them other things they could do."

For the second category — gang violence against the community — Lourdes took the lead. She'd known most of the gang members and leaders since they were children, had given them food to eat, a place to stay, a sympathetic ear. They trusted her, in large part because she always provided kindness without judgment.

Early on, the new team decided to focus on the children of the gang members first. But rather than conduct workshops or mediations, they offered services and community activities to start.

Soccer was one of them. There was an old municipal soccer field in the neighborhood of Chamelecón, long abandoned and in disrepair. Everyone called it "El Cementerio," because it was where MS-13 dumped bodies. The grass there grew shoulder-high, providing privacy for assaults and murders. The area was a hot spot for sexual assaults as well. The ravines around the field were clogged with garbage. It was a place most residents knew to avoid.

But it was also one of the only green spaces in the area. So over a period of weeks, Lourdes and her team reclaimed it. The first thing they did was deploy workers to clean up the trash. Lourdes and the others fanned out in the early morning with trash bags and cleared the garbage. When people stopped on the street to watch them, Lourdes and the workers asked them to join in too.

"This was a way to begin to change a social norm," she told me. "It made people think twice about throwing garbage everywhere."

Mowing the grass took coordination and attracted some attention, but there was no pushback. Even the gang members wanted their children to have a place to play soccer.

Once the field was cleared, Lourdes and her team planned an opening-day tournament. Her husband, Freddy, hired a band to play. Lourdes's sister, who ran a restaurant out of her house, supplied lunch. Lourdes created a tournament schedule and asked local kids to sign up.

On the day of the opening, she was nervous. Would MS-13 disrupt the proceedings? Would there be violence between the kids who showed up to play, many of whom were of the age when the local gangs began recruiting? Lourdes knew that in Honduras, the lines between who was and wasn't in a gang were often hazy for kids and early adolescents, and many of the kids didn't have much of a choice in the matter, anyway.

She couldn't exclude the gangs from the game, because that would mean excluding most of the community. As the sun came up and she whispered her morning prayers, she reminded herself that the purpose of clearing the field was to welcome *everyone*, even gang members and the children of gang members, to a new way. That was the point.

The morning was clear. Lourdes and Freddy brought in coolers filled with bottles of water, and Lourdes's sister lit a small burner to keep the rice and beans warm. They could see children standing shyly at the edge of the field, looking hopefully at the two battered soccer goals Lourdes's husband had requisitioned from the high school where he worked. The nets were frayed and full of holes, but there was enough twine left to stop the ball, or at least show that it had made it past the goalie.

At ten a.m., the band arrived — two trumpets, a drummer, and a tuba, its dented brass globe glinting in the sun. People milled around at the edge of the field until Lourdes gave the band the signal to begin. The opening strains of the Honduran national anthem, "Tu Bandera Es un Lampo de Cielo," rang through the air.

There was no grand speech about taking back the soccer field, no platitudes about community, no words of warning or shaming directed at the gangs, just Honduras's national anthem played before the tournament like it was the World Cup. When the music stopped, Lourdes and her husband consulted the tournament bracket, called the players to the field, and rolled out the soccer balls.

The day was a success. There was zero violence, just feet meeting ball, teammates shouting, cheering from the makeshift stands. Lourdes recognized senior gang leaders on the sidelines, there not to disrupt the proceedings but to cheer on their kids.

The strategy worked; there was no violence not because Lourdes and the team had changed people's minds but because they had changed the *purpose* of the space, and in so doing, they had shifted a norm.

Slowly but surely, the team's outreach efforts gained even more credibility and bore even more fruit. They made contacts out of people who would likely have killed them only weeks before.

Over time, they began to change gang members' behavior in other ways too. Customarily, outsiders who came from particular neighborhoods were shot on sight, because it was assumed they were in the employ of a rival group. Our workers in San Pedro Sula convinced the groups to use other criteria beyond where a person was from to distinguish friend from foe. For instance, did the person have tattoos indicating membership in a rival group? Why not first search his phone for known gang contacts?

Whenever there was a retaliation, it usually happened quickly and often started a war between gangs that resulted in injuries or death for those caught in the cross fire. Our workers suggested that the gangs give twenty-four hours' notice before a war started so residents had time to evacuate. And maybe this practice would become the new norm.

These might sound like small victories, but they were hard-won, and they began to yield results little by little. Over the next few months, step by step, killings began to decline. Retaliations went down. And the contagion slowed.

Within a year, killings in the areas of San Pedro Sula where we worked were down 90 percent. The city went from being the most dangerous city in the world to not even ranking in the top twenty. And over time, Lourdes, Lupe, and the team in San Pedro Sula began to reduce the levels of other overlapping syndromes, including femicide, sex trafficking, and violence against women. Soon with Lupe's guidance and partnership, Lourdes and her team convinced gang leaders to stop bringing young girls into the prisons to be "married" to incarcerated men, a practice that had previously been accepted and not questioned, a long-standing social norm. They ran workshops with young men in the neighborhood and partnered with women's groups working to help teenage girls extricate themselves from dangerous situations.

Just as they had changed the norms on the street, they were beginning to change norms in the home and in the street culture, reducing the incidents of sexual assault, domestic violence, and more.

Over the ten years following our organization's first visit to San Pedro Sula, our work spread to four cities in Mexico (Juarez, Tijuana, Culiacán, and Monterrey), three in Colombia (Cali, Medellín, and Barranquilla), and communities in El Salvador, Uruguay, Chile, and Argentina. The approach has also been applied in the Caribbean in Trinidad, Jamaica, and Puerto Rico.

Studies show reductions in violence in Culiacán, Mexico (down 90 percent), in Cali, Colombia (down 30 to 47 percent), and in San Salvador, El Salvador (down 64 percent). Communities in the Caribbean have also shown changes, with a 45 percent drop in violence in Trinidad and 58 percent fewer killings in Puerto Rico.

EVEN FEMICIDE

In 2019, Cure Violence Global partnered with UNICEF to adapt its approach to end gender-based violence, including femicide, in Honduras. According to a UNICEF report, from 2020 to 2021, the violence-interruption teams averted 1,770 highly volatile incidents involving women and young girls in twenty-five neighborhoods in San Pedro Sula and nearby Choloma, including everything from sexual assault to trafficking and exploitation. According to the same report, the lives of 501 women were saved. Violence interrupters also organized the relocation of fifty-two people, mostly women and children, to safer places. The report noted that in 2019 in Choloma, Honduras, thirty-eight women died as a result of violence. In 2020, that number dropped to thirteen, an outcome that was attributed to a committed team of violence interrupters.

In one such incident, a woman named Alma and her two children were kidnapped and held hostage by a gang that had killed her husband. A neighbor grew concerned and reported her suspicions to local violence interrupters. The interrupters transported the woman and children from the situation, provided them with temporary shelter, and then relocated them to safer permanent homes.

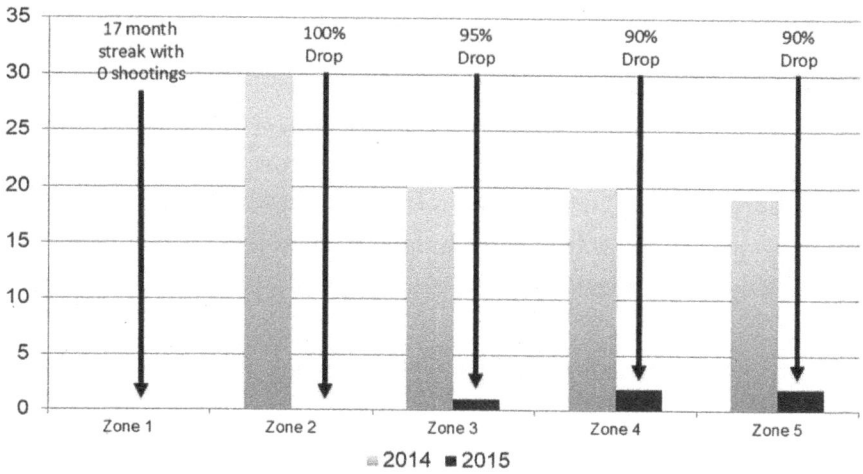

Cure Violence Sites in Honduras

WINNING STREAKS: THE ROAD TO ELIMINATION

Over time, the presence of the interrupters on the streets of San Pedro Sula became normalized; people expected them to be around just like EMTs and firefighters. It was no longer unusual for someone aligned with Lourdes's church to approach some of the most feared gang leaders and hardened street soldiers and attempt to broker peace or for someone in the community to seek out an interrupter to help peaceably resolve a conflict. This was a fundamental change in the street culture of violence.

In the following years, three of the zones in San Pedro Sula where Cure Violence's approach had been implemented enjoyed lengthy violence-free streaks. Zones one and four went fourteen months without a shooting, and zone three went *two years* without a killing.

As in Baltimore, these streaks became points of pride not only for the outreach workers and interrupters but for the residents. An area would go one month, two months, three, without violence, and suddenly the entire community was invested in keeping the streak alive. Signs would go up in store windows reading DAYS WITHOUT A

KILLING: 200, and the next day they would be changed to read DAYS WITHOUT A KILLING: 201.

The streaks even inspired some healthy competition. When a site in Brooklyn kept a streak of no killings going for thirty-two months from 2014 to 2017, outreach workers, interrupters, and community members in other neighborhoods wanted to beat it. The results — in New York City, in Philadelphia, in Los Angeles, in Washington, DC, in Baltimore's Cherry Hill and McElderry Park, in Cali, Colombia — were staggering. Everyone was committed to keeping the streaks going.

I'd seen something similar happen during my time at WHO working to roll back HIV in Africa. If one country was doing a particularly good job in reducing the number of new HIV infections, that success spurred other countries to follow suit. If Uganda showed great results, Rwanda, Burundi, and Ethiopia did not want to be left behind.

IT'S NOT JUST EPIDEMIOLOGY

As Cure Violence developed partners in several regions, I began to reflect on our staff and the workers. In addition to access, credibility, and trust, the best violence outreach workers and interrupters, the ones who could work in conditions others might deem impossible, shared something intangible, something that went beyond former group affiliations, past histories, knowledge of the problem, and extensive roots in their communities. It was a deep underlying caring.

Leon Faruq had it. Lourdes, Brent, Lupe had it. I could name hundreds, and there now are thousands. On paper, these people — a Black Muslim from Baltimore who spent most of his twenties in prison; a charismatic pastor in Honduras; a white musician with a master's degree; a woman who grew up in the streets and alleys of Chicago's West Side — have little in common. They speak different languages, believe in different things. But all of them, in their own way, bring deep inner and spiritual commitments to their work.

This intense dedication and commitment to the mission they all share helps ease the exhaustion and the heartbreak. It keeps them from succumbing to despair or numbness and from carrying too much of the pain and loss they see daily. For them, it is akin to a spiritual practice, this work of changing norms and building systems to eliminate violence in the most afflicted communities around the world and in their own communities at home.

CHAPTER EIGHT

INFECTIONS OF THE STATE

If we could read the secret history of our enemies, we should find in each one's life sorrow and suffering enough to disarm all hostility.

— Henry Wadsworth Longfellow,
Prose Works of Henry Wadsworth Longfellow

In the fall of 1991, Zainab al-Suwaij stood in line at the border of Iraq and Jordan, hoping the guard at the crossing couldn't read.

She had been in hiding for two months. She had been jailed for participating in a failed uprising against Saddam Hussein's Baathist regime and then escaped, and she suspected that her name was on a list of people who were to be executed on sight. And her name was not exactly obscure — her grandfather Hamid al-Suwaij was the ayatollah of Basra, one of the most powerful religious leaders in the country.

The bus ride to the border had been dusty and hot, the sun blinding overhead. For hours, she had listened to the quiet conversations of refugees from across the region — Palestinians, Kuwaitis, Kurds — on their way out of the country. She had watched the reddish sand of the desert disappearing under the bus, an unending expanse. In the distance, she knew, was the safety of Jordan. Approaching the checkpoint, she had felt a sudden desire to jump out of the bus and run until she reached the other side of the border.

But she didn't. When the bus stopped and the soldiers ordered everyone into makeshift wooden trailers to show their documents, Zainab merely tightened her head covering and complied. She had already been shot once and still had the stitches in her shoulder to prove it. What she was doing now — crossing the border to Jordan in broad daylight — was risky enough. But after escaping from prison and then spending two months in hiding, she felt she had no other choice. She would not go back to prison, and living in hiding was a kind of death; if she was ever going to live anything resembling a normal life, she would have to leave Iraq.

She stood in line with her aunt and her grandmother. The three of them had agreed that if Zainab was detained, the other two would go on without her. Now, nervously waiting in line, she felt as if the hundreds of American dollars she had sewn into the borders of her ornate silk fans had begun to flutter like butterfly wings.

At last, Zainab reached the head of the line. The guard was older than she was, in his mid-thirties. He had a black mustache, black slicked-back hair.

"Passport," he demanded.

Zainab handed it over. The guard glanced at the photo, then at her, then picked up a small box from his desk. Inside it were hundreds of index cards.

Zainab had seen these cards before. The previous winter, she and her fellow revolutionaries had freed political prisoners from a jail in Basra, and afterward, she had wandered through its halls, stepping over hundreds of index cards just like the ones the guard was examining. On each of them was a name — and a punishment Saddam Hussein's regime had chosen in the event of that person's capture.

The guard pulled a card from the stack. He held it next to her passport, comparing the spelling of the name. Then he looked up. His eyes were dark, with puffy circles beneath them, and his army uniform hung off his thin shoulders.

"We are in a rush to get to Amman," Zainab said, trying to keep the terror out of her voice. "Is something the matter?"

"It looks like you will be staying here with us for a while," the guard answered gruffly.

Zainab cocked her head and smiled. She decided to play dumb. "Will I be your guest?"

"In a manner of speaking," replied the guard. He turned the card toward Zainab.

On it was her name, followed by one word:

أعدم

Execute.

Zainab smiled again. She reached into the pocket of her abaya, retrieved a tight roll of American twenty-dollar bills, and folded a piece of paper around them.

"I have another document that might shed light on this matter," she said, willing her voice not to shake.

The guard took the money and casually slid it into a drawer in the desk.

Two hundred dollars — the price of a life in Iraq.

"Enjoy Amman," the guard said. Then he stamped her passport.

All the way back to the bus, Zainab kept a placid smile on her face. She knew that any moment, the guard could change his mind. He could send soldiers onto the bus to remove her. He could detain the vehicle at the border. She could still be dragged off to prison. She had liberated the inmates in one of Saddam's prisons and saw what had been done there.

The torture devices, the racks and pliers, the electric cattle prods.

The blood on the floors.

But no one followed her onto the bus. The bus was not stopped. At the border crossing, a bored-looking teenager waved them through. Zainab turned her head and watched as the boy's figure grew smaller and smaller, the hills behind him vanishing into a dusty desert haze.

Then she turned away and faced forward into the desert.

The events of the past hour finally hit her all at once. She felt anxious, relieved, cold, alive, hopeful, despairing. Night was falling; the landscape disappeared into darkness as the bus sped through the empty desert. But she kept her eyes focused on the distant horizon. Even though she believed she would never see her homeland again, she could not bring herself to look back.

Twelve years later, Zainab was back in Basra. But this time, she was there under the auspices of the US government.

In the decade-plus that she had been gone, Zainab had made it to the United States and started a family. And she had enrolled in a graduate program at Yale and formed a group, the American Islamic Conference, whose mission was to combat the negative stereotypes and misconceptions about Muslims following the September 11 attacks on the World Trade Center and the Pentagon.

Zainab had heard and was occasionally the target of the hate speech, the xenophobia, the slurs. She worked to counter them, often appearing on television to show angry and fearful Americans that not all Muslims were terrorists, that not all Muslims supported the bloodshed of 9/11, that many of them, like her, had found a welcoming home in the United States and supported its democratic ideals.

But she also knew that parts of the Muslim world — such as her homeland of Iraq — suffered under autocratic regimes and that autocracy was often linked to Islamic fundamentalism. She had been a freedom fighter, after all. She had fought in Kuwait and in the streets of Basra. She longed for her homeland to be free of the brutal dictatorship of Saddam Hussein, who had tortured and killed *hundreds of thousands* of her fellow Iraqis, led a *genocide* against the Kurds, and involved her country in *multiple wars*.

There was violence under Saddam. There would be violence to get him out.

But once he was gone, what was next?

That was where she thought she could help.

THE LARGER COMMUNITY

As we have seen throughout this book, violence, like any contagious disease, first begins to spread within a particular defined community, be it a family, a neighborhood, or an entire city.

However, not all violence is contained in individual neighborhoods or cities or even countries. Disease, after all, knows no borders. As epidemiologists do with infectious disease–control efforts, we must work the problem of violence at other levels as well. We must consider it in its many other destructive and larger forms, among them state and state-sanctioned violence, hate crimes by extremist groups, terrorism, war, and genocide.

When you look at violence through the lens of public health, all of these forms come into focus in the exact same frame; they are the most devastating variants or syndromes of the *same* disease.

These syndromes usually present at a different scale than shootings in Chicago or gang murders in Colombia, but as it is the same disease, it behaves according to the same rules of contagion: exposure, susceptibility, and transmission.

Organizations were able to stop the spread of violence in the hot spots of Chicago, Baltimore, Colombia, Honduras, and other places around the globe, and we can do that for political violence as well. But we must use the same understanding and tools that we use on the local level; we must detect locations and sources of spread, identify and reach the most susceptible, interrupt transmission, change norms, and educate the public on the means of transmission and what to do and not to do to prevent it.

"IT'S POLITICAL"

Over the past ten years, I and many others have grown more and more concerned about the extent and brutality of the violence taking place in so much of the world today. In the past decade, the world has seen increases in war and conflict: Russia's invasion of Ukraine, the war in Gaza, the armed conflicts in Africa, Asia, and across the Middle East. From 2019 to December 2024, the number of global armed conflicts *doubled*.

Even the world's most powerful democracies are experiencing unprecedented tilts toward violent extremism. In many countries, extremist groups and parties control the government.

These trends are not unrelated.

Political violence is a term I have some difficulty fully endorsing. Several times in response to our organization's work fighting violence, I've heard, "It's political, Gary." I disagree.

Yes, nearly any act of violence carries with it political implications, even very local violence. But politics does not cause violence any more than it causes any other infectious disease. The disease does not care who you vote for or what you believe in. It works through the brain. In my view, *political violence* remains a weak and sometimes distracting term for the most lethal forms of violence seen in human history.

However, epidemics can and do *take over* what we call politics. I saw that with HIV/AIDS in Kenya, where the country's leadership denied the epidemic existed even though it was causing terror and death throughout the country, and conversely in Uganda, where the country took over the epidemic. And I saw that with COVID in the United States, where lies and misinformation and denial led to the most COVID deaths of any country in the world. Like a dark cloud hovering over an entire populace, fear of a serious epidemic or pandemic disease overtakes a society, and that fear comes to define its politics, its policy, its leaders, and its norms. These are infections of the state, with deadly implications that extend far beyond politics.

The WHO defines this form of violence as "the deliberate use of power and force to achieve political goals." That definition may sound straightforward, but in reality, power and force can be used to infect a populace in many different ways by the state itself, by nonstate actors on behalf of the state, and by individuals or groups against the state. A repressive autocracy deploying its army to shoot protesters is an infection of the state. So is a state using its military to incite or support a civil war or invade a sovereign country.

A civilian-led militia occupying public lands and threatening to kill public officials is an infection of the state. So is a paramilitary group threatening marchers in an ethnic or gay pride parade. And so is the government deporting immigrants to foreign prisons and denying people lifesaving health care or disaster-relief services.

As Stathis Kalyvas, professor of government at the department of politics and international relations at the University of Oxford, writes, political violence can take a number of distinct forms, including interstate war, civil war, terrorism, political assassination, military coups, intercommunal violence, organized crime/cartels, ethnic cleansing, genocide, and state repression.

To boil this down, we can divide infections of the state into three strains:

1. Violence against the state from within or violence that undermines the state from within (e.g., terrorism, insurrection, civil war, assassination attempts, hate crimes, and extremist violence)
2. State violence against those within the state, including violence by individuals or groups on behalf of the state (e.g., state oppression, illegal or violent imprisonment or deportations, militias, famine, deprivation of health care, genocide)
3. State violence against another state (e.g., war and genocide)

These three strains of an infected state overlap and are commonly seen together. For example, violence against a religious or ethnic group infects the state by dividing and undermining it. When this occurs, events that started out on the local level can quickly escalate to the national level as the state itself gets involved on one side or another

Infection of the State

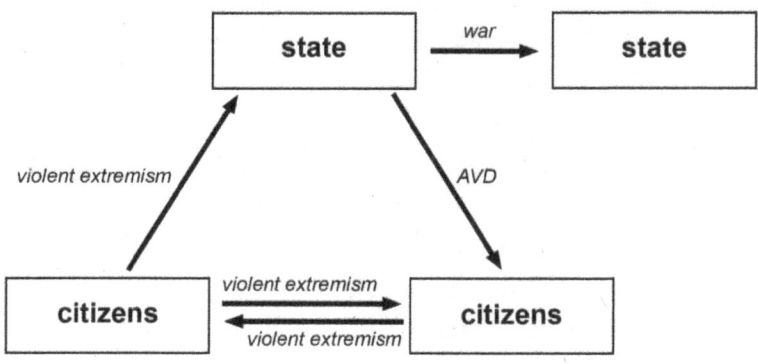

through legislation or deployment of the police or the armed forces. The chain of transmission can then extend across borders, infecting other states through any number of means: state-sanctioned threats, imprisonments or executions of dissidents, deportations, and armed invasions.

Zainab al-Suwaij came into contact with each of these lethal strains of an infected state. As a child, she lived in Basra, a city that was frequently bombed during the Iran-Iraq War (strain three, violence between nation-states). She lived under a brutal authoritarian government and knew people who had been tortured or killed by the state (strain two, state violence against the populace). As a young woman participating in an uprising against the government, she had thrown grenades at army tanks, had fired at soldiers before they could shoot her first (strain one, individual violence against the state).

Zainab's story shows us how transmission of disease crosses borders. The Iran-Iraq War lasted eight years, with one to two million killed or injured, many of them young people and children. Two years later came the Iraqi invasion of Kuwait, followed by two military responses to Iraqi violence by the United States, first in Kuwait and then in Iraq. These waves of violence splintered allegiances within the Iraqi state and helped create conditions for groups like al-Qaeda, which reinfected the US via the September 11 attacks. This in turn instigated new wars in Afghanistan and Iraq, leading to civil war and, eventually, ISIS (and other groups).

Just as with any other infectious disease, preventing a full-blown pandemic of violence requires us to step in and interrupt contagion as early in the disease process as possible.

STRAIN ONE:
VIOLENCE AGAINST AND WITHIN THE STATE

The first time Tony met skinheads, they terrified him.

It was 1982, and Tony was attending boarding school in Scarborough, England. He was what parents and teachers called a "troubled kid." Angry, rebellious, and outspoken, he found an outlet for his adolescent turmoil in punk music.

Tony came from a well-to-do family. His father was an English psychiatrist who had emigrated to Canada in the 1950s, seeking to escape his haunting memories of World War II. His mother was a retired flight attendant who stopped working to take care of her son. Theirs was, to all outside eyes, a loving home.

But inside, something was wrong. Tony spent most of his childhood idolizing his father. But when he was ten, Tony had walked in on his father with another woman. And after that, Tony's confusion, disillusionment, and fury curdled into self-hatred, shame, and pain. He started to defy teachers at school. He lashed out at his peers. His grades, once an impeccable parade of As, turned to Bs, then Cs, then Ds. Alarmed by the change in Tony's academic performance and by his increasingly disruptive behavior, his parents contacted the headmaster of his school, who suggested a regimen of corporal punishment at school: Whenever Tony acted out, he would get a beating. Whenever he got less than a B on an assignment or test, he would be hit.

The principal was a priest named Father Giardi. The first time Tony was sent to his office, it was because he had failed a math test. He leaned over a chair, and the principal said, "This is going to hurt you more than me."

Then he raised the yardstick over his head.

The beatings continued all that year and into the next. At first, each time, the principal hit Tony only once. Then it was twice. Then it was three times, four, five. At its worst, Tony braced himself for eight painful blows.

It wasn't the physical pain that bothered him the most. It was the powerlessness. The shame. The humiliation. The sense that something even more terrible was going to happen, and there was nothing he could do about it.

The punishment didn't work. Tony's grades continued to plummet. His behavior got more disruptive. He got angrier.

Fed up, his parents decided to send him to boarding school in northern England.

"This should straighten you out," his father said.

It didn't. Tony's rebellious streak ran afoul of the social hierarchies of British private schools. He was also an Irish Catholic in a school full of English Protestants. He got into fights with other kids about the Troubles and argued with his teachers about his schoolwork. His grades were deplorable. And he was angry. The powerlessness he had felt in the headmaster's office at his previous school, bent over the desk, waiting for the blows to rain down, only intensified. He was living in a foreign country, on his own, despised by nearly everyone.

The only thing that brought him solace was music. The raw, visceral rage of groups like Minor Threat and Black Flag thrilled him, and he attended as many shows as he could. He loved the energy of the crowd surging toward the stage, angry, sweaty, and flailing.

Still, even Tony was frightened of the skinheads he saw at shows, their scalps buzzed to the skull, their black pants pegged above shiny Doc Martens boots. They were aggressive and sneering and frequently threw punches. They lingered at the bars near punk clubs, smoking and choosing people to assault seemingly at random. They were older, bigger, and angrier than Tony was, and their anger seemed more violent and more hateful.

Back in Vancouver after his stint in boarding school, Tony was waiting in line one night for a Black Flag show when two skinheads sidled up to him.

"What size shoe do you wear?" they asked, pointing at Tony's Doc Martens, which were rare in Canada at the time.

Tony pretended not to hear. He edged away.

Then the doors to the venue opened, and Tony ran.

CONTAGION BY RECRUITMENT

Ten years after that first encounter, Tony McAleer had become fully enmeshed in the white-power movement in Canada. He shaved his head. He attended paramilitary exercises and training in an Idaho forest. He stocked his garage with guns and weapons in preparation for the coming race war.

In pictures, he was seen giving the Nazi salute. On television, he extolled the virtues of the white race. In print, he denied the Holocaust ever happened and urged his white compatriots to protect their families against minorities, foreigners, and Jewish people.

How did he go from fearing the skinheads to being one of them?

Whatever form it takes, violent extremism is transmitted through the same predictable mechanisms: recruitment, then copying group behaviors, and, eventually, obedience to the group.

One does not become a white nationalist ideologue overnight. Tony was not intentionally raised to be hateful. But he was raised to be scared, and he thirsted for a sense of belonging, acceptance, and love.

And the skinheads gave it to him. This is how recruitment operates. Often, extremists use stories — stories about which groups of people are inferior, about who did what and who deserves what in a society — to further weaken susceptible people's immune defenses. This is part of the system by which previously nonviolent people get infected. It is not unlike how people get swept up in cults, where there is also increasing isolation from inputs that might protect them.

What attracted Tony to the movement, at least at first, wasn't the swastikas, the Nazi salutes, the racial slurs. It was the friendship, the sense of belonging he felt after a fight when he was surrounded by his new friends in a bar or in someone's squalid apartment. It was the brotherly pats on the back he got as they recounted the kicks to the head they'd given and the punches they'd thrown.

Soon after Tony's encounter with the skinheads who wanted to rob him, he realized that they had friends in common. He saw them at concerts and became friendly with them. The skinheads were eager to hear about his time in England and his exposure to the skinhead scene there. Tony felt accepted and welcomed. He also felt protected; in a rough scene, it made sense to have the bullies on his side.

They bonded over the music, but in the early 1980s, punk music began to change. Bands like Skrewdriver — which released the single "White Power" in 1981 — inspired legions of followers to repeat their slogans and their story. Later, the punk scene began to splinter into factions, some of them overtly fascist or racist.

Tony loved this music and adopted its fashions, but the ideology came gradually. As Tony wrote in his book, his "embracing of the white supremacist philosophy was not the result of a single moment but rather a slide toward a normalization of the extreme."

At first, Tony was just donning a costume. They all shaved their heads. They wore the brown shirts of the Nazi storm troopers, the polished black boots with white laces of the National Socialist Party; they goose-stepped and slam-danced and spat at the stage. So Tony did the same, mirroring behavior designed to shock, to instill fear.

The first few times he beat someone, Tony hoped the victims weren't too badly hurt.

But over time, those twinges of regret faded.

And the things he did for shock value began to be things that he believed in, part of his identity. They weren't just things he did.

They were who he *was*.

At this time, the late 1980s and early 1990s, violent ideologies and stories were transmitted largely in person. White nationalists met each other through music or through meetups that carried considerable personal risk. Tony told me about how nervous he was as a teenager to strike up conversations with skinheads he saw in public and how he had to work up the courage to enter the white-power record store where he bought some of his first racist records. The progression from leftist anarchist to neofascist white-power propaganda leader took *years*, and it required some "skin in the game"; to be accepted, Tony needed the clothes, the attitude, *and* the actions. He had to be hit and hit back.

Today, however, budding white supremacists find one another online. Transmission of this disease once required years of direct exposure but it is now delivered via algorithm in a fraction of the time. Extreme ideas and hate spread as fast as an internet connection allows.

In the past decade, in the United States and abroad, beliefs that were once on the fringes of society have increasingly taken center stage in national politics. In addition, the same tools that extremist groups use to recruit new members — the internet, social media, algorithmic news feeds, and in-person rallies — are used by politicians to weaponize the same dynamics.

EXTREMISM, INTERRUPTED

The men and women with Bibles were screaming. The men and women with dyed pink hair and black leather jackets were screaming. And the petite Asian woman at the folding table handing out maps studded with the locations of progressive churches looked terrified.

"*All of you sinners are going to hell!*" yelled the group with Bibles.

"*Get these homophobes out of our safe spaces!*" yelled the group adorned with rainbow flags.

Then an older man in his sixties wearing a rainbow-colored T-shirt joined the fray.

"*Get the fuck out of here!*"

This was the situation Ryan Nakade found himself in June 2024. He was in Vancouver, Washington, working as a mediator for Cure PNW, a group of peace activists turned modified interrupters that aimed to counter violent extremism in and around the Pacific Northwest. The tensions on display were reminiscent of many situations Ryan had encountered in the previous few years.

There was the time the Proud Boys showed up to a drag story hour in Oregon City, wielding pepper spray and throwing punches. And the time that the Rose City Nationalists held up signs accusing people at an LGBTQ event in Pasco of being pedophiles. And the armed clashes involving advocates for racial justice, the police, and antifa during the 2020 protests in downtown Portland.

Ryan knew that nothing good would come of these groups screaming at each other. And he knew that the confrontation might quickly become violent if he didn't step in to interrupt it.

Ryan was, in some ways, an unusual presence at a Christian protest. The son of a Buddhist minister of Japanese descent, he'd grown up in a temple in Hawaii. Slight and shy, he was bullied relentlessly in high school, a violent place where parking-lot brawls were common and anti-Japanese slurs accompanied his weekly beatings. Ryan dropped out at sixteen and started spending his days online.

Ostensibly, he was studying for the GED. But in reality, he was disappearing down a series of internet rabbit holes — 9/11 conspiracy theories, Freemasonry, flat-earth science. Lonely, angry, and isolated, he began to train as an MMA fighter under the tutelage of a neighbor, a once-promising boxer who now spent his time training and inhaling the books of noted conspiracy theorist David Icke.

As a teenager, Ryan searched for direction, purpose, and acceptance. There was an emptiness in his life that neither his job as a dragon fruit farmer nor his hours in a community college classroom could fill. So he built up his body and listened to his neighbor's spiel about reptilian aliens and Jewish plots for world domination.

He veered from one obsessive pursuit to another, with no discernible goal. Eventually, Ryan decided to move to the mainland and enroll in a spiritual college in California. It took him several years to realize that the unaccredited institution was in fact a borderline cult and that his degree was largely worthless. But he had found love, a girlfriend whom he followed to Estonia, where he spent several months teaching English and martial arts. When the relationship ended, he returned to Hawaii and soon met the woman who eventually became his wife.

In 2016, Ryan landed in Portland, Oregon, where he lived on the $200 a month he earned from babysitting and doing yardwork, and struggled to find friends. In his free time, he read up on philosophy — Aristotle, Plato, Kant — and conspiracy theories. He didn't necessarily subscribe to the theories, but he felt a kind of kinship with those who did. Many of them were alienated, alone, and searching for meaning, just like he was.

In the wake of the 2016 election, Ryan and a friend decided to compile a Wiki of all the conspiracy theories they could find online and organize them in an easily searchable database, everything from the conviction that Hillary Clinton and other prominent politicians operated a pedophilia ring out of a Washington, DC, pizza parlor to the conspiracy theories of QAnon. It became clear to Ryan that these confusing and fringe beliefs were actually moving closer to the center of American life.

Ryan got to know quite a few people online who believed the world was flat and some who said that the Holocaust had never occurred. They weren't just online either. Ryan began to go to various events where holders of extreme views congregated — white-power rallies in Eugene, anti-abortion protests in Olympia, antifa gatherings in Portland. He wanted to see and learn what the people who attended such events were like and ask them more deeply what they believed and why.

He also came into contact with and then joined a group of Cure Violence workers who had established a new organization focused on learning about and interrupting the violence of hate groups in the Pacific Northwest. Members of the hate groups were hard to reach; their cultures were closed off, and they were suspicious of outsiders.

Ryan impressed the team with his openness, and his deep knowledge of various conspiratorial subcultures gave him a solid foundation on which to build relationships with people whose views he was interested in learning more about.

He didn't tell people they were wrong or that they were crazy. He just listened, with true curiosity.

In Vancouver on the day of the protesters' clash, Ryan used a technique he'd learned in mediation school, the leapfrog. He approached one of the Bible-carrying protesters, a quiet man in his sixties named John.

"Hi, John," he said. "I'd love to talk to you about what you and your group are protesting, but some of your friends are being a bit loud, so I can't really concentrate. Can you maybe get the big guy over there to calm down a bit and come talk to us over here?"

John left, and Ryan stepped back three feet. A large, muscled man wearing an American flag T-shirt approached him.

"How's it going," Ryan said. "My name is Ryan, and I own ten African pygmy goats. Wanna see a photo?"

This was a common opening gambit of his, meant to surprise and disarm. People usually said yes, and this protester was no exception.

The man peered at Ryan's phone, a smile appearing on his face.

"Nice," he said. "I like the little one."

"I noticed you were saying some interesting things about love," Ryan said. "A minute ago you said love between two men or two women was wrathful and vengeful. I'm interested in that. Can you tell me more?"

The man seemed surprised, perhaps even suspicious. But Ryan's question was so earnest, his face so friendly, that he answered, referring to various Bible verses, which he found quickly in his well-thumbed King James Version and showed to Ryan.

Ryan asked follow-up questions, prolonging the conversation. Then, gradually, more and more of the big man's fellow protesters began to congregate around him. One by one, Ryan picked off the louder members of the group and included them in the conversation.

No one was hurt that day in Vancouver or for the next several months after this encounter. It took ninety minutes, but eventually, Ryan led the majority of the protesters to a place across the street. His knees ached, and his mouth was dry, but no one was yelling anymore. No one was angry. Ryan had successfully intervened, stalled, and reoriented the situation. And in doing so, he derailed the violence that had been threatening to emerge.

As a result of interruptions like this as well as ongoing community outreach, Ryan has put together a network that is a diverse mix of white nationalists, ultraconservative Christians, antifa organizers, militant lesbian separatists, militiamen, and truthers of all stripes. He regularly speaks with people who are preparing for the apocalypse, for the coming race war, or for the Rapture. Some of his acquaintances talk about how the 2020 election was stolen. Others believe a cabal of lizard people control most of the world's most powerful governments.

All of them consider Ryan a friend — or, if not a friend, at least someone who does not judge them. Someone they can trust.

With nonthreatening diversions, Ryan can lower the temperature and draw potentially violent members of these groups away from situations that are edging toward violence. He told me his chief asset is a "pathological open-mindedness" — an almost automatic willingness to not only listen to people thoroughly but also draw them out. But his unique background and exposure to online extremism are also a big part of what makes him so effective.*

"In many ways, I was the exact poster child for someone who would be recruited into an extremist movement," he said. "I just went the other way."

Eventually, Tony, too, turned the other way. In 2005, he cofounded Life After Hate, an organization dedicated to helping people leave white supremacy and turn their lives around. In his book, he writes that "we need to learn to call out behaviours, call out ideology,

---

* Targeted Violence and Terrorism Prevention (TVTP) Report of Cure Violence Global to DHS, July 2025.

call out the activity, but we need to call the human being in. If dehumanization is at the core of this, then we need to rehumanize them. The way that we rehumanize people is through compassion. When we're compassionate to someone, we hold a mirror up and allow that person to see their humanity reflected back at them."

Between 2020 and 2024, Ryan and the staff of seven along with eight local community groups involved in Cure PNW, a Cure Violence Global pilot program to control extremist violence in the Pacific Northwest (which in 2020 was a national hot spot for extremism), recorded eight hundred and fifty interruptions, de-escalations, and other preventive engagements with high-risk persons. In those four years, according to ACLED data, the rate of extremist protests and protests involving rioters in the region dropped by more than half compared to the rest of the country.

STRAIN TWO: STATE VIOLENCE

The outbreak of violence that occurred on January 6, 2021, was world shattering in both emotional and political terms. The events of that day are well known. Tens of thousands of people assembled near the Washington Monument, on the National Mall, to protest the result of an election that those gathered had been led to believe, without evidence, was stolen.

"And we fight," they were told. "We fight like hell. And if you don't fight like hell, you're not going to have a country anymore."

They did as they were directed. They turned in the direction of the Capitol, and in just a couple of hours, hundreds of them stormed the seat of the US Congress, breaking through barricades. They reached the Senate floor, where some of them assaulted security personnel, frightening lawmakers, who had to run and hide, and threatened to hang the then–vice president. By the end of the next day, five people were dead, including a police officer. This was violence from the state and against the state.

Violent speech is an accelerator. It excites and normalizes. And when it flows from government, it can quickly infect the culture, particularly susceptible groups and individuals who adopt the narratives and begin to amplify them. The disease spreads in two directions: from state actors in positions of power and influence to the populace and the other way around, from the populace to government officials, creating loops of contagion. This is how a country can arrive at a political system taken over by this disease, fostered by it, enabled by it, and ultimately carried out in its spirit.

Violence initiated by a sitting administration is typically carried out by obedient followers who are already susceptible and primed for violence. As we have seen, the most susceptible are those with burning grievances and a felt need for relief. Many of the January 6 rioters likely craved that same sense of belonging Tony found when he was embraced by the skinheads. They were also told powerful stories, stories about rigged elections, about revenge, and about white and Christian exceptionalism. They were led to believe that they were fighting for what was right and even necessary.

This is how the machinery of state and media aids the spread of violence to a population of individuals who are not only highly exposed and susceptible but primed for violence through the scripts and behaviors they have internalized and a profound need for belonging and the approval of their leaders. And the state's leaders, in turn, achieve more power by granting their followers the approval they crave, power they use to incite more fear and obedience.

These factors are too often ignored or discussed only in superficial ways in our examinations of how violence infects the state at several levels. But they reveal clues as to what might be needed to stop the transmission of this disease.

PATHWAYS FOR THE TRANSMISSION OF STATE VIOLENCE

An authoritarian leader using his voice, influence, and platform to infect the populace is what epidemiologists might call an index case — not necessarily the first case of infection but the most prominent case detected by health authorities, the one that alerts them to an outbreak and from which contact tracing usually proceeds.

When this index case is at the highest level of power, the infected individual has access to multiple effective contagion pathways. This means more channels and opportunities to expose large numbers of susceptible people to infection and, in turn, a greater likelihood of widespread morbidity and mortality. This is how the index case becomes a superspreader of violence.

Though the particular circumstances might differ, the disease pathway is always the same. It is characterized by an infected leader* and a highly susceptible and exposed populace. The leader weaponizes violence or the threat of violence to intimidate the public and consolidate more power through control of media channels, businesses, and institutions of the state. With access to these *mass-contagion pathways*, an authoritarian leader infects the populace with lies, misinformation, distortions, and emotional speeches rooted in grievance, humiliation, and blame that tap into the vulnerabilities of susceptible individuals. It is mass contagion in plain sight.

And one of the most damaging parts of all this is that the dehumanization of others not only permits but activates the brain's systems to violence while also causing the moral disengagement.

The airwaves become conduits for normalizing violence. The institutions of government become vehicles for enacting it. And the legal system bends, out of fear of retribution or the pathology of obedience, to excuse or even condone it. The shift occurs when there is social reward for violence or when the biological system goes so out of whack that people *need* a dopamine high from using cruelty. Dopamine does not know right from wrong, good from bad, helpful from harmful. And the need for more dopamine can be insatiable.

Every arm of the state — from its leaders to its mid-level bureaucrats to special agents of the government to extremist groups and individual citizens — takes its cue from the violence at the state's core.

---

* Almost all the infected leaders acquired this infection years to decades prior, usually but not always in brutal and humiliating childhoods.

Dopamine Pathway in the Brain

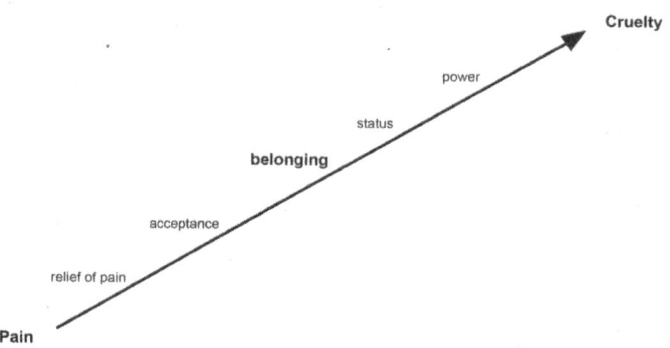

Scripts are copied and norms are molded, but at a certain point, the violence is no longer about politics or power. This is where the epidemic process takes over. The violence itself begins to act like a biological agent, spreading through the population like a plague. To slow or stop the spread, we need to interrupt it on every level, from the emotional stories that capture the public's imagination to the powerful leaders who wield those stories as tools for amassing even more power.

To many, the American experience has long been one of endemic violence targeted at one population after another, in some cases persistently, for the country's whole history. This includes the genocide and violent displacements of the Native American peoples by European colonialism and then by US policy. It includes the centuries of enslavement, lynchings, and disenfranchisement, the continued discrimination in housing, education, and health care, and the mass incarceration of Black people. It includes the abduction, deportation, disposition, and family separation of migrants, and it includes policies that restrict certain groups' access to food and medicine. Sadly, despite many attempts to improve and despite the progress that has been made, the United States continues to use state power to enact violence of different forms against nonmajority and vulnerable populations. When viewed through this lens, it should not surprise anyone that the United States has a high level of acceptance of violence and high rates of violence compared to other countries.

The American experiment was, in many ways, born from a long history of state violence in Europe, many carrying the infection with them. The disease has been with the nation from the beginning, recurring in the population throughout the centuries. And like many countries around the world, the United States is now facing one of its most threatening waves yet.

AUTHORITARIAN VIOLENCE DISORDER (AVD)

Currently, approximately *two billion people* globally live under autocratic rule. And this strain of state violence is still spreading. According to a 2022 report from the Institute for Democracy and Electoral Assistance, the number of countries with autocratic leaders doubled between 2016 and 2022, with citizens of those nations making up about 40 percent of the world's population.

The World Health Organization defines *violence* as "the intentional use of physical force or power, threatened or actual, against oneself, against another person, or against a group or community, that either results in or has a high likelihood of resulting in injury, death, psychological harm, maldevelopment, or deprivation."

Much of what happens in authoritarian states can be seen in this definition.

Living under the constant threat of state violence changes people. Citizens become afraid to speak openly in public and sometimes even in private. When working in Somalia, a military dictatorship under Mohamed Siad Barre, I censored letters I sent home, editing them to avoid any comment that could be interpreted as critical of the country or government. If I had dissatisfactions to air, I spoke only with the most trusted persons. When epidemic violence reaches this level of scale, we begin to see it as normal. For many in Malawi, malaria is normal. In Uganda, people with slim disease (AIDS) on the streets and in the hospitals became normal. In many authoritarian states around the world, violence from the state has become normal.

Authoritarian leaders and would-be authoritarian leaders know that repression and intimidation carried out at scale can be depressing and demoralizing. They count on exhaustion, disengagement, and normalization to weaken the public's immune defenses. In the public health field, this is called *epidemic fatigue*. When it sets in, the people can become fatalistic, making them even more susceptible to infection.

That's the natural history of violence at state level. It's how the epidemic becomes endemic, by a malignant "normality." In other words, this is no longer a matter of politics but a matter of this disease. It's an actual sickness masquerading as politics.

In my time at WHO, I again saw this endemic form of state violence firsthand; I worked in at least a dozen countries ruled by dictatorship or martial law. People disappeared, were imprisoned, were sometimes tortured. In one country, there were rumors of public executions. In another, you could be imprisoned or worse for *looking* at a building where the president lived.

We have seen this pattern play out all over the world — in Russia, China, Hungary, Turkey, several states in the Middle East, Africa, Latin America, and Asia. Increasingly, we are seeing it here in the United States.

In writing this book, I have come to name this strain of the disease *authoritarian violence disorder*, or AVD. This strain is by far the most malignant, contagious, and lethal mutation of violence in human history. It operates at a scale that can dwarf all other epidemics and pandemics, terrorizing and killing a country's own citizens as well as populations of other countries. It is what has resulted in world wars, widespread famines, and unthinkable genocides.

AVD naturally grows out of the other strains when conditions of high susceptibility are widespread, as occurred in Italy in the 1920s,

Germany in the 1930s and 1940s, and Cambodia and Uganda in the 1970s. No matter where or when it takes hold, AVD follows the same biological and physiological process as all other strains and contagions. Yet there exist at least two contagion pathways that almost uniquely apply in AVD.

The first is the complete immorality and deception in the form of degrading, threatening, and dehumanizing speech by the highly infectious authoritarian leader and his collaborators. The continuous lying and distortion often involves grand stories in which the targeted groups are portrayed as villains and those in power are painted as the victims. The lying doesn't just alter what is to be accepted as truth. It alters *how the brain takes in truth*, as the leader's rhetoric and stories are imprinted on those closest to him. It also confuses people to the point that *the moral ground and prior norms fall away*. People can no longer tell right from wrong. The only "truth" becomes us versus them; everything else is "too confusing."

The second pathway is cruelty and brutality, led by the same authoritarian leader. This includes both verbal and actual violence against weaker groups (or those made weaker), often ethnic or religious minorities, LGBTQ people, immigrants, and others outside the dominant group; bullying and intimidation to suppress press freedoms and individual rights; discrediting or oppressing anyone who threatens the leader's agenda; and deprivation of certain essential items, such as food and medical care.

In these *highly infected states* with continuous exposure, the violence is inflicted by the state on its own citizens. A government can kill more people in its own country than outside it, even in wartime, a phenomenon known as *democide*. And people can inflict more violence on their own neighbors and fellow citizens than on other countries' populations.

AVD is, to a certain extent, a countrywide mass shooting in slow motion.

Infections of the State

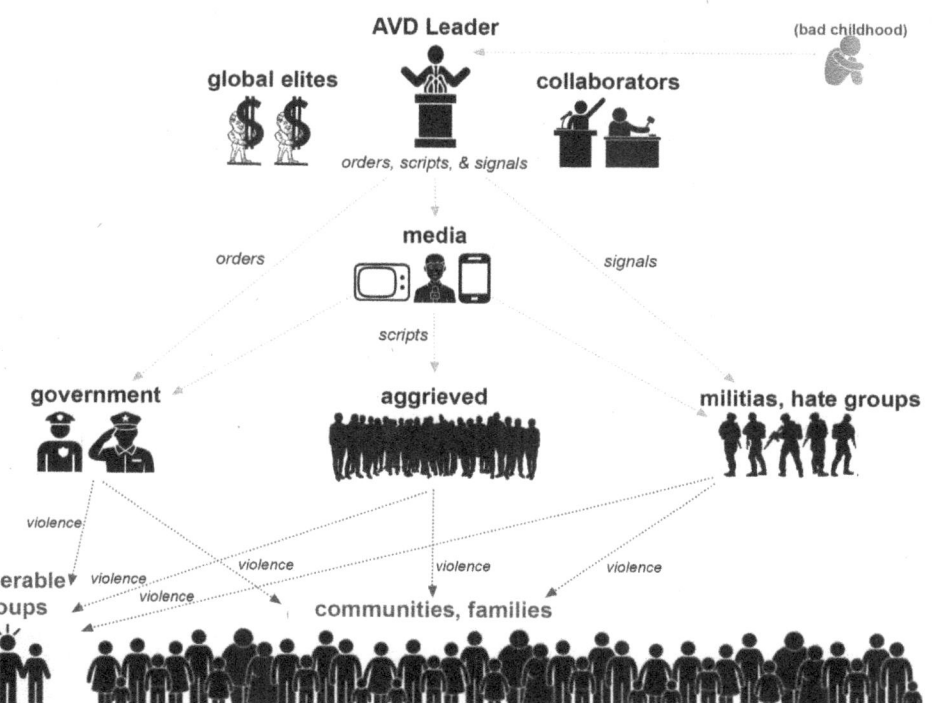

MORAL DISENGAGEMENT AND DOPAMINE HIGHS

The global pandemic we call World War II featured historically unique atrocities and horrors. In addition to the mass destruction and battlefield killings, millions of Jewish people and others were kidnapped and deported in railroad cars to death camps, where they were exterminated, factory-style, by poison gas and their bodies burned in crematoria ovens.

Philosophers, historians, social scientists, psychologists, psychiatrists, and, more recently, biologists and neuroscientists who have researched how this could have happened have focused on the psychology of the leaders: Mussolini, Stalin, and Hitler. Their findings reveal common threads that can illuminate the pathogenesis of authoritarian violence disorder.

Polish-Swiss psychologist and psychoanalyst Alice Miller wrote that "every dictator torments his people in the same way he was tormented as a child." This was certainly true for Hitler, who as a young boy was severely beaten and humiliated by his father. There are in fact compelling reports of most, if not all, index cases of AVD being heavily infected with violence early in life. Most were regularly humiliated, bullied, abused, beaten, or neglected as children, which, as we have learned, can create painful and lifelong wounds.

This is what we call *intergenerational transmission of violence*. The child's helplessness in the face of brutality is encoded in the brain, resulting in an insatiable need to inflict the fear and pain of one's own childhood on others.* Like an addict needing one more drink or shot of heroin to alleviate the suffering, people can become addicted to the dopamine rushes that cruelty provides. But it is never enough. The need for violence and cruelty becomes insatiable, as the addictive system of dopamine knows no bounds.

And yet, there is more to the story. When violence is present on such a massive scale, death and destruction occur not just at the hands of one autocrat but through the contagion. Mass violence requires people who are "just following orders" or who have been manipulated into believing, often after the fact, that the violence is justified. These people often appear normal, yet they are capable of carrying out acts of terrifying cruelty. Why?

History shows that obedience (which is not the same as loyalty) is often the silent engine of mass murder and other atrocities. And as well-known experiments by Stanley Milgram and Philip Zimbardo showed, under the right circumstances, it turns out to be fairly easy to elicit obedience from human beings. It is even easier in people who have what researchers refer to as *authoritarian personality tendencies*. These are people who reserve the utmost deference for leaders, prefer uniformity in culture, and display hostility toward those they perceive to be different or threatening. Many of them were

---

* Vladimir Putin's childhood shows an eerie parallel to the atrocities playing out in Ukraine today.

made susceptible by their upbringings, often parented in ways that taught them to value obedience over independent thinking. Most of us like to think of ourselves as immune to these instincts, but political scientist Matthew MacWilliams estimates that 18 percent of Americans score very high on the authoritarian scale, and another 25 percent are only a notch down; this is higher than in other countries surveyed.

When obedience is paired with grievance, pain, and need in certain people, they may even derive pleasure from acts of inhumanity; what began as following orders can become a high. Many involved know that what they are doing is not right. But it has become normalized, just part of a typical workday.

In 1854, when London physician John Snow discovered that the cholera outbreak plaguing the city was due not to "bad humors" in the air but to contaminated water from a particular water pump, he pulled the handle off that water pump to stem the outbreak. Similarly, it is unhelpful to attribute acts of mass cruelty and violence to bad humors or a lack of morality. To stem an outbreak of AVD, we must focus on ways to cut off the flow and contagion of violence.

THE EPIDEMIC-CONTROL APPROACH TO AVD

We can adapt the time-tested epidemic-control playbook to stop the spread of AVD just as we did for other syndromes of violence.

For authoritarian violence, this means using the following strategies:

1. **Educating the public on the disease.** Create awareness through widespread and highly visible messaging campaigns that emphasize the following:
    - Authoritarian violence disorder is a disease — a malignant syndrome of violence that can affect anyone and everyone under the right conditions.
    - Those conditions include exposure to constant lies, dehumanization, cruelty, fear, and obedience.

- To stop it from spreading, we must push back *at every point* of the violence and the cruelty. *At every level. Every time. Every single act* of violence at every level needs to be interrupted and condemned by everyone — in person, on social media, and elsewhere — regardless of group membership or political persuasions.

We've won or are winning most battles against infectious diseases *by changing the public's understanding of the disease*, not by condemning those infected but by putting the correct information into the public sphere at the right intensity.

I learned how to do this at WHO from Farag Elkamel, a UNICEF leader I hired to help combat the false stories and lack of understanding around AIDS. In language and images people could understand, we carefully explained how the disease was transmitted and how it wasn't and what to do and what not to do to be protected and stop the spread of the disease to others. We need to do the same for all violence, and as an emergency, for AVD.

It is critical for public health workers not to be political in this pursuit. Health is not a partisan issue. During my time with WHO and other groups fighting epidemics in various nations, our mission — to stop the epidemic — was more important than our views of a country's politics, policies, or leaders.

We need to adopt this mindset in the United States today. Though it can be hard to see past politics, it's critical that we do, and that the public views AVD — and all violence — as a contagion and a disease. We need to urge the public to focus on interrupting the violence, not on attacking the people infected by it, and remind them that neither violence nor dehumanizing language is acceptable. And we must stop imagining that authoritarian leaders or the people closest to them can change. They will not. Some have empathy disorders; as Elizabeth Mika points out, it is not that they *don't* care — they

can't. Further, they often have an addiction to power, greed, and cruelty that is insatiable.
2. **Active case finding.** We need to determine where the disease is spreading, who is spreading it at all levels,* how fast it is moving, and who is most affected. Those spreading the violence — political leaders, media personalities, extremist groups, and government entities, including the military and other armed groups acting outside normal rules — need to be recognized as active cases.

    Monitoring media, online forums, social media channels, and public rallies can help. The purpose of active case finding, a 24/7 activity for all diseases, is not to blame or punish but to enable and assist in the interruption of further spread at those points of contact.
3. **Interruption of spread.** Remember that AVD index cases are highly infected themselves. They do not actually cause the disease of violence, but they do accelerate its transmission, usually aided by media influencers and institutional power (e.g., government agencies, cooperating organizations, and oligarchs).

    To protect the population, we must reduce the exposure *and influence* of known spreaders. One way to do this is by limiting their exposure via media and social media platforms, public appearances, and institutional influences or power. Another option is to reduce their infectivity, in this case by *changing the way they are perceived.* This includes recognizing and condemning all dehumanizing speech and actions, not just by correcting lies and distortions but by *putting forward what is true.* For example, despite what superspreaders say, immigrants are *not* a danger to our country. They commit fewer crimes than American citizens and are of great value to our society.
4. **Outreach systems.** This is critical and not being done enough. We need both organized and ad hoc strategic outreach to key

---

* This includes superspreaders with large media platforms, government officials, and even family members who may be actively spreading the disease. Almost all activities, governmental and individual, can be done without promoting, encouraging, or inflicting violence.

officials who are in positions to influence leaders and others who are actively promoting, enacting, or enabling the violence. This means carefully selecting and recruiting credible messengers, including legislators who can help turn things around. Just as with local violence interrupters, they should be trained to reach out to people who may not want to be reached and taught to approach them privately, quietly, confidentially, and without judgment. And others need to support them in their efforts to push back against violent acts and verbally interrupt violent events.

5. **Community responses.** Shifting norms requires individual, group, and community responses to every single act of violence — we need to condemn violence at every level, every time. This includes resisting and objecting to dehumanizing speech, which causes functional and structural changes in the brain that increase susceptibility to infection. Leaders and influential figures of all ages, backgrounds, and political persuasions should be urged to voice opposition respectfully and very publicly.

    Social and political opinions matter. Individual voices matter. Voices from insiders and former supporters may matter the most. Leaders and enablers infected with AVD will keep chasing the dopamine high of violence and cruelty unless and until we push back.

    Local, regional, and national community responses, including fully nonviolent protests, boycotts, and dozens of other means of pushing back, have been shown in multiple studies to make a difference in the direction of state violence.

    There is good evidence that community interventions can influence the course of violence epidemics. Further, people who are ill, including those with AVD, may on some unconscious level *want* limitations such as enforcement of social and legal guardrails.

6. **Changing the story.** AVD is fueled by toxic and intentionally false narratives, stories of some groups being inferior to others,

less human than others, more of a threat than others. Stories drive violence and are driven by the violence. AVD index cases and their allies understand the power of these damaging and brain-manipulating stories and use them to collect and confuse followers. Think of Putin's story about Russian supremacy, his invoking historical ties with the expansionism of Catherine the Great, and claims Lenin "created" Ukraine to justify the violence in Ukraine. Or stories in the name of religion that justify killing.

Stories like these must be countered with true stories and new stories grounded in our shared values and shared humanity. Narrative frames need to be broadened or changed. There are a lot of possibilities for new stories in which our enemies are not each other. There are stories in which we don't need enemies at all.

7. **Isolation and Containment.** In some cases, it may be necessary to consider the public health strategy of some form of isolation or containment. Just as we temporarily isolate some highly infectious patients during other epidemics, we might have to reduce exposure to the violence of AVD via nonviolent legal means and enforce and further empower legislative and judicial guardrails on executive powers.

Containing an already powerful authoritarian index case is hard to do and requires courageous actions on the part of lawmakers, courts, institutions, and the population in the face of threats, intimidation, and pressure. These people and institutions need our support* in curtailing illegal or immoral acts of violence, such as a leader intentionally depriving targeted populations of food and medical care.

Using force to prevent these leaders from infecting the population is the backup to the backup option. What's true for policing in communities is also true for AVD: Force should be

---

* As with other diseases, we often have to provide help by developing mechanisms and systems to offer physical, financial, legal, and social support to people facing precarious conditions.

used to push back against violence only when there is no other option to safeguard the health and safety of the public.

8. **Providing an off-ramp.** In the very first sentence of the book *How Tyrants Fall*, political scientist Marcel Dirsus writes, "The most powerful tyrants on earth are condemned to live their life in fear." We tend to forget this, but these leaders are living in fear. And with good reason. About two-thirds of leaders with AVD are assassinated, imprisoned, or exiled. Authoritarian leaders have a pretty good idea of how such things usually go; think of Mussolini, Hitler, Gaddhafi, and Saddam. Violence, like all diseases, does damage to the afflicted.

It's a natural impulse to want to punish those responsible for cruelty, brutality, and the deaths and suffering of fellow human beings. It's normal to want to have them imprisoned, to seek vengeance and what we think of as justice. But there is no justice when it comes to diseases. There is only illness. And when people are ill, we work to treat them, no matter who they are or how many they have infected. But we must stop the spread.

This is the way of effective epidemic control.

STRAIN THREE: STATE-ON-STATE VIOLENCE

For most of history, we have viewed war through the lens of geopolitics and diplomacy. We think of countries invading one another due to broken treaties, a struggle for resources, or assassinations and power jockeying. But once we see violence as a contagion and a disease, we must begin to understand war and genocide as violence's most severe and lethal syndromes.

Wars do not exist in isolation from the other syndromes that lead up to or follow them. Other infections of state violence can escalate into war, and war can lead to everything from bullying to family violence, child abuse, community violence, and suicide. In fact, there is evidence that nearly every syndrome of violence is higher following exposure to war.

Violence Is One Disease

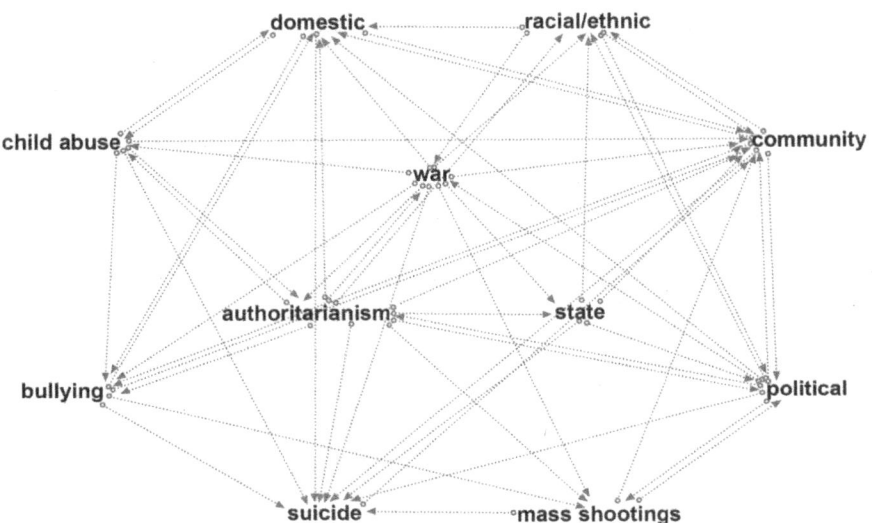

At this moment, *hundreds of millions* of people are living in an active killing zone or have narrowly escaped from one. Some escaped to conditions of famine or disease, others to places with continued violence. Many are in countries where they are resented, marginalized, or deported. Contagious diseases know no borders; this is true for cholera, TB, AIDS, and COVID, and it is true for violence.

Throughout history, wars have killed hundreds of millions and injured hundreds of millions more. They have demolished cities and destroyed entire civilizations and empires. These events are well documented. What the history books sometimes overlook, however, is the fact that in most wars, 50 to 75 percent of the dead and wounded are civilians.*

Further, these statistics of deaths and casualties don't capture the full extent of the infection; wars also transmit the disease of violence to survivors and even to populations and people removed from the front lines.

There are those affected by state violence and wars who become

---

* Sometimes that percentage is even higher, as we have seen in Ukraine and Gaza.

refugees, as occurred in Iraq, Syria, Sudan, Congo, and elsewhere. Even as victims of violence, they are among the infected, and some can spread the disease across borders as they flee their homelands in search of safety. Then there are the soldiers who return home to their countries carrying the contagion they have seen and experienced.

It is no coincidence that rates of family violence, community violence, violence in the home (including child abuse), ethnic violence, mass shootings, and suicide are all higher among persons who were involved in war; how could they not be infected with violence after so much exposure? And studies show that, more often than not, even after wars end, killings in those countries do not abate; in fact, homicide rates in those countries *increase*. This occurred in several Central American nations following civil wars and in South Africa after the end of apartheid.

One study examining homicide rates in 110 nations found that nearly half the countries that fought wars experienced substantial increases in rates of homicide after the wars ended,* a pattern dating back to 1900. There is no explanation for this other than the contagion mutating into different syndromes of the same disease, which remained active even when the nations were no longer fighting an enemy.

War is something we're all exposed to on some level, even if we have not lived in a war zone. It's part of the history of every country and of our ancestors. And, increasingly, it beams from our TV screens and overwhelms our news feeds in prominent, dramatic, and horrifying ways.

It is estimated that anywhere between 187 million and 230 million people have been killed or left to die by wars in the past century.

And the pandemic rages on — it is now in a potentially dangerous relapse.

The nuclear doomsday clock† is now measuring the countdown to

---

* This was true for large wars and small wars, for victorious as well as defeated nations, and for countries with improved postwar economies and worsened ones.

† The experts who set the clock cited climate change, the proliferation of nuclear weapons, instability in the Middle East, pandemics, and the incorporation of artificial intelligence into military operations as reasons for the latest change. The group said it was concerned about cooperation between North Korea, Russia, and China in developing nuclear programs. President Putin has also floated the idea of using nuclear weapons in his invasion of Ukraine.

the **end** of civilization in seconds, not minutes. The epicenters of war have changed, migrating from Europe in the 1940s to Korea in the 1950s to Southeast Asia in the 1960s and 1970s to Central America, Africa, and Asia in the 1980s and 1990s, to Ukraine, the Middle East, and Africa today, but the syndrome has not. Cold wars, civil wars, religious wars — *all follow the same logic,* the same disease process as other forms of violence. These syndromes are interconnected, overlapping, and morph from one form to another. It is one disease. Which means that if we have the tools to manage one form of it, we have the tools to manage all of them if we have the resources and will.

El Salvador's civil war, which began in 1979, is a good example of the intersection of war, displacement, deportation, gang violence, incarceration, and continued transmission. Fueled by fear and a story about the spread of Communism in Central America, the United States backed and joined with the Salvadoran government in their violent suppression of a coalition of leftist militia groups that were seen as a proxy for the Soviet Union. The United States provided one to two million dollars a day in recruitment (that is, contagion) funds and trained the military's counterinsurgent groups, known as death squads. This war displaced an estimated one million people, one-fifth of the population of El Salvador, and many of these refugees ended up in Los Angeles.

To survive in the violent neighborhoods of Los Angeles, the children of the displaced people banded together in groups that in time became some of the most powerful—and violent—gangs on the streets of inner-city Los Angeles and then, soon after, in California prisons.

Upon the cessation of El Salvador's civil war in 1992, many of these incarcerated Salvadorans were deported back to El Salvador as well as to Honduras, Guatemala, Mexico, and beyond, thereby establishing the gangs in Central America. And so the violence that began with the civil war of the 1970s and 1980s still rages on, untreated, to this day.

Like all major outbreaks, wars are not random; we can track direct chains of transmission back through time. World War I, called "the Great War" then, started with a single act of violence — an archduke and his wife murdered in Sarajevo by a Bosnian nationalist. This triggered one outbreak after another that rapidly infected nearly the whole of Europe. Austria-Hungary declared war on Serbia, activating a network of preset alliances and spreading the disease to five continents and over thirty countries, including Germany, Russia, France, Belgium, the Ottoman Empire, and, eventually, the United States.

Years of trench warfare, the destruction of dozens of cities, the killing of twenty million people, the economic devastation of Germany and much of Europe, and Germany's humiliation under the terms of the Treaty of Versailles all instilled in the survivors a sense of hurt and grievance, a smoldering national infection waiting to be reactivated.

After twenty years of relative dormancy, this disease reappeared with pandemic-level force in World War II. This time it was even worse, resulting in a death toll of more than eighty million people in over forty countries, many deaths occurring even after the index case committed suicide in his bunker.

Historians and politicians often discuss "forever wars." This is usually a series of epidemic waves, a continuous process of infection and spread. There are periods in which violence is endemic followed by — in the absence of a functioning system to prevent it — reactivations of the disease process.

In 1978, following the Somalia-Ethiopia war in the Ogaden region, a million people were forced to flee Ethiopia. The forty refugee camps discussed earlier were hastily erected throughout Somalia to house them. Around this time, after years of military dictatorship in Somalia, nonstate actors began to fight against the state, triggering a civil war that lasted over two decades, with new waves of violence emerging as various coalitions splintered into groups.

Viewed through this lens, Russia's February 2022 invasion of Ukraine should have been foreseen; this serious and interruptible reactivation of a wave of violence dated back to World War II and had been previewed by earlier outbreaks in Chechnya, Georgia, Moldova, and Crimea — all from the same disease source.

Consider the 1994 genocide in Rwanda, in which members of one ethnic group killed hundreds of thousands of members of another ethnic group, many of them previously friends and neighbors whom they'd known for decades. Grievances between the Hutu and Tutsi groups had lain dormant since the late 1950s and were reactivated following a Hutu uprising. Fueled by radio broadcasts dehumanizing the Tutsi and calling them locusts, Hutu militias — made up of ordinary citizens, farmers, and peasants — picked up their machetes and whatever else they had at hand and massacred close to a million Tutsi and forced millions of others to run.

Even when wars seem to be settled, at least in a political sense, it is common for some groups in the area not to agree with the terms, causing them to splinter off into warring groups or factions. We saw similar patterns in Chicago, where existing gangs frequently splintered into new ones. If our organization was on top of the situation, we could prevent violence from emerging, but if it happened too quickly, there would be a new outbreak that required a rapid response to keep it from spreading farther.

When a war breaks out, the problem is rarely that the violence one country inflicts on another catches the world off guard; it is that there wasn't a system already in place to interrupt it. When dealing with strains of violence as lethal as war, interruption often requires a continuous system of interaction to both and all sides. This is *not* the same as mediation or diplomacy, which often involves representatives of third-party nations that may have insufficient knowledge about and access to the leaders of the warring countries. And just as with community violence, family violence, or any other kind of violence, these interruptions must be conducted by people with preexisting access, credibility, and trust.

Georgios Kostakos, a cofounder of the Foundation for Global Governance and Sustainability, has worked in strategic planning for two UN secretaries-general, Kofi Annan and Ban Ki-Moon, and he understands this gap well. "The UN should have violence interruption clearly as part of its mandate," he told me. In his view, to prevent violence from spreading across regional and national borders, "there should be such global interrupter presence closer to the ground," in what he calls a preventive deployment. This is how epidemic diseases are managed.

Even mediation experts agreed in a comprehensive report based on confidential interviews with eighty-six leading professionals that existing mediation systems, including those of the United Nations, are insufficiently prepared, not well maintained, and do not have the right mediators and methods for most circumstances.

Whether unresolved grievances are between individuals or countries, if there is residual pain in the aftermath of a conflict, there is a need for an on-the-ground interruption system to reduce exposure and interrupt further spread. In Baltimore in 2015, Freddie Gray was killed while in police custody, sparking city- and nationwide unrest, but the neighborhoods in which the Safe Streets program operated remained peaceful. This was primarily because they had the infrastructure for interrupting violence *already in place*. This is also why the response to COVID was swifter and more efficient in parts of Asia than it was in the United States. It's not because Asia was the first to see the waves of disease coming; Asia was simply more prepared for the outbreak and had epidemic-control systems already set up in several countries.

The starkest example of a remitting and recurring epidemic of violence can be found in the Middle East. This region is a historical epicenter of violence, the "pinched nerve of the world," as negotiation expert William Ury called it recently. Not just centuries but millennia of exposure to violence and trauma has been transmitted vertically to generation after generation.

Through this lens, we can see Hamas's October 7, 2023, massacre of Israelis and the subsequent mass killing in Gaza certainly not as the beginning of a conflict but as the reactivation of a dormant — or perhaps not so dormant — disease. The state of Israel was founded by people fleeing violence from dozens of countries in Europe after having been exposed to violence for centuries. The country has been involved in seven wars and approximately a dozen violent conflicts in the nearly eighty years of its existence, a repeatedly unmanaged or undermanaged string of recurrences. The Palestinians too have experienced extensive violence and displacement during multiple conflicts with Israel, including an often violent fifty-year-long occupation of the West Bank.

As of this writing, Israel has been further infected with its own strain of authoritarian violence, its leadership weaponizing power to spread dehumanizing rhetoric across a hurting and aggrieved population. Since 2007, when Hamas took control of Gaza, the Palestinians have also been subjected to authoritarian governance; political opposition is suppressed, civil liberties are restricted, and perceived collaborators and dissidents are executed. The whole region — including Iraq, Lebanon, Syria, and more — is infected and is one of the main epicenters of the world's ongoing unmanaged violence pandemic.*

While researching this book, I was surprised to see studies in political and historical journals directly describing the phenomenon of war as a contagious disease. In a 1982 paper titled "The Contagion of Great Power Behavior," Jack Levy of the University of Texas showed that the likelihood of a new war was greater during an ongoing war. He noted that the "expansion of a war is characterized by contagion," and new actors were brought in "through an infectious process." As Dutch historian Jan Faber wrote, "The principal cause of war is war itself."

In studying wars from 1816 to 1980, Dutch researchers Henk W. Houweling and Jan G. Siccama found "patterns of time and space clustering similar to those of infectious disease outbreaks," and in a 1979 article titled "The Epidemiology of Peace and War," Francis A. Beer, professor emeritus of political science at the University of Colorado, wrote that the study of war "should follow epidemiology," noting that "epidemiology and the study of [war] developed along similar

---

* In a summit of international mediators that I participated in in June 2025, a map of the violence pandemic was put together. In its simplified form, it looked at the main unresolved conflict as being between China and the US, with Russia and Ukraine, Israel and Iran, and India and Pakistan seen as proxies. There is little effort being put into the resolution of issues between the US and China, as far as our group could determine.

lines, moving from magical, mystical ways of thinking to more scientific ones."

Most interesting was the work of Israeli political scientist Jonathan Fox, who found not only that wars were contagious but that religious wars were "a *particularly virulent strain*: even more contagious than other kinds." This is because religious wars are fueled by an inherent mechanism to amplify the contagion: stories.

Some religions carry a great deal of identity and emotion as well as powerful narratives about the origins of the universe, about the historical birthright of lands, about who counts as "us" and who counts as "them." Some religions have millions or billions of followers for whom encoding and transmitting these stories is a prerequisite for belonging to the group. In other words, religions can serve the same role as gangs, cartels, tribes, extremist groups, or countries do, infecting members with stories that pit one group against another.

In his book *Nexus*, Yuval Noah Harari discusses the role of stories as central to wars. Sunni-Shia conflicts in Iraq and elsewhere are an example, in that they are driven by differing fourteen-hundred-year-old stories naming the true successor of Muhammad, and he calls the conflict in the Middle East a "fight over a rock" — a reference to contradictory narratives regarding whether a particular holy site belongs to the Jews (who call it the Temple Mount) or the Muslims (who call it Haram al-Sharif). These are just a few examples of stories that have driven waves of violence over the centuries, from the Crusades to the "end-times" stories heard in several religions today.

These stories are ready-made vehicles for the transmission of violence. But they can also play an important role in interrupting it — religions also have stories of compassion, peace, kindness, and community.

In February 2006, three years into the Iraq War, one of the holiest shrines of Shiite Islam, the al-Askari Shrine, built in AD 944, was bombed; its famous and glorious golden dome was reduced to ruins. Sunni fighters were suspected, and thousands of Shia gathered near the mosque calling for retaliation.

Iraq's top Shia cleric, the grand ayatollah Ali al-Sistani, asked the people to remain calm. Notably, he called for a week of mourning (buying time). He then tackled the sectarian rhetoric head-on, rejecting it as an interpretation of Iraqi history (changing people's perspective) and decrying its dangers for Iraq's present and future (giving the people an off-ramp). Instead of a story about religion, he appealed to a story of Iraqi nationalism. He *changed the perspective*, shifted the frame. And it worked.

Similarly, religious leaders led or participated in most if not all the community responses after shootings in Chicago and Baltimore. For example, Cardinal George, a cochair of CeaseFire, led several of our community responses in Chicago and also mediated a critically important interruption among Latino groups. There are recent examples of bishops appointed by Pope Leo XIV showing up at ICE deportation proceedings, their solemn presence a form of protest against the brutal treatment of asylum seekers and refugees and possibly helped interrupt violence on the scene.

To interrupt violence carried out in the name of religion, we need to examine the stories more carefully — what they're really saying, who benefits from them, and whether the interpretations align with their true meanings. When there are too many stories with too many competing interpretations, it might be time to tell some new ones.

Wars are mass-infection events, spreading the disease across nations, continents, and oceans.

Unless they are interrupted.

THE SAME DISEASE

People, groups, governments, nation-states — all of them can be infected with violence. The mechanisms of infection may differ, the weapons may differ, and the collateral damage may differ, but the disease is the same.

In 2005, First Lady Laura Bush visited Cure Violence at the local office of our community partner in Chicago's Logan Square, the Alliance of Local Service Organizations.

This was the fifth year of her husband's presidency, and she was looking for ways to expand her national program to help at-risk boys and men, one of her signature national initiatives as First Lady.

Mrs. Bush arrived in a discreet black town car flanked by SUVs carrying Secret Service agents. When she emerged from the car, she was impeccably polite, warm, and gracious. After Mrs. Bush met the staff, we sat down at a square table. I made some introductory remarks, then ceded the floor to our workers, who described their daily efforts to reduce violence in Chicago. Throughout, the First Lady was attentive and very engaged.

She stayed with us for two hours. As she listened to staffers tell their stories, I couldn't help but think of the war in Iraq. The violence had escalated terribly. Every day there was news of IEDs, suicide bombings, and beheadings. Earlier, I'd seen an image on television of four or five young men, members of al-Qaeda, brandishing large guns and posing in front of tanks.

I recognized the expression on all their faces. I'd seen it before — in the eyes of child soldiers in Sudan, teenagers in West Garfield, and grown men in Baltimore. They were posturing but afraid.

Escorting the First Lady out to her car, I told her about the images and how I saw the peer pressure those young men were under as the same thing we were dealing with in Chicago; they just had larger weapons. Mrs. Bush responded, "I was thinking the same thing."

"It just doesn't look like that to most people from two thousand miles away," I continued. "We're so accustomed to seeing this problem through a different lens — *politics* or *terrorism* or *war* — that we can't see it as what it is: community violence." I paused, then added, "We have the tools to stop the spread of violence, but when it comes to global conflict, we don't use them."

It was through Mrs. Bush — and through the efforts of Karen Volker and myself — that Cure Violence was able to connect with operators at the US State Department and, eventually, Zainab al-Suwaij, who had formed the American Islamic Congress in Washington, DC. Zainab and I talked almost every day for two to three weeks. At first, she didn't think our approach could work in Iraq. Then she visited Chicago and came to believe the community approach could be replicable, even in a place where sectarian violence and tribal division reigned and where violence had been so normalized over decades of war.

She said she understood that gangs were similar to tribes, subcultures stressing loyalty and belonging, each with its own codes, norms, rituals, and territories.

Zainab had a lot of credibility and cover as her grandfather was very close to Ali al-Sistani, a great ayatollah of southern Iraq. She was someone even tribal leaders would listen to.

She set up a community program in Iraq based on our work, and in the first year of operation, the initiative, called Ambassadors for Peace (AFP), conducted over two hundred workshops involving over twelve thousand people, mostly tribal and religious leaders, women, and youth, to share the new thinking about violence and brainstorm how to apply advanced interruption and mediation methods to create a safer Iraq.

At the time, most sectarian conflicts were resolved through the tribal leaders. They had the access, trust, and credibility to represent their tribes and mediate disputes, and they had been doing so for hundreds of years. But Zainab was also uniquely situated to resolve conflicts. As the granddaughter of the region's most powerful imam, her name meant something. While her lineage might have afforded her access to spaces not always welcoming to women, Zainab also knew the social codes of Iraqi tribal power and how to work with them — she knew to flatter tribal leaders and appeal to their desire to appear powerful; she knew how to ensure that they saved face and sometimes even emerged as heroes for solving these conflicts.

She knew how to listen, knew how to let a leader vent, make threats, vow vengeance, and then cool down. She knew that allowing them to let off steam could lower the temperature.

These methods were straight out of the Cure Violence playbook. But Zainab also understood how to modify the approach for her culture. For instance, in the United States, we didn't use money as a tool in interruptions. In Iraq, money was a culturally important signifier of tribal diplomacy — in fact, many interventions were not considered legitimate if money did not change hands. Similarly, Zainab and her team recognized that imams were particularly powerful mediators in tribal politics, and they often involved local religious leaders directly in conflict interruption, far exceeding what the organization did in more secular societies in most circumstances.

In their first nine months in Iraq, Zainab and her local team successfully interrupted over two hundred sixty conflicts, one hundred seventy-five of which were considered high risk and likely would have resulted in a killing. After three years, AFP was able to reduce intertribal violence to *zero* in one of their focus areas in Basra. Overall, her work led to a 42 percent drop in killings in Basra and Sadr City as a whole.

At least as notable, Zainab was able to convince twenty-eight tribes to sign a pledge to end the widespread practice of using women and young girls as diplomatic currency. It was common in Iraq for conflicts to end with women and girls — sometimes as young as fourteen — being traded like property, essentially sold into slavery as part of the deal to end a long-running dispute. Encountering this practice, Zainab saw an opportunity: If she could change how tribal leaders viewed and used violence, couldn't she also change how they viewed and used women?

The first time a tribal leader proposed ending a conflict in exchange for three women, Zainab put her foot down.

"No," she said. "We are not doing that anymore."

And they didn't. With the signing of that agreement, she saved the lives of hundreds of women. She changed a norm, one leader at a time. She accomplished what Lupe and Lourdes had in Honduras, half a world away, in the shadow of another protracted war, in a different failed state, when they convinced gang leaders to stop bringing young girls into the prisons as offerings to incarcerated men.

Zainab recently told me the treaty on this still stands. People call what happens in Chicago *gang violence*, but are the gangs' concerns — face, funds, and females — really that different from those of the world's governments? When insurgent groups infect a country's government with violence, it's called *civil war*, but is there any fundamental difference between rival political factions and the *grupos* of Colombia? When Russia's authoritarian leader invades Ukraine, is it hard to make the comparison to a school bully who repeatedly beats up his weaker classmates? The scale of violence may differ dramatically, but the disease process is the same. *And so are the tools and methods for interrupting it.*

―――

There are several wars that have been averted using aspects of the epidemic-control approach (even if that's not what they called it) in hot zones like Northern Ireland, El Salvador, Mozambique, Liberia, Aceh, Indonesia, Colombia, and South Sudan. Most of these were negotiated by experienced mediators using the methods of interrupters.

The United Nations has done extraordinary work in trying to end these conflicts but has suffered in some cases owing to a lack of strong leadership and disagreements among member states with different interests and different ideas about whom to condemn and blame. The result has sometimes been interventions that show up too late.

One obstacle to faster intervention is philosophy. Not just the moralistic frame, but the sentiment I have heard uttered many times in discussions with mediators: The parties are "not yet ready" for peace.

Another obstacle is the fact that those best suited to serve as interrupters in geopolitical conflicts are often unwilling to do so. The United Nations doesn't have interruption workers and negotiators on the ground in all places needed.

And we do not yet have a system for dealing with AVD.

The United Nations was established "to end war," as President Truman stated in July 1945 after the end of World War II. The UN charter was signed by fifty-one countries, at the time representing 90 percent of the world's population. There have been remarkably few major deviations from adherence to the charter for all these years, but the Russian invasion of Crimea and then the rest of Ukraine changed everything. It was a massive break in the rule of law, and the United Nations is now trying to regain its bearings.

Following the Russian invasion, I helped form a group representing senior Russian, American, and British mediators with a large amount of experience in the region and in conflict resolution with the goal of finding very high-level officials or former officials who had credibility and access to President Putin. We desperately wanted former chancellor of Germany Angela Merkel to participate as one of these potential high-level interrupters. Merkel had a relationship with President Putin going back to their days in East Berlin, and the two had spent significant time together over the decades. When we spoke with her close colleagues in the party and the administration, however, we were repeatedly told that she was not available to help.

I presented a list of fifteen potential envoys to the Russian representatives of this group,* who confirmed that each would have access to and would be respected by the Russian president. We were confident enough in this plan that we even began drafting scripts. And yet we were not able to attract the attention or interest of these individuals.

Though our far too weak attempts to interrupt the war in Ukraine failed, we learned something important. Like the gang members in the United States, these leading international figures were primarily concerned about how getting involved in the mediation would look to the rest of the world and, in some cases, to the population back home. Getting these former presidents and senior parliamentarians and other leaders involved would have required the promise of political and physical safety as well as a way to save face. This turns out to be an important strategy when dealing with the leaders of warring nations — addressing their own fears.

---

* We had collected these names from current and former UN officials and those with knowledge of who had this level of access, credibility, and trust with President Putin.

BUILDING A PILOT SYSTEM FOR A REGION

In 2016, when the Syrian civil war was in its fifth year of relentless bombing, rising death tolls, displacements of people, and near total destruction of some cities, Cure Violence Global had already selected the Middle East as one of its three regions of focus.

To get involved, we would have to create a system for Syria on the fly, as nothing was in place. It had to reach the Syrian government and its backers (including those with close ties to the top political and military leaders), Syria's adversaries, and the communities in all three Syrian regions.

We partnered with the Stockholm International Peace Research Institute (SIPRI) and put together an international advisory team made up of sixteen people, including former ambassadors, special envoys, representatives of the European Union, and others with known access to persons very close to President Assad, the Kurdish leadership, selected European governments, and high-ranking officials in Syria, Russia, Jordan, Turkey, and the United States. This team served as an interruption table similar to those we had assembled in other situations. We called the new approach New Shape (from New Strategies for Health and Peace).

Karen Volker, our director of strategic partnerships, was leading this effort, and she screened potential nongovernmental community partners on the ground who already had broad reach in government-controlled, opposition-controlled, and Kurdish-controlled areas in Syria. Between 2017 and 2019, six hundred of their staff members were trained in epidemic control, leading to ninety-three interruptions of violence within the war zones.

The pilot showed we could set up the system. It showed we could reach people in a conflict zone and interrupt violence at community levels even during war. At the same time it showed that we could find and fully engage people who had the highest-level access to Kurdish leadership, to opposition leadership, and to those who were a step or two away from Syrian government. The effort was stymied by the conflicting priorities of the initial funders. However, both agreed on the potential. This was the first time that a strictly public health–based epidemic-control system had been used to reduce violence in a conflict zone. And it is a model for preventing violence locally while also working to influence leaders to end a war.*

A NUCLEAR INTERRUPTION

Washington, DC, 2017. Serious tensions had been building between the United States and North Korea for decades, and the newly installed US president had done little to tamp down tensions, responding to every North Korean missile test with threatening tweets; one of the most notable promised "fire and fury" if Kim Jong Un continued to test his intercontinental missiles. "Old lunatic," Kim responded, then claimed he possessed new missiles with the ability to reach New York City and stated he had successfully tested a hydrogen bomb that could be loaded onto an intercontinental missile.

Most of the world simply watched as the men at the helms of two nuclear arsenals traded threats. But in a house in Boulder, Colorado, a strategy for interrupting this brewing catastrophe was quietly being developed.

William Ury and I had been in several war-strategy sessions together over the years. He was one of the world's most experienced and respected negotiators, and if anyone could lead us out of this global disaster, it was William.

Things continued heating up, with some experts estimating a 50 percent chance of nuclear war, and William was alarmed to learn that no one in the US government appeared to be focused on this crisis. So, as he had done before, William pulled together a team,

---

* This effort lasted three years. It was funded by the Gates Foundation and later by the EU through Germany. Neither violence nor war is a priority of the Gates Foundation, but I was able to get pilot funds from a small humanitarian pot to show how this could be done. The EU delegation was focused on "Assad must go" rather than on interrupting conflict, and perhaps as a result of this ineffective framing, the killing continued for about ten more years. However, we learned such a system could be set up, and similar exercises are now being considered in areas where there is a more lasting infrastructure.

of which I was a member. I saw this situation as an urgently needed basic violence interruption. I also believed that underneath their bravado, the two leaders didn't really want to start World War III. Like the gang members and tribal leaders we met in chapter 6, they likely wanted someone to say, "You don't have to do this." It soon became clear that these two leaders resembled the gang members in other important ways too — they both wanted to appear powerful, to be heard, and to be respected and feared. They wanted off-ramps that would allow them to save face and claim victory without having to fire a single missile. So William and his group decided to help give them off-ramps.

"I want everyone in this room to write Trump's victory speech," Ury told the assembled team. "Then I want everyone to write Kim's."

Trump's hypothetical speech practically wrote itself: *We made the greatest deal, a deal that had never been done before. We solved the problem, the biggest problem. Obama couldn't do it. But I could.*

Kim's was a bit more of a puzzle. But once we realized that he craved respect and international recognition above all, we thought it might be useful to convey to Mr. Kim that there was no need to start a war because in fact *he had already won*. Mr. Kim's victory speech began to take shape: *We have already proven that we've won. There is no need to start a war with the United States because now they fear us.*

Now that we had a potential message, we needed to deliver it.

This did not happen overnight.

William led efforts with the team to develop contacts on both sides, orchestrating several visits to the White House to plant the seeds with people in Trump's inner circle, including his daughter Ivanka. He spoke to Trump's confidants of the "historic" peace announcement the two men might hold in the region. A mock-up photo was even created and field-tested.

Finding trusted massagers to approach Kim was next on the agenda. For this, William enlisted the help of Jonathan Powell, a British diplomat and one of the most experienced mediators in the world, and Glyn Ford, a former European parliamentarian who had been on mutual exchange trips to North Korea and who was familiar and credible to people close to Mr. Kim. Nobody could have been better.

The Pyongyang delegation emphasized to Kim's most trusted handlers that opening talks could legitimize North Korea on the world stage. Trump's advisers were told that the president was essentially being handed the opportunity to make the biggest diplomatic deal in decades.

In early 2018, Kim gave a speech that sounded eerily familiar: "Our republic has at last come to possess a powerful and reliable war deterrent. In no way would the United States dare to ignite a war against me." *We have already proven that we've won. There is no need to start a war with the United States because now they fear us.*

Trump's transformation was equally striking. The man who had threatened Kim with "fire and fury" now called him an "honorable man" and his "friend." In June, the impossible became reality — the two leaders met in Singapore, grinning and shaking hands in a somewhat familiar photo that seemed to defy the usual laws of international relations.

The crisis that brought the world far too close to nuclear war was not averted using the typical diplomatic tools of back-channel negotiations, handshakes, and photo ops. Instead, it took highly trusted, highly credible messengers. Strategic planning. Changes in perspective. Intensive, continued effort — a full-court press. And neutrality, confidentiality, and best practices.

William and his team did not and would never claim credit for averting this or any other catastrophe on their own. But through careful preparation and persistent outreach to those closest to Trump and Kim, a potentially cataclysmic clash between two of the world's most volatile and seemingly unpredictable leaders was interrupted, and the world stepped back from a disastrous abyss.

Reducing fear, satisfying needs, and assuring the physical and social safety of those who are infected with, threatening to use, or actively using violence might not always feel right. But it can be an effective means of stopping the dangerous progression and spread of this malignant disease.

EPILOGUE

A WORLD WITHOUT FEAR

It always seems impossible until it is done.
— Nelson Mandela

In my years helping to manage epidemics, I've witnessed a lot of death and suffering from starvation, illness, and other crises that often follow violence. In San Francisco, over two-thirds of TB patients were refugees fleeing violence in Central America and Southeast Asia. In Somalia, refugees suffering from TB, malaria, measles, pneumonia, or cholera were fleeing the violence between Somalia and Ethiopia. HIV/AIDS became more concentrated in Central and East Africa than anywhere in the world, largely due to its spread during the violence that occurred when Tanzania attempted to remove a dictator from Uganda.

My work took me to epicenters of many diseases, and I still feel the effects of these experiences — not just the pain and suffering but the fear. But it's the violence that scares me the most. And the only way I know to deal with this fear is to work to better understand what we are up against — and to work with others to stop it.

With this new understanding comes a new opportunity, the same opportunity humans had when they discovered the mechanisms of other invisibly transmitted diseases.

And people throughout the country and the world are now seizing that opportunity.

Ending a disease that's been with us for all of human history might seem impossible. This was also what we thought about other epidemics before we figured out how to eliminate them.

But now we know how to put epidemic diseases in the rearview mirror. We have done it many times, in many places, and for many diseases with even fewer means of intervention than we have with violence.

In just the past fifty or so years, we have not only rid the earth of millennia-old diseases and reduced child deaths by 50 percent, we've also immunized billions of children, dramatically turned the corner on HIV/AIDS, TB, and malaria, and almost eradicated polio. Some of the greatest killers of all time are either gone or are on their way out. At one point, nobody thought any of this was possible.

Of course, there is no vaccine for violence as there is for some diseases. But as we have shown in the communities, cities, and countries discussed in this book, there are effective and proven strategies for containing and interrupting the spread of violence, strategies that result in large reductions and long streaks of elimination.

That's our goal — elimination, one step short of eradication.

Elimination means "reduction of incidence of a disease to zero in a defined geographic area with active measures to prevent its 'reestablishment,' or reduction of transmission to a predetermined very low level at which the disease is no longer a public health problem and ideally is not transmissible to other communities."

This is a reasonable and doable goal for every community, city, and country. I realize it might not seem that way. However, throughout history, whenever we were faced with impediments to public health, we worked around or through them. This is what we did for smallpox, plague, and many other diseases. Put simply, epidemic control works.

It's tempting to assume that human interventions can't keep up with the pace at which an epidemic can progress, but every infectious disease in history has had a big head start in this race. We are usually way behind before we get going, and the situation often looks hopeless.

For HIV/AIDS, by the time we launched a global response of any significance, over one-third of the adults in several major cities of Africa were infected with a disease that had 100 percent mortality.

Within just four days of our team being alerted that cholera had returned to Somalia, seven hundred people just outside the capital city of the north were infected, and the disease was rapidly spreading across twelve more refugee camps.

However, in both of these cases (and many others), we caught up — and then pulled ahead.

Global campaigns can be mobilized fast.

The WHO Global Programme on AIDS initially consisted of one full-time person, one part-time assistant, and an Apple computer, but it grew to a staff of four hundred, staffers who set up national programs in one hundred and twenty countries in just three and a half years. Similarly, the global campaign against child deaths, the international alliance for global vaccination access, and multiple other worldwide efforts to stop epidemics and make people safer and healthier began as the ideas of small groups but led to hundreds of millions of lives being saved.

We have won this race over and over. And we will do it again.

The tools we need to eliminate violence already exist, but they have been hiding behind a fundamentally incorrect diagnosis of the problem itself. For too long, we have viewed violence as hopeless, immoral, political, ideological, inevitable, and unsolvable. Most of these explanations are judgments and excuses. And this has resulted in the misguided strategies of punishing, retaliating, and mistreating the problem and the people who have it or just letting the violence go on, deeming it hopeless, as was the case for many diseases, often for centuries.

That's not what we do in public health. It's not what we do in epidemic control. And it's not what we do for our communities and our families.

It's time to deal with this problem better. And smarter.

What is encouraging is that we have not only the tools but also the models for the systems we need. What is even more encouraging is that we haven't yet put them all together. Therefore, there is the opportunity for much more impact and scale when we do. Here are some reasons for optimism.

1. **We know how to control epidemics.** Thanks to the hard work and successes of many leaders, groups, and organizations, we have tested and used the playbook and methods successfully across many different contagious and epidemic diseases. These are the methods of effective interventions to control and eliminate infectious diseases.
2. **We have local, citywide, regional, and global examples and models** showing us how to set up systems, networks, and infrastructures that put the epidemic-control playbook into motion. This is how the successes happen at scale — through application and ongoing learning.

    We are already starting to apply some of these systems to address global, regional, and local syndromes of violence.
3. **Some epidemics can be reversed through behavior change alone.** Violence is one of these. When the new understanding of TB as a contagion became clear in the nineteenth century, behavior changes alone — in this case, isolating active cases, increasing ventilation, spending more time outdoors, and improving nutrition — caused the number of cases to rapidly plummet. Similarly, before there were any medical treatments

for HIV, the Ugandan program was able to reduce new infections by 75 to 85 percent, *also through behavioral changes alone.* We have shown this works for violence.

4. **Solutions with strong results have been shown to work for every syndrome of violence**, even when just part of the playbook is used. The syndromes of violence are so many that we tend to view them and treat them separately. But as with most diseases, the different strains of violence overlap, so we can now look at them together, not just for their common exposure profile but as a new set of resources for use across sydromes, i.e. for the whole field of violence control, that have up to now been underutilized.

   There are now many examples of 50 percent or more reductions in violence syndromes, and among some of the research, significantly greater reductions. Further, in my experience with epidemics, when you get to 50 percent, you are at a tipping point where getting much closer to zero new disease events mainly requires more intensity, continued effort, better monitoring, and adjusting — all doable through serious and sustained campaigns.*

   Further, you may recall that it took just two big moves — focusing on the most active cases and adding the right outreach workers — to reduce TB infections in San Francisco by 50 percent and, over time, by more than 80 percent.

   Similarly, we were able to lower the rate of new HIV infections in Uganda by 70 to 85 percent with just two added interventions: massive public education and community-based norm change.

5. **Violence is not a human universal.** Violence is not endemic in every or even most communities, cities, countries, or cultures.

---

* Sometimes the last 10 to 15 percent requires additional interventions, as for tough or tough-to-find cases of TB and cholera, and some regions require more resources or containment.

And cultures of violence can be changed. It's important to be aware that there are several countries with extremely peaceful cultures; there are examples on every continent.

Cultures are not fixed; they consist of norms that communities shape through their decisions, responses, public education efforts, outreach, and expressions of approval or disapproval. Through continued vigilance, peaceful societies successfully prevent and stop the spread of violence.

How the community responds and is guided to respond is the big factor. For instance, if a community shooting or mass shooting occurs in a peaceful country, community responses and actions ensure the violence doesn't spread further. Uganda responds immediately to every new case of Ebola, and most countries respond quickly to new cases of TB; similarly, dozens of communities now rapidly respond with concern and objection to new cases of violence. A community acting visibly and swiftly to prevent further spread of violence and to heal those who are suffering makes all the difference.

THE PLAYBOOK

In researching for *The End of Violence*, I reviewed books, chapters, reports, studies, and evaluations from researchers, policymakers, practitioners, and community leaders in fields as diverse as epidemiology, infectious disease, political science, child health, refugee health, psychology, sociology, criminology, anthropology, childcare, parenting, policing, veterans' affairs, women's health, human rights, trauma care, child protection, neuroscience, medicine, and history. It's important to study violence from every angle and in all its different syndromes, from domestic abuse to war to suicide. Each of these fields has its own specialists, its own vocabulary, its own literature, and its own methods. And each is in a different stage of research, development, and understanding.

And for each syndrome of violence, I found examples of successes that were achieved using one or more elements of the epidemic-control approach. These methods went by other names, like *home visitation*, *threat assessment*, and *deradicalization*. But in each case, the results moved us closer to control and elimination. Here's where I've found epidemic-control practices in effect already, with a look at how we can better apply all the knowledge and experience from one syndrome to another and to the whole field. As in many cases, only a part of the playbook has been used. Let's look at the syndromes already benefiting from the parts they are using.

> **Active case finding.** The practice of finding and focusing on those at highest risk and those already showing signs of acute disease has been a component of successful approaches to reducing community violence, violence against women, bullying, election violence, prison violence, child abuse, violent recruitment, and war while also being central to pilot programs in reducing violent extremism and mass shootings.
>
> In schools, teachers and counselors serve as active case finders, but they could be better trained in best practices for defusing situations and preventing and responding correctly to bullying and other forms of violence.
>
> Family members, friends, classmates, and neighbors can also play a large role in alerting other parents, community leaders, and mental-health workers to prevent mass shootings and suicides as well as community violence, domestic violence, hate crimes, and more. If these services are truly confidential and trusted, there should not be hesitation.
>
> **Outreach with credible messengers.** Trusted messengers who have existing relationships with good access and credibility have been effective in interrupting and reducing community violence, child abuse, prison violence, and some state violence, including (as we have seen) violent extremism in the Pacific Northwest, sectarian conflict in Iraq and Syria, and a potential nuclear war.

In cases of war and other infections of the state, choosing messengers with the most credibility, access, and trust is not as common a practice as it might be. For these interruptions to work, we need the right messengers, people who preserve both confidentiality and neutrality and who can work without judgment in the interests of involved parties while interrupting the disease spread. The interests of the parties and the interests of the disease must be separated.

Case-management and intervention protocols. When we detect someone who has contracted a highly infectious disease, we follow case-management protocols. For those with active cases, the goals are specific treatment, care, and prevention of spread. For some diseases, like measles, the only treatment is skilled supportive care and temporary isolation. For TB, we immediately initiate a drug regimen and trace the infected person's contacts, looking for other infected people, at which point they, too, will undergo treatment and contact tracing.

For patients with the most acute cases of violence, the methods of interruption described in chapter 6 have been adapted to community violence, gangs, tribes, and cartels as well as for conflict zones and prisons. This system has decreased retaliations by up to 100 percent and correlates with less violence for the whole community.

For those with less acute infections, there are now many examples of treatment protocols for violence; they focus on providing behavior change and emotional and social support while preventing further spread. For example, individual case-management methods include cognitive behavioral therapy, motivational interviewing, mind-body approaches, peer support, and other therapies that reduce the underlying susceptibility, heal the wounds of past exposure, and decrease the chance of new disease or relapse. These case-management protocols have been effective with war veterans and people exposed to community and gang violence.

Less well known is that similar protocols have been shown to be effective for active cases (perpetrators) of domestic violence, for prisoners and former prisoners, and even for some persons with potentially violent psychopathy.

These methods could be more effective still if they targeted the greatest spreaders, were more selective in the choice and training of messengers, and involved more intensive, persistent, and creative attempts to reach such persons.

Community responses and norms. We already know how to interrupt a drunk driver's attempt to get behind the wheel. When a friend or close colleague says, "Give me the keys, friend," they are making it clear that they object and disapprove of the behavior. Similar conversations are now occurring in communities around the country about using violence. (For example, "You plan to do what?")

Comprehensive and community-wide norm-changing programs that guide new behaviors have been used to reduce domestic violence and bullying and are part of community-violence reduction. Visible objection, disapproval, and condemnation of recent, ongoing, or expected violence is central to changing norms and behaviors.

It is now very common to see community-wide responses in the wake of violent events such as instances of police violence and mass shootings. Protests against authoritarian violence and other infections of the state, now seen worldwide, can be effective expressions of disapproval and condemnation when nonviolent themselves. The size of these responses is relevant to the success. They are often directed at the specific leader rather than at the specific acts of violence, cruelty, or deprivation the leader and others infected are spreading and that must all be stopped.

Community meetings and decisions, bystander trainings, parent trainings, and other forms of skills training and support can make it more safe and effective for people to interrupt behaviors and changes norms. Examples in the book include the work of Lupe and Lourdes in Honduras and Zainab in Iraq in changing norms about violence against women and girls. Family-violence support systems and hotlines have been successful in changing norms and reducing intimate-partner violence in India, South Africa, Uganda, and the United States.

Legislation has been very helpful in shifting the norms around gun violence, domestic violence, and child abuse, especially in Europe after World War II, where corporal punishment of children was outlawed in several countries and investments were made in public education and parenting training to reduce abuse of children. This is now a global initiative of WHO because of its importance and because of its relevance to future violence in many forms, including state violence.

However, community, country, and global norm change supported by much stronger public education efforts need to play a bigger role in interrupting community violence, violence against women, police violence, war, genocide, and tyranny. And it needs to be incremental in some cases, a series of small shifts that build toward fuller transformation.*

Public education and training. Public education campaigns have been a crucial part of effective responses to HIV, cholera, smallpox, COVID, and many other disease-control campaigns. Here, the key is to clearly explain *how the disease works*. People need to understand a disease in order to know what to do and what not to do. People need to know that violence is contagious and that they can do something about

---

* Examples of small steps include expecting and regularizing interrupter efforts, sticking to ceasefire agreements, and stopping the separation of families in deportations.

it, and they need to know what they can do. We need universal training on this.

With epidemics, there will always be lies, conspiracy theories, and misinformation. As Farag Elkamel, a communication expert for UNICEF in the Middle East, once told me: Don't try to silence the noise, just insert 4 to 5 percent of truth about the facts that matter most. This approach can be applied to violence as well.

The most successful initiatives to curb school bullying utilize many core tenets of epidemic control. In Norway, for example, a nationwide initiative put anti-bullying messaging at the center of the public education system at nearly every level. Systematic, data-focused, and supported at every level of government, the Olweus Bullying Prevention Program is credited with reducing bullying by up to 50 percent and has been adopted in many countries. Public education has also been key to reducing domestic violence and preventing suicide by, among other methods, raising people's awareness of hotlines as a place where support can be provided confidentially.

Yet despite its power to change attitudes, behaviors, and norms, public education is being greatly underutilized for every form of violence and for most other epidemics as well. It could be deployed to much greater effect, particularly for political violence and other infections of the state.

Isolation only when necessary. As a communicable disease officer in San Franciso, I had the authority and the responsibility to isolate patients with TB temporarily if necessary. This was not punishment but an important public health practice for stopping transmission if it was the only way to ensure that a person would not infect others. I had to do this only four or five times for persons who would not adhere to the treatment regimen no matter what our outreach staff did. (Most of these very few patients had drug-resistant TB, an even more serious form of the disease.) They were isolated for just one month or so, until they were not infectious and we were assured they could be effectively supported at home.

Just as COVID patients can protect their family members by isolating themselves for a few days, domestic abusers can be removed from their families to stop the disease from spreading to the rest of the household. This method has been less frequently used for other violence syndromes, with the exception of community violence, where it has been abused, and for some infections of the state. Isolating patients is a method of containment we should consider only when all other options have been exhausted and not for the purpose of punishment but for the health and safety of the public.

PATHWAYS TO ELIMINATION: ALL THAT'S LEFT TO DO

Violence has been with us a long time — all of our history. But we now find ourselves at a critical juncture. Over one hundred countries have deteriorated in measures of peace in the past ten years due to this violence pandemic.* However, we can now take advantage of all the new science combined with the time-tested methods of epidemic control to interrupt its spread — and turn back its course. We no longer need to allow violence to continue its uncontrolled spread.

What we need now is local as well as a global understanding of violence as a disease and knowledge of how it is spread. We need to be more aware of the effects of exposure to ourselves and others, and work to limit it. And be aware of our own and others' susceptibilities from pain, grievance, and unhealthy norms — and provide care. Then we need to do whatever we can to stop the spread. There is too much

---

* Global violence is growing, with increases in the number of conflicts, surges in state-based armed conflicts (the highest numbers since the end of World War II), rises in political violence, and authoritarian rule.

pain in the world, and most of us aren't attending to it well. We can help each other heal.

We need to actively use the basic definition* and new language† of the problem, then use our new understanding to sharpen our focus on the disease itself, recruit others, and develop networks and systems at the community, regional, national, and international levels that focus on violence reduction and sustain the work over time.

We can do this. We've done it before for other epidemics.

With sufficient implementation of case finding, outreach, community responses, intervention, and public education, we have a pathway to use to take us from a culture in which violence is a malignant normal to one in which it is a rare event.

I began doing this work not knowing what would come of it. I stepped into a world fraught with violence, unsure of what I would find, just as many readers of this book might have.

What I found is great hope.

I have seen pain and suffering, but I've also seen lightness and beauty. And I've seen the growing successes. And the more I studied how our minds work, the more I understood that our capacity for harm is far outmatched by our abilities and commitment to turn this problem around. And to heal.

In these years working with epidemics, including violence, I've met so many people with so much to teach. And who taught me so much.

The more I dug, the more I found. And there is still much to learn.

---

* The intentional use of physical force or power, threatened or actual, against oneself, another person, or a group or community that either results in or has a high likelihood of resulting in injury, death, psychological harm, maldevelopment, or deprivation (World Health Organization).
† Progress will accelerate when we use epidemic language like *epidemic, contagion, transmission, spread, exposure, susceptibility, behaviors, norms, interruption, elimination, health,* and *care*. New words change the way we see and manage a problem and lead to a new way ahead. (Nelson, et al; Giesecke; Anderson and May; and Kuhn).

Each answer I uncovered led to more questions. And although one book can reveal only so much, a lot of the work ongoing in our communities and throughout the world is already succeeding. The science, the experiences, and the people all fill me with optimism and even excitement for what can be done next and what we might discover while creating this new peaceful world.

We can create a world where women can walk down the street or be at home without fear. Where minority populations are treated well and are not at risk. Where children play without danger. Where ongoing wars and conflicts are stopped and become a thing of the past because conflicts are detected and potential violence interrupted early. A world where authoritarian leaders are removed from power or never get there and where the people of Ukraine and Russia and Gaza and Israel and Sudan and elsewhere feel safe and protected. And where family members, friends, and neighbors take care of one another and themselves, and have no reason to fear violence anymore.

We have never had as much knowledge, understanding, and experience in healing this disease as we do now.

We can re-create the world without violence. And faster than we think.

We can put this epidemic behind us.

ACKNOWLEDGMENTS

My mother and father undoubtedly formed the way I see and feel things and likely what became this book. Their concerns, inquiries, pleasures, and challenges became mine. Mom, who remains the biggest influence of my life, showed her caring and her own suffering for anyone in difficult circumstances, and I absorbed it—the blessings, concerns and the fears. Once when I was leaving home in Chicago to return to WHO, she asked, "You're going back to Europe, aren't you? If you only knew what it took for us to get out of there." She carried the pain of her immigrant ancestors, but I didn't hear it until later, as she shielded us.

Dad was not only a scientist but a deep lover of biology and a real-world naturalist. I got from him not only the awe of science but of the natural world. And the conflict of being *indoors* (lab—or this book) versus the peace and freedom of being *outdoors*. This conflict affected the progress of this book. I am beyond fortunate to have had their kindness and tolerance of my being away, and to have grown up in a peaceful home.

My loving wife, Marla, has been the blessing of my life in many ways, helping through our daily discussions with her insights and questioning, as well as through her spirit, support, and love. She is sharp and can dissect details as well as see the whole, the holes in my thinking, and can tell me when there are other ways of looking at things. She has somehow put up with my lifestyle, work, obsessions, and me. And she has been there for guidance and support during the challenges, conflicts, and opposition to what this work was thought to be doing to the existing order and the existing thinking. Marla has helped me get through this. Marla is a natural spirit, and her studies of spiritual teachings are valuable to us both. It is easier to write the details of a book than to express the whole of our life, as our time together gives life more meaning than a book or work. I also want to recognize the important influence of Marla's thoughtful parents, Inez and Warren.

I am grateful for a precious family including my treasured brother, Huey Freeman, an author before me, and his lovely wife, Katherine, my nephew, Matt, nieces Betsi, Linda, and her loving and amazing husband, Chris—and Selene(!) and dear Michala. I am close to and get support from my loving cousins Cindy, Andrea, and Sandy, Jay, Anita, and Bruce and my cousins-of-sorts Aaron and Harper, Ryan and Belinda, Rebecca and Perry, Austin and Izzie, Peyton and Tatum, Marla's cousin Kim Rosenthal and Jakob Hedrich, and my loving in-laws Mark and Cathy, Matt Anderson and Mary Waguespak, and Michael and Amanda Anderson.

I've been grounded for decades by Glen Joffe, my best friend, since we were ten years old, when I rang his bell for revenge for unintentionally hurting my brother—he talked me out of it for the first violence interruption I knew. Like the Cain and Abel story with a better ending. Glen and his wife, Claudia Morgan, keep me sane, and gave important feedback to this book. Special friends and colleagues, Eve and Fred Ozer, Randi Fiat and Stephen Sayadian, and Jane Ferguson and Bruce Dick, have kept me inspired and supported for this book.

Special thanks to Diane and Richard Weinberg, who became close friends, as well as friends of the project; for introducing us to others, for Diane's work on mindfulness training for our staff, and both for their generosity; and to the Charlotte and Michael Newberger family including Tamar and Robin Newberger, Andy Schaprio and David Sacks, who invited us into their home to introduce us to friends and supporters, as well as their own generous support.

I am beyond grateful to Dr. Sandy Gove, much more than a highly valued colleague and close personal friend, who was in Somalia before

ACKNOWLEDGMENTS

me, and requested I go there to address the TB problem. This was the start of my on-the-ground training in Africa and of my career abroad, which probably would not have occurred if not for her. Dr. Gove, serving in Somalia at the same time, was the medical advisor to the Refugee Health Unit. As an infectious disease epidemiologist, she later worked at WHO to develop practical tools for health care for children and adults including for emergency management for Ebola and COVID abroad. Sandy contributed very substantially to my career and this book, to help me get as much right as I could.

I've been fortunate to have had many great teachers and mentors, a few stay in my mind all the time: Dr. John Mills, then chief of infectious diseases at SFGH, accepted me as a fellow, taught me to approach these diseases intellectually, with curiosity and practically, and famously taught us when you find something in research that's the opposite of what you thought it was, it's usually true *and* important, also a key insight of Thomas Kuhn in *The Structure of Scientific Revolutions*. Dr. Mills advised me that leaving San Francisco for Mogadishu would be the biggest mistake of my life and was right.

Phil Hopewell, chief of pulmonary SFGH, a world expert in TB taught it to me, and through it, how to do epidemic control. And as he and many have said, "If you know how to do TB, you can do any epidemic - because of how the disease works." Phil also helped with sections of this book regarding the data, and Janice Louie, the current TB director, helped as well. It is this work with Phil that was our (and the) first experiences of "experimenting" with credible messengers to reach TB patients and their contacts.

Dr. Daniel Tarantola, who had led the campaign to eradicate smallpox from Bangladesh and was head of all disease control for the Western Pacific including China, was my boss, mentor, teacher, and most trusted and also joyful guide at the World Health Organization. One of the most capable professionals the world has ever seen. I was lucky he agreed to take me in, within minutes of our first meeting. I checked in with him before and after every one of dozens of country missions. Daniel taught me how to work effectively with countries and their governments from measurements to impact, from persons to global, with humor, love, and great sense.

Other important teachers and colleagues at WHO include the late Jonathan Mann, the founder of the Global Programme on AIDS, Jim Chin, the director of surveillance, Peter Piot and David Heymann, probably the two leading epidemiologists then and today, and Manuel Carballo, the lead social scientist at WHO.

Too many to count, I want to especially thank colleagues from WHO: Adjua Amana, Ben Nkowame, Bob Hornik, Christine Norton, Clinton Nyamaryakunga, Don Sutherland, Dorothy Blake, Eric Brenner, Eric Van Praag, Faraq Elkamel, Faustin Yao, John Wickett, Kathleen Cravero, Kathleen Kay, Manuel Carballo, Mariela Baldo, Michel Carael, Nina Forencic, Naphthali Agata, Paul Delay, Peter Aggleton, Peter Eriki, Rudi Wabitcsh, Rob Moodie, Roy Widdus, Sam Okware, Tony Burton, Warren Namara, and Werasit Sittitrai. And my main indispensable assistant—Elizabeth (Lilou) Matt!

My endless respect and admiration goes to Dr. Jonathan Mann, the founder and director of the Global Programme on AIDs, also a mentor who became a friend, someone decades ahead of his time; and to Mike Merson, the director of GPA following Dr. Mann, who I am grateful to for keeping me while the rest of the senior leadership was changed.

Somalia colleagues, influencers, and teachers include coworkers in the Refugee Health Unit, most notably Abdi Kamal Ali Salad, the RHU director to later join WHO; Hussein Maalin Mursal, who worked most closely with me on TB at the RHU, later to join Save the Children; Abdi Rahman, the medical director of Bo'o; Ahmed Mohammed Magan, the RHU director who later joined UNICEF; Mohammad Warsame, to join UNHCR; and the thousands of CHWs and TBAs, the credible messengers of Somalia. From the Somali people I learned a deep love, caring, gentleness, brotherhood, storytelling, and an ease of life in both a very tough climate and other circumstances. I saw how people smile and enjoy themselves despite it all. I have also been greatly influenced by these unique and outstanding leaders in

ACKNOWLEDGMENTS

refugee and global health—Helene Gayle, Ronnie Waldman, and Mike Toole, who I have known from those years.

There are hundreds who have worked directly with CeaseFire and Cure Violence for over twenty-five years, including field teams of hundreds, now thousands, to tens of thousands—with possibly millions involved and reached in communities. Here I'm including the work of all of the organizations doing not just our work, but similar work under the successful banner—and movement(s) now called community violence intervention (CVI) and by many countless local names.

In addition to those mentioned in the book, I want to highlight those who helped build this house and played close roles with me and who I learned so much from—focusing here on Chicago and then the first groups of cities and countries: These include the central staff of over twenty years who made it through the storms together—Brent Decker, Candice Kane, Camerron Safarloo, Charlie Ransford, Charles Mack, Cheryl Lewis, Chico Tillman, Ricardo (Cobe) Willams, Daria Zvertina, Debbie Eison, Eddie Bocanegro Elena Quitana, Frank Perez, Frank Sanchez, Guadalupe Cruz, Jalon Arthur, Joyce Love, Jeryl Levin, Josh Gryniewicz, Karen Volker, Kathy Buettner, Kyen Phaovanij, LeVon Stone, Lori Toriscano, Lourdes Henriquez, Rosales, Marcus McAllister, Marlita White, Mata Zeimer, Melody Lewis Engram, Miguel Arcos, Mohammad Asideh, Mohammad Alshurafa, Norman Kerr, Pat Broughton, Raul Gonzales, Shannon Cosgrove, Shiela Regan, Tim Metzker, Tina Johnson, Tio Hardiman; and in essential roles holding us together in the central office, Amanda Geppert and Anna Kate Lewis and the true superstars Derba Pitts-Browne and Danielle Russel; and more than gratefully our current CEO, Dr. Monique Willams (!).

I want to especially highlight Joyce, Candice, Brent, Norm, Cobe, Tio, Lupe, Frank, Daria, Elena, Jalon, and Karen V for their outsized—and larger than life—roles in the success of this work.

I would like to especially recognize the enormous role of our success and the success of so many communities and cities in the United States of Ricardo (Cobe) Williams, serving as the director of US programs. His personal and determined attitude, sincere relationships, and relentless efforts to make this work a success has benefitted dozens if not hundreds of communities and dozens of cities. His efforts have been central and essential. His life story and work is available in his own book, *Interrupting Violence*.

Way more than thanks and acknowledgement are due to our very essential friends and major heroes Laurie Glenn and Reverend Robin Hood—who were our key political, communication, strategy, and community eyes, ears and intelligence service—needed constantly to weather the storms of opposition.

Some of the thousands of superstars in the field were Alfonso Prader, Calvin Hunt, Demeatrius Whatley, Evans (Chip) Robinson, James Highsmith, John Lofton, Rick Jackson, Tim White, Karl Bell, Rick Jacslon, Rodney Phillips, Tony Raggs, Marilyn Pitchford, Patrick Halloway, and Tony Pickens. I ask those who are still around to pass my apologies on to all too many greats to mention here.

People who invested in the idea of this approach who were the first to say "this makes sense" or "let's try it" were Phil Lee, HHS; Shay Bilchik, DOJ; Jim Mercy, CDC, who grounded me on multiple occasions on the science to date as well as contacts throughout the city and the country; Ada Mary Gugeneim, CCT, the first Chicago funder; Susan Lloyd, also a pioneer at MacArthur Foundation; Marjorie Craig Benton, who made countless key connections for me; and Senator Lisa Madigan, who made the first community success possible. Very special gratitude to David Wilhelm for sharing his expert political wisdom and guidance (including at a pivotal moment, "Would you rather overdue or underdo it? "); Jon Levine (who believed reducing violence was "doable" before most and pushed us on Chicago when the demand was more elsewhere); and to the many-times program-saving legal work of Scott Lassar, former US Attorney, recently at Sidley Austin; and Oscar David; Winston Strom, who saved us—and our workers many times from sometimes unjust challenges to the workers.

Board chairs and board leaders over the years include Francis

Cardinal George, Marjorie Craig Benton, Kakul Srivastava, Jack Edwards, John Cammack, Judge Sheila Murphy, Leon Andrews, and at this writing, Jermey Kaufmann.

Thank you, First Lady Laura Bush, for agreeing to be an honorary board chair, which brought so much additional credibility to the idea and the work; I am so grateful. And thank you to President Geroge W. Bush for honoring the work at a State of the Union Address.

Thank you to board members over the year: Al Sommer, Alethas Maybamk, Andrea L. Zopp, Andrew Zolli, Ann and Bruce Strohm, Caryn Rosen Adelman, Charlie Beck, Charlotte Newberger, Dan Ratner, David Jaworski, David Kanis, David Wilhelm, Doug Rowan, Eric Goosby, Erica Atwood, Fatimah Muhammad, Fred Tuomi, Gary Kachadurian, Gigi and Michael Pritzker-Pucker, Harriet Edeman, Howard Draft, the world-renowned Imogen Heap, Jeff Frazier, Jenny Molina, Jody Weis, Joan and Bob Feitler, Jonathan Levine, Kahlil Gibran Mohammed, Kathleen Yosko, Laurie Robinson, Lee Hill, Leon Andrews, Lisa Witter, Mary Heidkamp, Merri Dee, Mike Crowley, Oscar David, Paul King, Rev. Marshall Hatch, Richard Fishman, Rima Salah, Ron Serpas, Scott Lassar, Steve Salzman, Susan Bissel, Susan Scrimshaw, Tanarra Schniedier, Thomas MacLellan, and Tracy McClendon-Cole.

Foundations supporters that both made the work happen and also frequently saved the day include AAA-ICDR, Advocate Christ Medical Center, Blue Cross and Blue Shield, Charles E. Marks Jr. Charitable Trust, Chicago Community Trust, Chicago Department of Public Health, Chicago White Sox Charities, Circle of Service, Conant Family Foundation, Core, Crown Family Foundations, Field Foundation, Irvin Stern Foundation, LaSalle Adams Fund, Leafglen Foundation, Lloyd A. Fry Foundation, MacArthur Foundation, McCormick Tribune Foundation, Michael Reese Health Trust, National Recreation Foundation, Oprah Angel Network, Polk Brothers Foundation, Pritzker Pucker Family Foundation, Robert R. McCormick Foundation; and our backbone, the nation's largest and most innovative foundation I have known, the Robert Wood Johnson Foundation; the Sherwood

Foundation, Smart Family Foundation, The Just Trust, Toms Shoes, and the University of Chicago Biological Sciences.

Government funders include the CDC, Chicago Department of Public Health, Cook County Office of Judicial Advisory Council, Cook County State's Attorney, US Department of Homeland Security, US Department of Justice (several branchers), Illinois Criminal Justice Information Authority, Illinois Department of Corrections, Illinois Department of Human Services, Illinois State Police, and Illinois Violence Prevention Authority.

We had strong support for the US Department of Justice under several administrations starting with Shay Bilchik, and continuing and strengthening with AG Eric Holder, Laurie Robinson (later an incredibly helpful and guiding board member), Jim Burch, and Theron Pride and Thomas Abt, who remain important leaders in this field.

Generous international funders include Bernard van Leer; Bill and Melinda Gates Foundation; Interamerican Bank (IDB); Leafglen Foundation; The German Government (GIZ), representing the European Union (EU); US State Department; UNICEF; UBS Optimus, Zurich; The World Bank; and for the Latin America work USAID/CONVIVE; USAID/CARI Honduras; UNICEF Fundación GC1; Juárez, Mexico—FICOSEC; Culiancán, Mexico—GC1 Foundation and IDB Bank; Alvalice, Cali, Colombia.

Private philanthropy and philanthropists including AJ Goulding, Anne and Bruce Strohm, Art Winter, Daniel and Genevieve Ratner, David and Paula Hellman and Steiner, Fred Tuomi, Henry Crown Company, Jack Begley, Jeremy Kaufman, Karen Ware, Lorie Leleux, Mark and Nancy Ratner, Michael Cera, Michael and Gigi Pritzker Pucker, Sam Fuchs, Scott Lassar, Stacy Ratner, and Steven Sacks,

Some of the key people in this funding world included or still include Ada Mary Gugenheim, David Hiller, Donald Stewart, Dorothy Gardner, Helene Gayle, Jane Lowe, Julie Stasch, Julie Wilen, Laura Leviton, Maisha Simmons, Mark Connoly, Michael and Gigi Pritzker Pucker, Nicki Stein, Pauli Seitz, Risa Lavizzo-Mourey, Sandy Guthman, Terry Mazany, and specifically for the Latin

America work, Mark Connolly, Nancy Zuniga, Miguel Calderon, Ana Leveron, Arturo Luján, Antonio Briones, Alejandra Vidal, Juan Camilo, Julieta Robleda, and Karen Ware.

Some people of *unusual impact* at these foundations in the early years and with long lasting impact: Risa Lavizzo-Mourey, Jane Lowe, Maisha Simmons, Polly Seitz, Ada Mary Gugenheim, Susan Lloyd, Gigi Pritzker Pucker and Michael Pucker and their daughters, Abby, Jessy, and Maggie, and Julie Wilen.

I'm incredibly grateful for the help of great friends and colleagues Christine Norton and Mark Connolly from WHO and UNICEF who paved our way in Central America and the Caribbean relentlessly.

We got a lot of support from Congress led by Senator Dick Durbin, and Congressmen Danny Davis and Mike Quigley, and Congresswoman Jan Schakowsky.

State Senators Lisa Madiagan and Representatives Susana Mendoza, Karen Yarbrough, Linda Chapa LaVia, and Harry Osterman. There were many more, excuse my memory. These heroes formed what was known as the "CeaseFire Caucus"

Community leaders Jeff Bartow, Autry Phillps, Patricia Watkins, Camen Reyes, Maggie Pagan, Mary Nelson, Mildred Wiley, Jackie Reed, Leona Spann, David Cassel, Carmen Reyes, Tracie McClendon-Cole. Again, so many more, with apologies.

Health directors and health leaders David Satcher, Helene Gayle, Josh Sharfestin Leana Wen, John Fairley, Oxidis Barbot, Tom Friedan, Mary Bassett, and Karen De Salvo made life easier for the work and their cities.

Mayors Lori Lightfoot, Brandon Johnson, Sheila Dixon, Stephanie Rawlings-Blake, Catherine E. Pugh, Bernard C. Young, and Brandon M. Scott; Mitch Landrieu, Mike Bloombrg, Bill DeBlasio, and AG Keith Ellison, who stepped up enormously.

Some of the reporters who gave this new idea the chance to break through and/or fought for it—Annie Sweeny, Bruce Dowd, Clarence Page, David Heinzman, Glenn Reedus, Jeremy Gorner, Jerome McDonnell, Jim Dwyer, Joe Nocero, John McComrick, Lois Beckett,

Mary Mitchell, Nick Kristof, Rex Huppke, Sanjay Gupta, and Tina Rosenberg, and the incredibly inspiring Nick Kristof.

Thank you so much to Alex Kotlowitz and Steve James with the support of Gordon Quinn, of Kartemkin Productions for making the award-winning film *The Interrupters* on our work, which gave the work great exposure, and gave the world a lasting very great film for anyone to see.

I'm in great debt (but I paid it off over fifteen years) to the University of Chicago Pritzker School of Medicine and the University of California San Francisco for the best biological, medical, and physician training I could imagine. These institutions teach deep biology, physiology, and practical medical care. Both with smart, creative, interesting, and enjoyable people to explore under pressure invisible forces in a person and problem.

Special appreciation and thanks to the University of Illinois at Chicago which housed our work through both Ceasefire and Cure Violence years, especially for accepting to hire persons with difficult past histories that not every university did, and in going further by offering free educational benefits. And special thanks to Dean Susan Scrimshaw for inviting me to UIC and Dean Paul Brandt Rauf for keeping it going with heart, and to Curtisteen Steward for over fifteen years of making it work. Special thanks to Darcy Evan for intelligent strategic guidance in so many directions and Wayne Weibel for making it happen.

UCSF, SFGH, and U of C special friends and teachers cochief resident Jim Leach, Dave and Connie Wofsy, Michael Okada, Ernie and Debbie Mhoon, Kanu Chaterjee, Jafar Al-Sadir, and Julie Oyler.

Some of the researchers who taught us a lot by studying the work and those of others in the field include Patrick Toland, Nancy Guerra, Kathy Christoffer, Andy Papachirsotrs, Daniel Webster, Sheyla Delgado, Jeff Butts, Tracy Villancourt, Jennifer Whitehill, Shani Buggs, Sherry Towers, Caterina Roman, Ed Maguire, Robert Muggah, Ed Maguire, and Wes Skogan.

Many contagious researchers, some mentioned in the book: Rowell

Hausmann, Eric Dubow, that preceded Eric Dubow, Jacqueline Campbell, Madelyn Gould, Chalotte Watts, Evelyn Toaszewski, Jacqueline Campbell.

Teachers to me about war and civil war: William Ury, Hrair Balain, Peter Galbriath, Matt Waldman, John Paul Lederach, and, about the UN including ongoing discussions of what it needs to be, the Peace Reflection Group (PRG) of the Foundation on Global Government and Sustainability led by Georgios Kostakos including Amb. Francis M. O'Donnell, Charles Petrie, Douglas Gardner, Gay Rosenblum-Kumar, Henk-Jan Brinkman, Ingeborg Breines, Kerstin Leitner, Mats Karlsson, Michael Askwith, Michael Heyn, Paola Bettelli, Patrice-Ariel Francais, Peter Schumann, Ryan Jordan, Stephen Browne, Suvira Chaturvedi, Sukehiro Hasegawa, Victor Angelo, Vladimir Zhagora, and Yoriko Yasukawa.

I'm deeply indebted to the spiritual teachings of the late Rabbi Dr Douglas Golhamer, a uniquely accomplished scholar and inspiring teacher grounded in the ancient languages and original texts, a teacher of Kabalistic prayer, and friend, and with much gratitude as well to his life partner in all things, Peggy Bagley, Rabbi Shari Chen, and synagogue friends, colleagues and supporters Ken and Rabbi Charlene Brooks, Laura and Mark Schwartz, Bill Donets, David Freireich, Chris Malwitz, and others.

I have also had the opportunity to learn from the Tibetan Lama Sogyal Rimpoche, who told me directly when bothering him about methods and practices, that "View" is more important than methods. His first words of his teachings were about "spaciousness."

The Vietnamese monk, Thich Nhat Hahn, told me directly when I was questioning him about a particular global conflict, "We can't get to understanding and solution until we are closer." Reminding us again of why the onsite community "staff" and others makes the most sense.

THE BOOK

I wrote a book on this topic ten years ago but stopped because I didn't understand the brain processes that cause the contagion. When I got through that to some satisfaction and put it in the IOM proceedings, I was still left with, how do we possibly understand the cruelty of authoritarianism, tyranny, and genocide. This took longer to study.

To make this book happen then, it meant starting over when I had the good luck to be approached by the creative and leading literary agency, Idea Architects (IA), and benefit from their extraordinary assistance and guidance. And to then be introduced to the expertise and wisdom of Little, Brown and Company, an imprint of Hachette Book Group, to take this book the rest of the way and make it happen with even more brilliant expertise added.

My enormous thanks to Idea Architects and its personally helpful and wonderfully tenacious founder and CEO Douglas Abrams for taking on this project, and to Rahcel Neuman and Lara Love Hardin who originally gave the critical and enjoyable first call asking, "Where's your book?"

I was extremely fortunate to have Jordan Jacks of IA meet with me almost weekly for about three years as we interviewed people together. Jordan helped me make what otherwise would have been a boring science and concepts book (they told me), to include the real stories of people in the field. Jordan is a master of this work and was incredibly enjoyable to spend this time with.

Lucking out big-time, my editor at Little, Brown was Talia Krohn, who must be the best in the field—most hands-on—and most patient editor in human history. And it was probably needed in my case. Talia patiently sorted and resorted to make the book smooth and understandable, and allowing it to flow and read like a book, something I would have never been able to do. Talia beyond grasped the number of sciences that had to be worked with, and added her own deep knowledge, research, and critical thinking—brilliantly—as we went along. I asked for too much but could not have asked for more—or even imagined such impressive help in so many ways.

This book also benefitted very greatly from multiple reviews by Dr. Gove, mentioned above, an expert epidemiologist who knows well Somalia and WHO, and the infectious diseases mentioned.

ACKNOWLEDGMENTS

Chalie Ransford, the senior director of science and policy at Cure Violence Global, the senior professional in the organization for scientific expertise, as well as its use in communication for paradigm shifting, played a uniquely central role in this book's making. His professional expertise in the field as a whole, and his critical thinking have been essential to multiple aspects of the book from beginning to end. This includes the history of the work across sectors, scientific research, communication, perspective taking on the field, and even cocreating the images.

Brent Decker, our chief program officer, prominently featured in the book for good reasons, reviewed, revised, and added to the chapter on interruption and specifically the section on how interventions are done.

Thank you especially Dr. Monique Williams, our current CEO, for your critical input and for facilitating program staff to contribute their expertise and knowledge and perspective at this time, as well as your own invaluable thinking and leadership.

I am extremely grateful for the review of the infectious disease sections by Dr. Joel Ernst, professor of Medicine, Infectious Disease, and Global Health at UCSF, colleague and resident with me a time ago, and by the reading and review of neurobiology by Dr. Adam Wayt, a professor at Northwestern University, an expert in social psychology and cognitive neuroscience (and former board member). Both Joel and Adam taught me a lot as well as brought me up to date in these fields.

Etienne Krug and Alex Buthcart, the directors of the Violence Prevention Office at WHO. Tracy Vaillancourt and Sherry Towers contributed through their expertise in violence, as did Nealin Parker, of Search for Common Good (formerly at BDI), and her highly talented team and those at Moonshot—specifically on violence extremism and political violence, Karen Volker who is now guiding countries around the world with her innovative and important global initiative at URI, added to the "What You Can Do" section; Leslie Landis, Kathleen Cravero, and Susan Bissell gave important input into the section on success in interpersonal and domestic violence, and my colleagues at PRC and Everett Ressler; the HDPI network including Jim Brasher, and Caorlyn Willams, provided important input on war and civil war.

PEOPLE INTERVIEWED FOR THIS BOOK INCLUDE, WITH MY SINCERE THANKS:
Alex Butchard (WHO), Amy Sommers, Brent Decker, Catherine Fine, Connie Rice, Dan Ratner, David "MooMoo" Fitzgerald, Elena Quintana, Elgin Maith, Etienne Krug (WHO), Guadalupe Cruz, Josh Scharfstein, Karen Volker, Kathleen Monahan, LaDonna Redmond, Linda Toles, Lourdes Henriquez, Marilyn Pitchford, Norm Altman, Norman Kerr, Patrick Halloway, Rosa Lara, Ryan Nakade, Steve Salzman, Tio Hardiman, Tony McAleer, Tony Pickett, Tony Raggs, Tracy Vaillancourt, Wayne Wiebel, William Ury, and Zainab Al-Suwaij.

GLOSSARY

active case: Someone who is clinically ill and capable of transmitting the disease to others; some people may be less obviously symptomatic but still capable of transmitting to others.

agent of disease: A factor whose presence or absence is necessary for the disease to occur.

amygdala: A region of the brain closely associated with fear, emotions, and motivation.

authoritarianism: In politics and government, the repression of individual freedom of thought, civil liberties, and political action. Power is concentrated in the hands of a single leader or a small elite who make decisions without regard for the will of the people.

authoritarian violence disorder: An extremely contagious and lethal strain of violence, led by an index case in a highly infected populace.

Signs and symptoms include regular use of lies, dehumanization, fear and expressed hatred of ethnic, religious, or other out-groups, especially immigrants and (in the West) non-white persons, pushed by one or more primary spreaders of grievance; the groups to be attacked are often broadened. Deportation camps are common.

biology: The science of life and living organisms and their structure, function, growth, and evolution; includes all animals, plants, bacteria, and viruses and the relationships between individuals in the life course.

bullying: Habitually seeking to harm or intimidate those perceived as vulnerable.

carrier: An individual who harbors a specific infection or disease without visible symptoms of it; may show symptoms later when there is activation or relapse of the disease. In the case of violence as well as several contagious diseases, a carrier can transmit the infection without showing the full disease symptoms; an individual who incites violence may be considered a carrier or catalyst.

cluster: An aggregation of cases of a disease that are closely grouped in time and place.

communicable disease: A disease that is spread from one person to another through any of a variety of mechanisms.

community health workers: Public health workers, both professional and paraprofessional, who typically come from the community they serve and have support; essential for epidemic control as well as for a functioning health system.

community violence: Violence within communities, typically involving interpersonal or group disputes; more broadly, it includes family violence as well as mass shootings, violence in schools, local bullying, et cetera.

contact: Someone with proximity and exposure to an active case; for violence, the proximity may be physical, social, or both.

contact tracing: The public health process of identifying, assessing, and managing people who have been in contact with an infected individual, usually an active case, in order to prevent further spread.

contagion: Transmission of a disease from one individual to another through direct contact or indirect exposure.

contagion accelerators: In the case of violence, major and widespread media attention; lies, especially constant lies; dehumanizing and hate speech; pro-violence norms; obedience; peer networks; religion; stories, including religious stories; threat and fear.

contagious disease: A disease capable of being transmitted from one individual to another.

culture: The way of life of a people, including their attitudes, values, beliefs, arts, sciences, modes of perception, and habits of thought and activity.

disease: A deviation or interruption of structure or function of a part, organ, or system of the body as manifested by characteristic symptoms and signs causing morbidity and mortality.

A disease can be acute or chronic, stable or unstable, early stage or late, lethal or nonlethal, and communicable or noncommunicable and can involve any organ or system or a combination of organs or systems.

dopamine: A neurotransmitter tied to motivation, emotional regulation, and motor control. Dopamine pathways function as a reward system that reinforces dopamine-releasing behaviors and motivates individuals to seek them out again.

dormant: Inactive state following infection; can be activated days, months, or years later; considered the mechanism of latency. The term is commonly used interchangeably with *latency*.

dose: Refers to the amount of exposure that can be quantified.

elimination of disease: An effort that focuses on the reduction of incidence of a disease *to zero in a given geographic area*, with active measures to prevent its reestablishment after elimination. It can also denote reduction of case transmission to a *predetermined very low level* at which the disease is no longer a public health problem.

endemic: A disease or problem in a relatively constant or steady state; usually or always present.

epicenter: Area of concentration of an epidemic; area of active spread within itself and from it.

epidemic: Spreading rapidly and extensively and infecting many individuals at the same time in an area or population.

GLOSSARY

epidemic disease: A disease that meets the criteria of being at higher-than-normal level of incidence with infectivity or transmission; occurs in waves based on exposure and susceptibility.

epidemic wave: Typical curve seen on graphs charting levels of a disease over time; usually demonstrating exponential increases, plateaus, and decreases following patterns based on exposure and susceptibility.

eradication: Permanent reduction of the worldwide incidence of infection caused by a specific agent to zero as a result of deliberate efforts; intervention measures are no longer needed.

exposure: Instance of being subjected to an action or influence; exposure to a contagious disease is the principal and necessary risk factor for infection.

genocide: Any act committed with intent to destroy, in whole or in part, a national, ethnic, racial, or religious group. This includes actions meant to cause physical harm, measures to prevent births, cause deprivation, and forcibly removing children from their families.

hate speech: Public speech that expresses hate or encourages violence toward a person or group based on race, religion, sex, sexual orientation, disability, et cetera.

herd immunity: Relative term for disease transmission slowing as a result of reduced susceptibility, reduced transmission/spread, and reduced exposure in the population. Several mechanisms can be in play, including mask-wearing, hand-washing, peer pressure, vaccination status, or immunity from prior disease (the last is not effective for violence).

host: Individual in whom an infection lives; a potential infected person.

host factors: Biological, physiological variables within the host that leads to susceptibility or resistance (relative or total immunity). Host factors affect likelihood of infection, progression to disease, and severity of disease.

immunity: Resistance to infection; in the case of violence, an individual's level of immunity is frequently increased through exposure to protective factors and decreased through exposure to risk factors. For violence, this can include the effects of peer or group norms.

incubation period: The interval between initial exposure and first appearance of symptoms. In the case of violence, the incubation period varies widely; individuals can be exposed to violence but not exhibit any violent behavior until a significant amount of time has elapsed.

index case: Identified source; commonly thought of as the first case, but in practice it is the first or most prominent case detected or being investigated for the purposes of determining scope or potential of past, ongoing, or future spread.

infection: Entry of an agent of disease into the body. An infection can be either apparent (the person shows signs of illness) or unapparent (the person shows no signs of illness).

infectious agent: The agent associated with the cause of the disease, which may indicate its important or defining characteristics.

infectivity: The ability to establish an infection, measured by the ratio of the number of people who become infected to the total number exposed.

interruption: Preventing and stopping disease transmission; for violence, this includes new episodes of violence or possible retaliation in response to prior episodes.

isolation: Separating sick people with a contagious disease from people who are not sick.

latency: The state in which the immune system keeps the disease under control. The person doesn't feel sick and cannot spread the infection. This state can change if the disease is activated or if the person's immune status changes.

mirror neuron: A class of neurons that both see and do; essential for mimicry and replication of behaviors as well as empathy.

moral disengagement: Rationalization of behavior by disconnecting one's moral standards from one's actions. A mechanism of susceptibility to contagion and progression of the disease of violence.

morbidity: A rate or incidence of a disease; also refers to the state of illness and suffering short of death.

mortality: Lethality, death, fatality.

mutation: A permanent transmissible change in the genetic or other biologic characteristics of a disease; could be a change in genetic, functional, or structural form causing a different expression of the same basic disease.

norms: What is seen as a model, pattern, or standard of behavior. Situational; varies by culture and time. Guides expectations and behaviors of others.

pandemic: Epidemic widely spreading in several regions of the world, usually affecting a large number of people.

pathogenesis: Biologic mechanisms of disease progression within an individual; what occurs between exposure to infection and disease in a host.

propaganda: In the case of violence, lies that facilitate state-violence syndromes.

protective factor: An aspect of personal behavior, environmental exposure, or inborn or inherited characteristic that is associated with a decreased occurrence of disease.

relapse: The return of signs and symptoms after a period of remission; can pertain to an individual, community, or any syndrome. Can also apply to a community, country, or global phenomenon (for example, civil war) or any syndrome (for example, domestic violence). Prevention of relapse is a main basis for sustained systems and early detection.

remission: Latent disease with no signs and symptoms; person may be in a carrier state, undiagnosed.

replication: Mechanism by which the disease reproduces in the body; a biologic process. For violence, brain copying and imprinting as well as norms, approval and disapproval, acquisition, and attention.

reservoir: Where an infectious disease resides, as in water, animal hosts, or human carriers. For violence, there are no reservoirs outside of man, which makes elimination possible if treatment and interruption of spread can be brought to sufficient scale.

risk factor: Aspect of personal behavior, environmental exposure, another infection, or an inborn or inherited characteristic that is associated with increased occurrence of disease.

sign: Manifestation of a disease, usually objective and visible from observation or examination.

spread: The movement of an infectious disease from one person to another or from vector to a host. In the case of violence, one type of violence can spread to multiple cases of the same type, such as in suicide clusters, or it can spread and result in other syndromes, such as child abuse leading to later occurrences of intimate-partner violence.

susceptibility: Level of immunity or resistance to a disease. Susceptibility varies depending on mediators and cofactors such as time, context, and biological circumstances.

symptom: Subjective experience of a disease or condition.

syndrome: A set of signs and symptoms expressing the main criteria of a disease, with some varying characteristics. For violence, there are several syndromes; as with other diseases, a person with one syndrome can transmit a different syndrome.

transmission: Any mechanism by which an infectious disease is spread from a source to an individual. Violence can be transmitted horizontally, from individual to individual, and vertically, through intergenerational transmission.

treatment: Management and care of a patient's disease in an attempt to cure or heal; does not always require medications.

vector: A nonhuman carrier that can transmit an infectious agent from one host to another; not relevant for violence.

vertical transmission: Ordinarily this means transmission from one generation to the next—for example, from mother to baby in utero or through breastfeeding—but it is used here to refer to violence spread from one generation to the next by any means.

violence: The intentional use of physical force or power, threatened or actual, against oneself, another person, or a group or community that either results in or has a high likelihood of resulting in injury, death, psychological harm, maldevelopment, or deprivation (World Health Organization).

violence interruption: The process of slowing disease spread by stopping violent events, commonly performed by trained workers.

violent extremism: The use of violence to achieve political, religious, or ideological goals. Includes terrorism and other forms of politically motivated violence.

war: A syndrome of violence in which nation-states are involved with other nation-states or entities; a strain or mutation of violence usually associated with high levels of contagion, transmission, morbidity, and mortality.

ACTION PLAN

WHAT YOU CAN DO TO END VIOLENCE NOW:
Action Plan for Individuals, Families, and Communities

1. EDUCATE YOURSELF

Violence is an illness — an actual contagious disease. There should be no animosity for those who have caught the contagion. It's how this disease works.

Still, you don't have to accept it, and you can help cure it in your family, community, and country.

2. EDUCATE OTHERS

- Help those around you to understand that violence is contagious and discuss how one violent event leads to another in the home, the community, and the country. Discuss things to do together to interrupt and stop the spread of this violence.
- You can talk to anyone about violence, because *almost everybody is against it*.
- When talking to someone about violence, avoid focusing on who is to blame or why someone did it. This is not a partisan issue — don't talk politics. *Focus on the violence*.
- Remind people that the reason for violence is not because

people are evil, but because people are copying, following, or hurting. Nobody really wants to be violent or be around violence.
- Communicate clearly and patiently. Engage people who do not always share your point of view on everything.
- *Join or start a campaign* with signs, leaflets, posters, billboards, or online. Spread messages like "Stop the violence" and "No violence allowed here." *Establish violence-free zones.*
- Counter lies about immigrants or any other group being scapegoated. Pay particular attention to language that is dehumanizing, as this creates a permissive environment for violence.

3. SPEAK OUT AND PEACEFULLY PROTEST AGAINST VIOLENCE

- Condemn *every act* of violence whenever and wherever you see it — in the home, on the street, in your community, on social media, anywhere. *Encourage others* to do so as well. If possible, join with others of different faiths or political allegiances to speak out jointly against the violence.
- Denounce not only physical acts but also threats, intimidation, hate, and dehumanizing of others. *These all matter.* All spread like a contagion.
- Show that the community is united by having different groups *stand up together.*
- For political and state violence (including hate, threats, dehumanization, incitements, *and deprivation* aimed at certain groups) by the government, directly or indirectly, speak out through:
  - Letters and social media posts
  - Peaceful public demonstrations (Realize that an authoritarian will try to incite violence in order to justify more violence and take more power. It is essential that these

public demonstrations against violence are themselves nonviolent!)
  - Your vote
- Push back wherever violence is occurring, whether it's at the highest levels of the state or at the community or personal level. State the damage that was done or is being done to the person, the community, and the country. Stand up for people. Show your objection and humanize: "These are people like you and me, and we all deserve dignity and respect."
- Support groups that provide economic or legal protection to victims of violence.

4. BE PREPARED TO RESPOND TO CONFLICTS (WITH CAUTION) TO PREVENT THEM FROM ESCALATING TO VIOLENCE

- If you are aware of a conflict that may escalate to violence, *make sure you are safe*. If you feel threatened, walk away. Always be careful not to make a situation worse.
- *Calm people down:* If you know those involved and they trust you and it seems safe, you can say, "Okay, that's enough for now," or "Let's hold off," or "Let's cool down." Lower the voices; help someone walk away.
- *Distract:* Change the subject, divert people's attention.
- *Get help:* If there is a dangerous or ongoing problem, get professionals to the scene. Know whom to call — violence interrupters, safety outreach services, mental-health workers. Hotlines, such as suicide hotlines, can help stop mass shootings and other events, especially if there is trained outreach.
- *Be proactive:* Often we are aware that violence is brewing before it happens. Do not assume that it is inevitable. Do you know anyone who can influence the situation to keep it from escalating to violence? Is there someone who could speak with credibility to those involved and get them to change their thinking about the acceptability of violence?

- *Look close to home:* Be aware of what your children or grandchildren are doing; find out if they are involved in violence in a gang or affected by bullying at school. Pay attention to whether they are scared of violence or glorifying it. Talk to them and, if needed, get them help.

5. HELP A PERSON IN NEED

Outreach systems are important for violence reduction in a community. If you know or are aware of people who are showing signs of being violent, suicidal, or even excessively lonely:

- *Reach out, be a friend, listen, and care.* Emotional change and behavior change are possible with the right help and support. Violence is contagious, but so is caring and helping.
- Many people prone to violence are dealing with other things that contribute to whether or not they act violent. *Try to understand what these factors are.* See if you can get them help from trusted community social services that can treat them or provide the necessary assistance. Many are simply confused or are following orders so that they can belong. (Note: The need to belong is extremely powerful and can motivate people to do things they otherwise would not consider doing.) There are confidential ways to get people the support they need.
- *Protect and support* those who are being attacked verbally or physically in your community; help with their physical safety, social safety, financial safety, or through your brotherhood or sisterhood. Speak up for them so that they know they are not alone.

6. GET INVOLVED IN YOUR COMMUNITY AND MORE BROADLY

- *Consider what you can do in your community.* Can you help locate those who might be having trouble or organize or participate in community responses? You may not be able to do these, but recognizing the need is a start. What is needed in your community or city? What can you do? What can you do with others? What do you need training in? Where do you need help from others? There are programs operating in many cities to help people in need.

- *Work with an existing group in your community.* The organization does not need to be one that is dedicated to violence; as we have seen throughout the book, organizations that focused on health, housing, immigrant rights, or community development were tapped and eager to lead a movement against violence in their cities and in their country.

7. JOIN OR START A COMMUNITY GROUP OR COMMUNITY-LED MOVEMENT

Every city and community needs a violence-prevention program, just as it needs police departments, fire departments, schools, and health services. Every city should have a Mayor's Office and Health Department Office of Violence Prevention. These offices should have the assistance and guidance of professional training.* Violence-prevention activities include public education messaging through visible materials on the street and on social media and community responses to local, city, and national events. In community meetings, discuss what syndromes of this epidemic are of greatest concern to the members of the organization and the community it serves. Is it bullying in the schools, shooting on the streets, children who have been hurt in their homes, detecting potential suicides or mass shooting events, or even the national situation? Start with one or two of these, and *ask the following questions:*

- Do we have the best program models to address them? Models exist for every size, shape, strain, and syndrome of violence.
- Are there specific people we are concerned about, and is there someone who can reach out to them and help? Are some

---

* This can be provided by Cure Violence Global or any of the groups noted under Solutions: Community Violence Intervention (CVI) people bullying or spreading hate? Are there people threatening violence who are being ignored?

- Are there specific places of concern where there seems to be a lot of danger or violent activity? Cleanups could help "recapture" these spaces. Are the schools and workplaces experienced as safe? Are there services we should be bringing in to help us organize and make plans? Could we use some bystander training? Do we have people who can lead or coordinate our efforts?
- Are we making sufficient statements and objections to the violence on social media? Are we letting our voices be heard as a community as well as individually? Are we responding to threats within our community and to our community, including threats from the government?
- Is there more that faith leaders and members could be doing in the community to speak out against the violence?
- What is our connection to the other communities in the city and across the country? Can we merge or connect our campaigns against the violence with those in other cities? Can we align on messaging or share materials and ideas?

8. REMEMBER THAT VIOLENCE IS NOT INEVITABLE — AND IT IS STOPPABLE

It is up to each of us to do what we can to ensure that it does not happen in or around our homes, communities, and country. We all walk around with our own circle of influence. Let's use it to be the antidote to violence. Together we will eliminate violence at home, in our communities, and in our country.

9. TAKE CARE OF YOURSELF

Consider your own experience with violence, hate, rage, and your potential to do violence. Find your own peace. Consider your needs and those of your family, and whether you or they could benefit from any outside support or help — like Cognitive Behavioral Therapy, mindfulness, or trauma care.

Don't ever forget to take care of yourself, and seek support from friends, family, and anyone who can be helpful.

Keep in touch.

REFERENCES AND RESOURCES

>See Solutions By Syndrome
>For AVD and inflections of the State, also see:
>Ash Center for Democratic Governance and Innovation: https://ash.harvard.edu/.
>Bridging Divides Initiative: https://bridgingdivides.princeton.edu/.
>Gene Sharp, "198 Methods of Nonviolent Action," https://commonslibrary.org/198-methods-of-nonviolent-action/ https://commonslibrary.org/civil-resistance-tactics-in-the-21st-century/.
>Harnessing Our Power to End Political Violence (HOPE): https://www.endpoliticalviolence.org/guide.
>Search for Common Ground Peacemaker toolkit: https://www.sfcg.org/peacemakerstoolkit/.
>World Health Organization, Violence Prevention: The Evidence (WHO, 2010).

NOTES

INTRODUCTION
Gary Slutkin, "Is Violence 'Senseless'? Not According to Science. Let's Make Sense of It and Treat it Like a Disease," *Health Progress* 97, no. 4 (2016): 5–8.

Violence as a Contagious Disease
Gary Slutkin, "Violence Is a Contagious Disease," in *Contagion of Violence: Workshop Summary* (National Academies Press, 2013).
Gary Slutkin, "Reducing Violence as the Next Great Public Health Achievement," *Nature Human Behavior* 1, no. 25 (2017).
Johan Giesecke, *Modern Infectious Disease Epidemiology*, 3rd ed. (CRC Press, 2017).
Roy M. Anderson and Robert M. May, *Infectious Diseases of Humans: Dynamics and Control* (Oxford University Press, 1991).

CHAPTER ONE: ASSESSMENT AND DIAGNOSIS
The Harmful Effects of Harsh Punishment, Excessive Policing, and Mass Incarcerations
Alexandra Natapoff, *Punishment Without Crime: How Our Massive Misdemeanor System Traps the Innocent and Makes America More Unequal* (Basic Books, 2018).
Alex S. Vitale, *The End of Policing* (Verso, 2018).
Danielle Sered, *Until We Reckon: Violence, Mass Incarceration, and a Road to Repair* (New Press, 2019).
Emily Bazelon, *Charged: The New Movement to Transform American Prosecution and End Mass Incarceration* (Random House, 2019).
John Pfaff, *Locked In: The True Causes of Mass Incarceration—and How to Achieve Real Reform* (Basic Books, 2017).
Karl Menninger, *The Crime of Punishment* (Viking Press, 1968).
Michelle Alexander, *The New Jim Crow: Mass Incarceration in the Age of Colorblindness* (New Press, 2012).

Crime Bill
The Crime Bill (Violent Crime Control and Law Enforcement Act of 1994) was the largest anti-crime bill of its kind in US history and included ten billion dollars for prison construction around the country as well as multiple sentencing enforcements. The Violence Against Women Act (VAWA), however, was also included in this bill.
"Fifty Years of Building Solutions, Supporting Communities and Advancing Justice," US Department of Justice, https://www.ojp.gov/ojp50/1994-violent-crime-control-and-law-enforcement-act#:~:text=Media%20Inquiries,1989%20Drug%20Courts.

Characteristic Epidemic Waves, Clustering, and Transmission Characteristics of Infectious Diseases

Adam Kucharski, *The Rules of Contagion* (Basic Books, 2020).

Kenrad E. Nelson and Carolyn Masters Williams, eds., *Infectious Disease Epidemiology: Theory and Practice*, 3rd ed. (Jones & Bartlett Learning, 2014). A gold mine of characteristic epidemic curves and cluster maps for infectious diseases can be found here.

CHAPTER TWO: MAKING SENSE OF "SENSELESS VIOLENCE"

A Terrible Halloween

"Pregnant Mother Shot Dead, Victim of Random Halloween Violence," ABC News, November 1, 2007, https://abcnews.go.com/US/story?id=3805774&page=1.

Violence and Poverty

Paul Collier, *The Bottom Billion: Why the Poorest Countries Are Failing and What Can Be Done About It* (Oxford: Oxford University Press, 2007).

Author's conversation with Paul Collier, Northwestern University, Evanston, 2011 or 2012.

There is a strong literature on the relationship between violence and inequity and mistrust in government that won't be covered here. I liken this relationship to the connection between cholera and dirty water, or crowding and TB: Dirty water without the cholera bacteria does not cause cholera, and crowding without the TB bacillus does not cause TB. For all of these transmissible disorders, specific exposure is required and is dose-dependent, and we can reduce and reverse the disease processes by interrupting the contagion.

The Early History of AIDS in San Francisco

AIDS in One City: The San Francisco Story, National Endowment of the Humanities, 2020, https://www.neh.gov/article/aids-one-city-san-francisco-story.

J. M. Luce, "A Strange New Disease in San Francisco: A Brief History of the City and Its Response to the HIV/AIDS Epidemic," *Annals of the American Thoracic Society* 10 (2013): 143–47, doi: 10.1513/AnnalsATS.201208-039PS.

Past Misunderstandings of Infectious Disease

Theodor Rosebury, *Microbes and Morals: The Strange Story of Venereal Disease* (Viking Press, 1971); see especially chapter 14, "Disease, Sin, and Punishment."

Wolfgang Behringer, *Witches and Witch-Hunts: A Global History* (Polity, 2004).

Geoffrey Marks and William K. Beatty, *Epidemics* (Scribner, 1976).

F. Gonzáles-Crussi, *A Short History of Medicine* (Modern Library, 2007).

Tatsuo Sakai and Yuh Morimoto, "The History of Infectious Diseases and Medicine," *Pathogens* 11, no. 10 (2022): 1147.

Tuberculosis in the History of Medicine

"History of World TB Day," CDC, December 5, 2024, cdc.gov/world-tb-day/history.

Karen Dobos and Marcela Henao-Tamayo, "How an Ancient Disease Is Outsmarting Modern Medicine," *SciTechDaily*, April 1, 2025.

Ray M. Merrill et al., "Explanations for 20th Century Tuberculosis Decline: How the Public Gets It Wrong," *Journal of Tuberculosis Research* 4 (2016): 111–21.

R. Y. Keers, *Pulmonary Tuberculosis: A Journey Down the Centuries* (Baillière Tindall, 1978).

Richard M. Burke, *A Historical Chronology of Tuberculosis* (Charles C. Thomas, 1938).

Dr. Robert Koch, Discoverer of the Etiology of Tuberculosis
The 1905 Nobel Prize in Physiology or Medicine was awarded to Robert Koch "for his investigations and discoveries in relation to tuberculosis," https://www.nobelprize.org/prizes/medicine/1905/summary/.

Ritu Lakhtakia, "The Legacy of Robert Koch: Surmise, Search, Substantiate," *Sultan Qaboos University Medical Journal* 14, no. 1 (2014): e37–41.

CHAPTER THREE: YOUR BRAIN ON VIOLENCE
The Visual Experience of Violence
Richard L. Gregory, *Eye and Brain: The Psychology of Seeing* (Princeton University Press, 1997).

L. Rowell Huesmann and Lucyna Kirwil, "Why Observing Violence Increases the Risk of Violent Behavior in the Observer," in *The Cambridge Handbook of Violent Behavior and Aggression*, ed. David Flannery et al. (Cambridge University Press, 2007).

L. Rowell Huesmann, "An Information Processing Model for the Development of Aggression," *Aggressive Behavior* 14 (2011): 13–24.

Exposure: Bobo on the Brain
Albert Bandura et al., "Transmission of Aggression through Imitation of Aggressive Models," *Journal of Abnormal and Social Psychology* 63, no. 3 (1961): 575–82, https://doi.org/10.1037/h0045925.

Other important work by Dr. Bandura, the founder of social learning theory:

Albert Bandura, "Influence of Models' Reinforcement Contingencies on the Acquisition of Imitative Responses," *Journal of Personality and Social Psychology* 1 (1965): 589–95.

Albert Bandura, *Aggression: A Social Learning Analysis* (Prentice Hall, 1973).

Albert Bandura, *Social Learning Theory* (Prentice Hall, 1977).

Mirror Neurons and Mirroring
Marco Iacoboni, "Neural Underpinnings of Prosocial and Antisocial Behavior," in *Contagion of Violence: Workshop Summary*, ed. Institute of Medicine and National Research Council (National Academies Press, 2013), 29–34.

Giacomo Rizzolatti et al., "Functional Organization of Inferior Area 6 in Macaque Monkeys. II. Area F5 and the Control of Distal Movements," *Experimental Brain Research* 71 (1988): 491–507. Experiments like Rizzolatti's were not performed on humans because they required putting implants directly in the brain to record electrical activity.

G. di Pellegrino et al., "Understanding Motor Events: A Neurophysiological Study," *Experimental Brain Research* 91, no. 1 (1992): 176–80.

M. Gentilucci et al., "Functional-Organization of Inferior Area-6 in the Macaque Monkey: Somatotopy and the Control of Proximal Movements," *Experimental Brain Research* 71, no. 3 (1988): 475–90.

In recent years, pioneering research at Caltech with epileptic human patients awaiting brain surgery has allowed researchers to further analyze how our brains code concepts within particular neurons and neural networks. For an overview, see Rodrigo Quian Quiroga et al., "A Single Brain Cell Stores a Single Concept," *Scientific American*, February 1, 2013.

Marco Iacoboni, *Mirroring People: The Science of Empathy and How We Connect with Others* (Picador, 2009).

Uri Hasson and Chris D. Frith, "Mirroring and Beyond: Coupled Dynamics as a Generalized Framework for Modelling Social Interactions," *Philosophical Transactions of the Royal Society B* 371, no. 1693 (May 2016): 20150366.

For a broader discussion, see Slutkin, *Contagion of Violence* (National Academies Press, 2013), 73, 78.

For the most up-to-date analysis in humans and other species, see Luca Bonini et al., "Mirror Neurons 30 Years Later: Implications and Applications," *Trends in Cognitive Sciences* 26, no. 9 (2022): 767–81.

Mirroring Aggression

Nina Bai, "Mirroring Aggression: Watching Counterparts Brawl Fires Fighting Neurons in Mice," *Stanford Medicine Magazine*, no. 2, June 2, 2023, stanmed.stanford.edu/observer-neurons-mirror-fighters/.

Pascal Molenberghs et al., "Is the Mirror Neuron System Involved In Imitation? A Short Review and Meta-Analysis," *Neuroscience and Biobehavioral Reviews* 33, no. 7 (2009): 975–80.

L. Rowell Huesmann and Leonard D. Eron, "Cognitive Processes and the Persistence of Aggressive Behavior," *Aggressive Behavior* 3, no. 10 (1984): 243–51.

For a brief overview of Huesmann's research, see his statement before the Federal Commission on School Safety, "The Ecology of Schools: Fostering a Culture of Human Flourishing and Developing Character," Eisenhower Office Building, Washington DC, June 21, 2018, www2.ed.gov/documents/press-releases/201806-fcss-rowell-huesmann.pdf.

Activation of Latent Infectious Disease

The emergence of the HIV/AIDS epidemic was widespread enough, especially in Africa, to affect the overall prevalence of TB in the world and change the direction of the TB curve upward; see G. Slutkin, J. Leowski, and J. Mann, "The Effects of the AIDS Epidemic on the Tuberculosis Problem and Tuberculosis Programmes," in *The Global Impact of AIDS: Proceedings of the International Conference*, March 8–10, 1988.

R. E. Chaisson and G. Slutkin, "Tuberculosis and Human Immunodeficiency Virus Infection," *Journal of Infectious Diseases* 159 (1989): 96–100, https://academic.oup.com/jid/article-abstract/159/1/96/897158?redirectedFrom=fulltext.

Dopamine, Social Reward, and Violence

Rewards for social approval or other cues of belonging to social networks (e.g., positive reputation, consensus) are mediated by dopamine-like reward pathways.

Adriana Galván, "Adolescent Development of the Reward System," *Frontiers in Human Neuroscience* 4, no. 6 (2010): 1–9.

Elizabeth A. Reynolds Losin et al., "Own-Gender Imitation Activates the Brain's Reward Circuitry," *Social Cognitive Affective Neuroscience* 7, no. 7 (2012): 804–10.

Keise Izuma et al., "Processing of Social and Monetary Rewards in the Human Striatum," *Neuron* 58, no. 2 (2008): 284–94.

Roy F. Baumeister and Mark R. Leary, "The Need to Belong: Desire for Interpersonal Attachments as a Fundamental Human Motivation," *Psychological Bulletin* 117, no. 3 (1995): 497–529.

Sören Krach et al., "The Rewarding Nature of Social Interactions," *Frontiers in Behavioral Neuroscience* 4 (2010).

Stephen J. Watts and Thomas L. McNulty, "Delinquent Peers and Offending: Integrating Social Learning and Biosocial Theory," *Youth Violence and Juvenile Justice* 13, no. 2 (2014): 190–206.

Recommended book on dopamine, pain-pleasure pathways, and relationships

Anna Lembke, *Dopamine Nation: Finding Balance in the Age of Indulgence* (Dutton, 2021).

Fascinating and important new book on dopamine addiction and revenge
James Kimmel Jr., *The Science of Revenge: Understanding the World's Deadliest Addiction — and How to Overcome It* (Harmony, 2025).

Dopamine and Aggression
Jared J. Schwartzer and Richard H. Melloni Jr., "Anterior Hypothalamic Dopamine D2 Receptors Modulate Adolescent Anabolic/Androgenic Steroid-Induced Offensive Aggression in the Syrian Hamster," *Behavioural Pharmacology* 21, no. 4 (2010): 314–22.
Jared J. Schwartzer et al., "Prior Fighting Experience Increases Aggression in Syrian Hamsters: Implications for a Role of Dopamine in the Winner Effect," *Aggressive Behavior* 39, no. 4 (2013): 290–300.
Thorben Schlüter et al., "MAOA-VNTR Polymorphism Modulates Context-Dependent Dopamine Release and Aggressive Behavior in Males," *NeuroImage* 125 (2016): 378–85.
Thorben Schlüter et al., "The Impact of Dopamine on Aggression: An [18F]-FDOPA PET Study in Healthy Males," *Journal of Neuroscience* 33, no. 43 (2013): 16889–96.

Social Pain and Violence
Rejection hurts in the same way as physical pain, and people feel they have to relieve it. This was discovered through observations of patients with brain lesions who reported feeling pain but couldn't identify its location or knew the location where something was wrong but didn't report it as pain. For those who felt pain, it was relieved by Tylenol, even in the case of social pain.
N. I. Eisenberger, M. D. Lieberman, and K. D. Williams, "Does Rejection Hurt?: An fMRI Study of Social Exclusion," *Science* 302 (2003): 290–92, doi: 10.1126/science.108913.
N. I. Eisenberger, "The Neural Bases of Social Pain: Evidence for Shared Representations with Physical Pain," *Psychosomatic Medicine* 74 (2012).
Naomi Eisenberger, "The Pain of Social Disconnection: Examining the Shared Neural Underpinnings of Physical and Social Pain," *Nature Reviews Neuroscience* 13, no. 6 (2012): 421–34.
Heather J. Ferguson et al., "Neural Empathy Mechanisms Are Shared for Physical and Social Pain, and Increase from Adolescence to Older Adulthood," *Social Cognitive and Affective Neuroscience* 19, no. 1 (2024): nsae080.
K. D. Williams, C. K. Cheung, and W. Choi, "Cyberostracism: Effects of Being Ignored over the Internet," *Journal of Personality and Social Psychology* 79 (2000).

CHAPTER FOUR: EXPOSURE
Predicting Itself
Johan Giesecke, *Modern Infectious Disease Epidemiology*, 3rd ed. (CRC Press, 2017), 4–7 (an excellent description of the differences between noninfectious and infectious epidemiology).
Ben Cowling, *Household Transmission of Influenza* (WHO, January 2016), media.tghn.org/medialibrary/2016/03/3_Cowling.pdf.
Chandini Raina MacIntyre et al., "Respiratory Viruses Transmission from Children to Adults Within a Household," *Vaccine* 30, no. 19 (2012): 3009–14.
George W. Comstock, "Epidemiology of Tuberculosis," in *Koch Centennial Memorial, 1882–1982* (American Lung Association, 1982), 13–14.
Yang Yang et al., "The Transmissibility and Control of Pandemic Influenza A (H1N1) Virus," *Science* 326, no. 5953 (2009): 729–33.
Roy M. Anderson and Robert M. May, *Infectious Diseases of Humans: Dynamics and Control* (Oxford University Press, 1991).

Reducing Exposure: Wayne's Approach and Results

W. Wayne Wiebel et al., "Risk Behavior and HIV Seroincidence Among Out-of-Treatment Injection Drug Users: A Four-Year Prospective Study," *Journal of Acquired Immune Deficiency Syndromes and Human Retrovirology* 12 (1996): 282–89.

For more discussion of Wayne's work and our work at GPA in IDUs see *Global Report on AIDS, 1987–1995 — Final Report* (World Health Organization); also see Hema Bashyam, "Susan Allen: Confronting HIV in Africa," *Journal of Experimental Medicine* 205 (2008): 1000–1001, doi:10.1084/jem.2055pi.

Exposure and Dose

For almost all infectious diseases, the dose-response relationship is an important predictor of infection and of disease progression. The dose-response relationship of exposure to violence and the likelihood of infection and disease with violence confirms its contagious nature.

Richard Spano et al., "Are Chronic Exposure to Violence and Chronic Violent Behavior Closely Related Developmental Processes During Adolescence?," *Criminal Justice and Behavior* 37 (2010): 1160–79. The study showed vicarious exposure to be highly relevant; the trajectory of chronic vicarious victimization has an independent effect on the trajectory of chronic violent behavior. As a result, violence-prevention initiatives that focus strictly on reducing victimization are excluding a sizable proportion of youth who are indirectly exposed to violence, and they underestimate the effects of violence in the community on chronic violent behavior.

Degrees of Exposure (Physical and Social)

Nathan Collins, "One Brain Area Processes Time, Space and Social Relationships: Physical and Emotional Distance Overlap in the Brain," *Scientific American*, July 1, 2014.

Matthew Schafer and Daniela Schiller, "Navigating Social Space," *Neuron* 100, no. 2 (2018): 476–89.

Meng Du et al., "How Does the Brain Navigate Knowledge of Social Relations? Testing for Shared Neural Mechanisms for Shifting Attention in Space and Social Knowledge," *NeuroImage* 235, no. 15 (2021): 118019.

Violence and PTSD

The literature on PTSD for drone operators is variable. Some studies show yes. Other studies show less PTSD in drone operators than in soldiers in combat and no increased incidence of violence.

Rajiv Kumar Saini et al., "Cry in the Sky: Psychological Impact on Drone Operators," *Industrial Psychiatry Journal* 30, no. S1 (2021): S15–19.

Wayne Chappelle et al., "An Analysis of Post-Traumatic Stress Symptoms in United States Air Force Drone Operators," *Journal of Anxiety Disorders* 28, no. 5 (2014): 480–87.

Video Games and Media

I did not attempt to cover this topic with the completeness it deserves. Here are some key sources:

Davin Dupee et al., "Stanford Researchers Scoured Every Reputable Study for the Link Between Video Games and Gun Violence That Politicians Point To. Here's What the Review Found," *Fortune*, May 2, 2023.

Mengyun Yao et al., "Violent Video Games Exposure and Aggression: The Role of Moral Disengagement, Anger, Hostility, and Disinhibition," *Aggressive Behavior* 45, no. 6 (2019): 662–70.

Simone Kühn et al., "Does Playing Violent Video Games Cause Aggression? A Longitudinal Intervention Study," *Molecular Psychiatry* 24, no. 8 (2019): 1220–34.

Violent media is thought to have effects, at least in the short term, on decreasing empathy and increasing aggression. Dr. Rowell Huesmann, who has done extensive research on this topic, presents convincing evidence for a larger and important effect — as a real exposure. He reports from a long-term longitudinal study that "childhood exposure to media violence predicts young adult aggressive behavior for both males and females. Identification with aggressive TV characters and perceived realism of TV violence also predict later aggression. These relations persist even when the effects of socioeconomic status, intellectual ability, and a variety of parenting factors are controlled."

L. Rowell Huesmann et al., "Longitudinal Relations Between Children's Exposure to TV Violence and Their Aggressive and Violent Behavior In Young Adulthood: 1977–1992," *Developmental Psychology* 39, no. 2 (2003): 201–21.

L. Rowell Huesmann, "The Impact of Electronic Media Violence: Scientific Theory and Research," *Journal of Adolescent Health* 41, no. 6 S1 (2007): S6–13.

Exposure Depends on Who You Know

Andrew Papachristos et al., "Tragic, but Not Random: The Social Contagion of Nonfatal Gunshot Injuries," *Social Science and Medicine* 125 (2015): 139–50.

Ben Green et al., "Modeling Contagion Through Social Networks to Explain and Predict Gunshot Violence in Chicago, 2006 to 2014," *JAMA Internal Medicine* 177, no. 3 (2017): 326–33.

Time and Space

Georg Northoff and Zirui Huang, "How Do the Brain's Time and Space Mediate Consciousness and Its Different Dimensions? Temporo-Spatial Theory of Consciousness (TTC)," *Neuroscience and Biobehavioral Reviews* 80 (2017): 630–45.

Transmission Within and Between Disease Syndromes

A good summary of over fifty studies appears in Gary Slutkin, "Violence Is a Contagious Disease," in *Contagion of Violence* (National Academies Press, 2013), 103–5.

Andrea L. Roberts et al., "Witness of Intimate Partner Violence in Childhood and Perpetration of Intimate Partner Violence in Adulthood," *Epidemiology* 21, no. 6 (2010): 809–18.

Christopher W. Mullins et al., "Gender, Streetlife and Criminal Retaliation," *Criminology* 42, no. 4 (2004): 911–40.

Claire V. Crooks et al., "Understanding the Link Between Childhood Maltreatment and Violent Delinquency: What Do Schools Have to Add," *Child Maltreatment* 12, no. 3 (2007): 269–80.

Deborah Reitzel-Jaffe and David A. Wolfe, "Predictors of Relationship Abuse Among Young Men," *Journal of Interpersonal Violence* 16, no. 2 (2001): 99–115.

Miriam K. Ehrensaft et al., "Intergenerational Transmission of Partner Violence: A 20-Year Prospective Study," *Journal of Consulting and Clinical Psychology* 71, no. 4 (2003): 741–53.

M. S. Gould, "Suicide Clusters and Media Exposure," in *Suicide Over the Life Cycle: Risk Factors, Assessment, and Treatment of Suicidal Patients*, ed. Susan Blumenthal and David J. Kupfer (American Psychiatric Association, 1990).

Nancy G. Guerra et al., "Community Violence Exposure, Social Cognition, and Aggression Among Urban Elementary School Children," *Child Development* 74, no. 5 (2003): 1561–76.

Robert H. DuRant et al., "Exposure to Violence and Victimization and Fighting Behavior by Urban Black Adolescents," *Journal of Adolescent Health* 15, no. 4 (1994): 311–18.

Sandra M. Stith et al., "The Intergenerational Transmission of Spouse Abuse: A Meta-Analysis," *Journal of Marriage and the Family* 62, no. 3 (2000): 640–54.

Scott H. Decker, "Collective and Normative Features of Gang Violence," *Justice Quarterly* 13, no. 2 (1996): 243–64.

Shari Barkin et al., "Exposure to Violence and Intentions to Engage in Moralistic Violence During Early Adolescence," *Journal of Adolescence* 24, no. 6 (2001): 777–89.

Simha F. Landau, et al., "A Time-Series Analysis of Violent Crime and Its Relation to Prolonged States of Warfare," *Criminology* 26, no. 3 (1988): 489–504.

CHAPTER FIVE: SUSCEPTIBILITY
Mass Shootings

For this account of Dylan Klebold's last morning, and of the Columbine tragedy more generally, I relied primarily on Dave Cullen's excellent account of the event, *Columbine* (Twelve, 2009) and Sue Klebold's memoir, *A Mother's Reckoning: Living in the Aftermath of Tragedy* (Crown, 2017). I also referred to the section in Andrew Solomon's *Far from the Tree: Parents, Children and the Search for Identity* (Scribner, 2013) describing his interactions with Klebold's parents.

Best source for overview and updating of mass shootings, including susceptibility factors, is the Violence Prevention Project's database: https://www.theviolenceproject.org/.

Sherry Towers et al., "Contagion in Mass Killings and School Shootings," *PLOS One* 10, no. 7 (2015): e0117259.

Mass Shootings and Veterans

A CBS News analysis shows 26 percent of mass shooters have military service or training. Only 7 percent of the US population have military backgrounds, so a disproportionate number of alleged mass shooters are veterans; see https://www.msnbc.com/opinion/msnbc-opinion/michigan-north-carolina-shootings-veterans-mental-health-rcna234788.

Susceptibility (to an Infectious Disease)

Notably, finding and treating people with susceptibilities to infections results in less disease. This is what happened on a community level in Tanzania after it was shown that genital ulcers (sores) increased the risk of male-to-female transmission by a factor of ten to fifty and of female-to-male transmission by a factor of fifty to three hundred, prompting estimates that genital ulcer disease (GUD) "may be responsible for a large proportion of heterosexually acquired HIV infections in sub-Saharan Africa." Treatment of GUD resulted in a 42 percent drop in new HIV infections. I mention this to encourage you to look at social pain — social "sores" — as something to be taken seriously, detected, and treated.

H. Grosskurth et al., "Impact of Improved Treatment of Sexually Transmitted Diseases on HIV Infection in Rural Tanzania: Randomised Controlled Trial," *Lancet* 346, no. 8974 (1995): 530–36.

João Dinis Sousa et al., "The Impact of Genital Ulcers on HIV Transmission Has Been Underestimated — a Critical Review," *Viruses* 14, no. 3 (2022): 538.

R. J. Hayes et al., "The Cofactor Effect of Genital Ulcers on the Per-Exposure Risk of HIV Transmission in Sub-Saharan Africa," *Journal of Tropical Medicine and Hygiene* 98, no. 1 (1995): 1–8.

Alcohol and Susceptibility

Alcohol is one of the most significant influences on susceptibility in the acute activation, likely because of disinhibition, both social and through effects on the frontal lobe. I have never attended a single World Health Organization meeting (or any international meeting) that has not discussed the role of alcohol in activating acute cases of violence and in the spread of the contagion in groups. In the United States, this is almost never discussed in policy circles. But work has been done in other countries to limit alcohol consumption for this purpose, to great effect. It is likely the most common accompanier of acute violence activation, for homicides, and is a risk factor for intimate-partner violence (in terms of use by perpetrator and victim) as well as for suicides. Policies for alcohol restriction have been successful in reducing killings.

Alvaro I Sánchez et al., "Policies for Alcohol Restriction and Their Association with Interpersonal Violence: A Time-Series Analysis of Homicides in Cali, Colombia," *International Journal of Epidemiology* 40, no. 4 (2011): 1037–46.

Peter R. Giancola, "Executive Functioning and Alcohol-Related Aggression," *Journal of Abnormal Psychology* 113, no. 4 (2004): 541–55.

Timothy S. Naimi et al., "Alcohol Involvement in Homicide Victimization in the United States," *Alcoholism, Clinical and Experimental Research* 40, no. 12 (2016): 2614–21.

Epidemic Control in Refugee Camps

Report to the Refugee Health Unit (RHU), United Nations, 1986.

Refugee Health Unit, Somali Ministry of Health, *Guidelines for Health Workers in Refugee Camps*, 4th ed., July 1987.

Social and Cultural Norms and Susceptibility to Violence

Alfred L. McAlister, "Acceptance of Killing and Homicide Rates in Nineteen Nations," *European Journal of Public Health* 16, no. 3 (2006): 260–66. These cultural or normative differences — for example, "the moral justification" — varied greatly between countries and regions and correlated well with rates of violence, McAlister wrote. This is relevant because differences in homicide rates are commonly thought to be due to economic inequality or effectiveness of police or the criminal justice system.

Dov Cohen et al., "Insult, Aggression, and the Southern Culture of Honor: An 'Experimental Ethnography,'" *Journal of Personality and Social Psychology* 70, no. 5 (May 1996): 945–59.

Clinical Screening Scores

Right now, clinical screening scores are based primarily on exposure. Ideally, susceptibility would also be included.

Jason E. Goldstick et al., "Development of the SaFETy Score: A Clinical Screening Tool for Predicting Future Firearm Violence Risk," *Annals of Internal Medicine* 166, no. 10 (2017): 707–14.

CHAPTER SIX: INTERRUPTING SPREAD

Public Education and Behavior Change

Robert C. Hornik, ed., *Public Health Communication: Evidence for Behavior Change* (Routledge, 2002).

M. Silva et al., "Learning from the Past: The Role of Social and Behavior Change Programming in Public Health Emergencies," *Global Health: Science and Practice* 10, no. 4 (2022): e2200026.

Active Case Finding and Outreach: Tuberculosis in San Francisco

San Francisco Annual Report 2024, https://www.sf.gov/resource--2024--tb-reports-and-publications.

Amy S. Tang et al., "'Think, Test, Treat TB' in Action: An Innovative Primary Care and Public Health Partnership to Improve Tuberculosis Prevention and Care," *New England Journal of Medicine Catalyst* 8 (2024).

G. Slutkin, G. F. Schecter, and P. C. Hopewell, "The Results of 9-Month Isoniazid-Rifampin Therapy for Pulmonary Tuberculosis Under Program Conditions in San Francisco," *American Review of Respiratory Disease* 138 (1988): 1622–24.

Gary Slutkin and Charles Ransford, "Violence Is a Contagious Disease: Theory and Practice in the USA and Abroad," in *Violence, Trauma, and Trauma Surgery: Ethical Issues, Interventions, and Innovations*, ed. Mark Siegler and Selwyn O. Rogers Jr. (Springer Nature Switzerland AG, 2020), 67–85

Community Responses to Violence

Examples of community actions, including responses to shootings or other violent actions, and efforts to change norms are presented throughout this book. Public education, community responses, and outreach are overlapping inputs and interventions for behavior change and norm change, and intensity or dose is highly relevant to interpreting spread and predictive of success.

Patrick Sharkey, *Uneasy Peace: The Great Crime Decline, the Renewal of City Life, and the Next War on Violence* (W. W. Norton, 2018).

Erica Chenoweth and Maria J. Stephan, *Why Civil Resistance Works: The Strategic Logic of Nonviolent Conflict* (Columbia University Press, 2011).

Gene Sharp, *The Politics of Nonviolent Action* (Porter Sargent, 1973).

Interrupting Spread

The story of China Joe's interruption and other descriptions of the work can be found in Nicholas D. Kristof and Sheryl WuDunn, *A Path Appears: Transforming Lives, Creating Opportunity* (Alfred A. Knopf, 2014).

Chicago

Wesley Skogan et al., *Evaluation of CeaseFire-Chicago* (National Institute of Justice, Office of Justice Programs, 2008).

The Department of Justice funded the first seven years of CeaseFire work (2000–2007) with a ten-year baseline, using four different methods in eight communities employed by four different universities. It showed reductions in violence across all evaluated sites, including decreases in shootings ranging from 41 percent to 73 percent, declines in the density of violent hot spots by up to 40 percent, and, in five sites, a complete elimination of retaliation killings, with 50 percent reductions in two sites. Confidential interviews of participants indicated meaningful behavioral change: 59 percent intervened to stop a conflict, and 60 percent persuaded someone not to use a gun. In addition, 89 percent to 99 percent of participants with personal challenges reported having received effective help, addressing an average of 88 percent of their identified problems. Staffers were considered the most important people in their lives after their mothers.

CeaseFire Final Report: An Evaluation of Gun and Non-Gun Violence in 47 Chicago Police Beats: 1999–2009 (Cure Violence, 2012), https://cvg.org/wp-content/uploads/2025/05/2012-CeaseFire-Final-Report_Thuy-Tran.pdf.

The CeaseFire program in Chicago between 1999 and 2009 was associated with statistically significant reductions in gun-related homicides and shootings, particularly in beats with larger staff presence. A residual lag effect may also persist in beats after the program ends, and staff size matters; beats with larger CeaseFire teams had greater reductions in gun violence than those with smaller teams.

Charlie Ransford et al., "An Examination of the Role of CeaseFire, the Chicago Police, Project Safe Neighborhoods, and Displacement in the Reduction in Homicide in Chicago in 2004," in *Youth Gangs and Community Intervention: Research, Practice, and Evidence*, ed. Robert J. Chaskin (Columbia University Press, 2010). The sharp decline in homicides in Chicago in 2004 (25 percent citywide in one year) was driven by coordinated efforts: CeaseFire, improved police strategies, and Project Safe Neighborhoods. CeaseFire zones expanded from five to twenty-five communities that year and had an average drop of 50 percent.

David B. Henry et al., *The Effect of Intensive CeaseFire Intervention on Crime in Four Chicago Police Beats: Quantitative Assessment* (Robert R. McCormick Foundation, 2014).

"The 7-11 Hit: Evaluation of Impact on Shootings" (University of Chicago, 2016). A rapid-phase (7-11 HIT) intervention showed a 48 percent decrease in shootings in a five-week period.

Deborah Gorman-Smith and Franklin Cosey Gay, "Residents and Clients' Perceptions of Safety and CeaseFire Impact on Neighborhood Crime and Violence," University of Chicago, School of Social Service Administration (2014). Cure Violence workers were effective because of their credibility; their mentoring, job guidance, and personal support reduced involvement in violence, relieved isolation, and offered people a broader sense of possibility.

Franklin Cosey Gay, "Empowering High-Risk Males Through Street Outreach" (thesis, University of Illinois Chicago, 2019), https://hdl.handle.net/10027/23652. This qualitative study shows how CVG outreach workers helped high-risk young men move away from violence by using their own life experience and credibility.

C. Ransford et al., "The Relationship Between the Cure Violence Model and Citywide Increases and Decreases in Killings in Chicago (2000–2016). Cure Violence Report," Cure Violence Global, 2016. There is a strong correlation between CeaseFire's operation in Chicago and reductions in shootings and killings. Periods of expansion or reinstatement of the program coincided with sharp declines in violence, while interruptions or staff reductions aligned with corresponding increases.

Baltimore

Daniel W. Webster et al., "Estimating the Effects of Safe Streets Baltimore on Gun Violence: 2007–2022," Center for Gun Violence Solutions, Johns Hopkins Bloomberg School of Public Health, 2023. A 32 percent (on average) reduction in homicide was seen during the first five years of Baltimore's five longer-running Safe Streets sites. Three of these sites — McElderry Park, Belair-Edison, and Lower Park Heights — saw reductions ranging from 28 percent to 48 percent, while one site, Sandtown-Winchester, experienced an increase (previously described as due to other factors). All eleven sites had fewer shootings, with reductions ranging from 29 percent to 84 percent.

Daniel W. Webster et al., "Evaluation of Baltimore's Safe Streets Program: Effects on Attitudes, Participants' Experiences, and Gun Violence," Center for Gun Policy and Research, Johns Hopkins Bloomberg School of Public Health, 2012. Major reductions in violence in several Baltimore neighborhoods, including a 56 percent drop in homicides and a 34 percent decline in nonfatal shootings in Cherry Hill. In McElderry Park, there were no homicides during the first twenty-two months of implementation.

Shani A. Buggs, Daniel W. Webster, and Cassandra K. Crifasi, "Using Synthetic Control Methodology to Estimate Effects of a Cure Violence Intervention in Baltimore, Maryland," *Injury Prevention* 28, no. 1 (2022): 61–67. McElderry Park showed strong initial homicide reductions — 62 percent after three years and 48 percent after five years — though these effects lessened over time, whereas Cherry Hill maintained consistent declines in both shootings and homicides.

Adam J. Milam et al., "Changes in Attitudes Toward Guns and Shootings Following Implementation of the Baltimore Safe Streets Intervention," *Journal of Urban Health* 93, no. 4 (2016): 609–26, https://doi.org/10.1007/s11524-016-0060-y. Forty-three percent of the measured attitudes showed improvement compared to only 13 percent in the control area. Participants exposed to the program — such as seeing "Stop Shooting" signs or interacting with outreach workers — were more likely to adopt nonviolent views on handling conflicts. Overall, the findings suggest that community-based interventions like Safe Streets can meaningfully change norms and reduce the acceptance of violence among high-risk youth.

CHAPTER SEVEN: NORMS AND SYSTEMS
Integrating Systems: The Four Pillars

Note that all of the cities mentioned rely on all four of these pillars. The construction and strengthening of each pillar has worked differently, depending on the city, and credit for the development of the systems should be given to the city's leadership as well as the communities. David Muhammad and the National Institute for Criminal Justice Reform (https://ovpnetwork.org/wp-content/uploads/2023/09/OVP-Report_V15_90823.pdf) have developed and expanded a nationwide network of mayors' offices. The first hospital-based work in Chicago, Oakland, and other cities grew into a nationwide movement under the leadership of Fatima Muhammad and the Health Alliance for Violence Intervention (HAVI).

Hospitals and Health Care

Health Alliance for Violence Intervention, thehavi.org.

Gary Slutkin et al., "How the Health Sector Can Reduce Violence by Treating It as a Contagion," *AMA Journal of Ethics* 20, no. 1 (2018): 47–55.

Charles Ransford and Gary Slutkin, "Seeing and Treating Violence as a Health Issue," in *The Handbook of Homicide*, ed. Fiona Brookman et al. (Wiley-Blackwell, 2017).

Kyle R. Fisher, "Prevention Professional for Violence Intervention: A Newly Recognized Health Care Provider for Population Health Programs," *Journal of Health Care for the Poor and Underserved* 31, no. 1(2020): 25–34.

For more information on hospital-based programs and results from the first CVG hospital-based program, see Yalaunda M. Thomas et al., "Violence Prevention Programs Are Effective When Initiated During the Initial Workup of Patients in an Urban Level I Trauma Center," *American Journal of Men's Health* 16, no. 5 (2022). "Six percent (n = 18) of subjects in the treatment group and 11% (n = 33) in the control group returned with a new injury, yielding a total reinjury rate of 8.5%. Most patients returned only once with another violent injury. Individuals who did not receive Cure Violence services were nearly twice as likely (odds ratio = 1.94; 95% confidence interval = 1.065, 3.522) to return with a violent reinjury."

Ansh Goyal et al., "Screening for Youth Firearm Violence Exposure in Primary Care," *AJPM Focus* 3, no. 1 (2023): 100146.

Douglas Evans and Anthony Vega, *Critical Care: The Important Role of Hospital-Based Violence Intervention Programs* (Research and Evaluation Center, John Jay College of Criminal Justice, City University of New York, 2018).

New York City

Greg Berman and Emily Gold, *From Chicago to Brooklyn: A Case Study in Program Replication* (Center for Court Innovation, 2011). Save Our Streets (SOS) Crown Heights adapted Chicago's CeaseFire model to Brooklyn to reduce shootings and change community norms around violence; effective replication depends on maintaining the core principles while adapting to new environments.

John Klofas et al., SNUG Evaluation, Center for Public Safety Initiatives, Rochester Institute of Technology, July 2013, rit.edu/liberalarts/sites/rit.edu.liberalarts/files/documents/our-work/2013-10.pdf. In New York State, Cure Violence led to declines in killings in Albany (46 percent), Niagara Falls (40 percent), and Yonkers (47 percent) and declines in shootings in Albany (18 percent), Harlem (24 percent), and Yonkers (54 percent).

Rachel Avram et al., "Do Cure Violence Programs Reduce Gun Violence? Evidence from New York City," Cornell University arXiv, submitted June 4, 2024, arxiv.org/html/2406.02459v1.

Jeffrey A. Butts et al., "Effectiveness of the Cure Violence Model in New York City," John Jay College of Criminal Justice, CUNY, 2015. In the Cure Violence sites of East New York, Crown Heights, and West Harlem from 2010 to 2013, homicide rates fell by 18 percent; in comparable areas, the rates rose by 69 percent.

Sheyla A. Delgado et al., "The Effects of Cure Violence in the South Bronx and East New York, Brooklyn," John Jay College of Criminal Justice, CUNY, 2017. In the South Bronx, gun injuries declined by 37 percent and shooting victimizations by 63 percent, while in East New York, gun injuries fell by 50 percent—far greater than the small changes seen in the comparison neighborhoods. Statistical analyses confirmed a significant break in the trend of gun-related injuries in both intervention sites, indicating that these declines were unlikely to have occurred without the program. Surveys of young men in the same communities also revealed sharp decreases in support for using violence, with norms favoring nonviolence improving significantly in Cure Violence areas. Overall, the findings suggest that Cure Violence not only reduced shootings and injuries but also helped transform local attitudes toward conflict and retaliation.

H. Seoh et al., "Implementation of the Cure Violence Model with Enhancements in NYC," *Injury Prevention* 21 (2015). Six Cure Violence programs achieved strong results over a one-year period, demonstrating both reach and impact in high-risk communities. Between July 2013 and June 2014, the programs engaged 202 high-risk participants, conducted 588 conflict mediations, and led 92 community events reaching over 14,000 residents. Each site went at least 70 consecutive days without a shooting, and one program achieved an entire year—367 days—without a single shooting.

Los Angeles

California Board of State and Community Corrections, "GRYD–CalVIP 3 Local Evaluation Report," Sacramento: California Board of State and Community Corrections, December 2023, https://www.bscc.ca.gov/wp-content/uploads/2024/06/GRYD-CalVIP-3-Local-Evaluation-Report_FINAL_12.2023.pdf.

Nicole Santa Cruz, "Jordan Downs in Watts Marks Three Years Without a Homicide," *Los Angeles Times*, August 28, 2014.

Honduras

Instituto Igarapé, "Homicide Monitor: Distribution, Dimensions and Dynamics of Lethal Violence in the World," https://igarape.org.br/en/issues/citizen-security/homicide-monitor/.

Ana Gonzalez-Barrera et al., "DHS: Violence, Poverty Are Driving Children to Flee Central America to U.S.," Pew Research Center, July 1, 2014, pewresearch.org/short-reads/2014/07/01/dhs-violence-poverty-is-driving-children-to-flee-central-america-to-u-s.

Global Study on Homicide 2013 (United Nations Office on Drugs and Crime, 2014).

Global Status Report on Violence Prevention 2014 (World Health Organization, 2014).

Charles Ransford et al., "El Modelo Cure Violence: Reducción de la Violencia en San Pedro Sula (Honduras)" ["The Cure Violence Model: Violence Reduction in San Pedro Sula (Honduras)"], *Revista CIDOB d'Afers Internacionals* 116 (September 2017): 179–204.

"Reducing Violence and Preventing Femicides in Honduran Communities," UNICEF Honduras, August 15, 2024, unicef.org/honduras/historias/reducing-violence-and-preventing-femicides-honduran-communities.

Other Latin America and Caribbean Studies
Columbia (Cali)

C. E. M. León, M. I. Muñoz, and J. C. G. Benavides, "Informe Final de la Evaluación de impacto del Programa Abriendo Caminos de la Fundación Alvaralice," 2020, https://www.alvaralice.org/wp-content/uploads/2020/12/Informe-Final-de-la-Evaluaci%C3%B3n-de-Impacto-del-Programa-Abriendo-Caminos-de-la-Fundaci%C3%B3n.pdf.

Mexico (Culiacan)

"Más Vida," Informe Anual (2023), https://cvg.org/wp-content/uploads/2023/11/Culiacan-final-report-2022.pdf.

Mexico (Juarez)

Evaluación de impacto al program Del Barrioa la Comunidad 2016–2018 (Obervatorio Ciudadano, Ficosec, May 2019), cvg.org/wp-content/uploads/2025/05/Digital-Barrioalacomunidad.pdf.

Trinidad and Tobago (Port of Spain)

Edward R. Maguire, Megan T. Oakley, and Nicholas Corsaro, *Evaluating Cure Violence in Trinidad and Tobago* (Inter-American Development Bank, 2018), https://publications.iadb.org/publications/english/document/Evaluating-Cure-Violence-in-Trinidad-and-Tobago.pdf.

CHAPTER EIGHT: INFECTIONS OF THE STATE
State Violence

Cindy A. Sousa, "Political Violence, Collective Functioning and Health: A Review of the Literature," *Medicine, Conflict, and Survival* 29, no. 3 (2013): 169–97.

Stathis N. Kalyvis, "The Landscape of Political Violence," in *The Oxford Handbook of Terrorism*, ed. Erica Chenoweth et al. (Oxford University Press, 2019), 10–33.

Tony and Ryan: Violent Extremism and Interruption

Tony McAleer, *The Cure for Hate: A Former White Supremacist's Journey from Violent Extremism to Radical Compassion* (Arsenal Pulp, 2019).

Ryan Nakade and Jack G. R. Wippell, "Building Trust and Preventing Violence in Ideologically Polarized Communities: Lessons from Two Years of Practice, *Peace Review* 37, no. 1 (2025): 1–12.

Cure PNW; Armed Conflict Location & Event Data (ACLED), U.S. and Canada https://acleddata.com/region/united-states-and-canada; CVG.org Results and Impact https://cvg.org/wp-content/uploads/2025/05/2025.05.08-CVG-Evidence-Summary.pdf

AVD
See Further Reading for extended references.

Hitler's Childhood
Robert S. Robins and Jerrold M. Post, *Political Paranoia: The Psychopolitics of Hatred* (Yale University Press, 1997) 276–81.

Alice Miller, *For Your Own Good: Hidden Cruelty in Child-Rearing and the Roots of Violence* (Farrar, Straus and Giroux, 1983).

Dehumanization and Violence
Andrea Scalabrini et al., "Spontaneous Brain Activity Predicts Task-Evoked Activity During Animate Versus Inanimate Touch," *Cerebral Cortex* 29, no. 11 (2019): 4628–45.

Lasana T. Harris and Susan T. Fiske, "Social Groups That Elicit Disgust Are Differentially Processed in mPFC," *Social Cognitive and Affective Neuroscience* 2, no. 1 (2007): 45–51.

Mario F. Mendez, "A Functional and Neuroanatomical Model of Dehumanization," *Cognitive and Behavioral Neurology* 36, no. 1 (2023): 42–47.

Obedience
Milton Leitenberg, *Deaths in Wars and Conflicts in the 20th Century* (Center for International and Security Studies at Maryland, June 20, 2006), https://cissm.umd.edu/research-impact/publications/deaths-wars-and-conflicts-20th.

Stanley Milgram, *Obedience to Authority: An Experimental View* (Harper & Row, 1974).

Philip Zimbardo, *The Lucifer Effect: Understanding How Good People Turn Evil* (Random House, 2007)

On Violence Permeating Borders
Cecilia Menjívar and Andrea Gómez Cervantes, "El Salvador: Civil War, Natural Disasters, and Gang Violence Drive Migration," Migration Policy Institute, August 29, 2018, migrationpolicy.org/article/el-salvador-civil-war-natural-disasters-and-gang-violence-drive-migration.

War Scholars on War as a Contagious Disease
Jonathan Fox, "Is Ethnoreligious Conflict a Contagious Disease?," *Studies in Conflict and Terrorism* 27, no. 2 (2004): 89–106, https://doi.org/10.1080/10576100490275085.

Jack S. Levy, "The Contagion of Great Power War Behavior, 1495–1975," *American Journal of Political Science* 26, no. 3 (1982): 562–84, https://doi.org/10.2307/2110943.

Henk W. Houweling and Jan G. Siccama, "The Epidemiology of War, 1816–1980," *Journal of Conflict Resolution* 29, no. 4 (1985): 641–63, https://doi.org/10.1177/0022002785029004007.

Francis A. Beer, "The Epidemiology of Peace and War," *International Studies Quarterly* 23, no. 1 (1979): 45–86, https://doi.org/10.2307/26002.

War and Civil War
Barbara F. Walter, "Does Conflict Beget Conflict? Explaining Recurring Civil War," *Journal of Peace Research* 41, no. 3, 2004: 371–88.

Paul Collier, Anke Hoeffler, and Måns Söderbom, "Post-Conflict Risks," *Journal of Peace Research* 45, no. 4 (2008): 461–78.

Virginia Page Fortna, *Does Peacekeeping Work? Shaping Belligerents' Choices After Civil War* (Princeton University Press, 2008).

Joakim Kreutz, "How and When Armed Conflicts End: Introducing the UCDP Conflict Termination Dataset," *Journal of Peace Research* 47, no. 2 (2010): 243–50.

John Paul Lederach, *The Pocket Guide for Facing Down a Civil War: Surprising Ideas from Everyday People Who Shifted the Cycles of Violence* (independently published, 2024). I especially recommend this book, which is based on the author's decades of experience in dozens of countries and written in response to our times.

John Paul Lederach and Angela Jill Lederach, *The Moral Imagination: The Art and Soul of Building Peace* (Oxford University Press, 2005).

John Paul Lederach, *When Blood and Bones Cry Out: Journeys through the Soundscape of Healing and Reconciliation* (Oxford University Press, 2010).

On Current International Mediation Methods

Matt Waldman, "Peacemaking in Trouble: Expert Perspectives on Flaws, Deficiencies and Potential in the Field of International Mediation," Belfer Center for Science and International Affairs, Harvard Kennedy School, October 2024, belfercenter.org/research-analysis/peacemaking-trouble-expert-perspectives-flaws-deficiencies-and-potential-field. International mediation is just one of many of the existing systems and methods being applied to violence interventions. This extraordinary study is based on interviews with eighty-six leading mediators and specialists and ten expert colloquia. Matt Waldman co-led the mediation group working on the Russia-Ukraine violence referred to in the text and continues in this capacity. The study shows that many of the mediators themselves see the shortcomings of their approach.

Continued and Increased Contagion of Violence Postwar

D. Archer and R. Gartner, "Violent Acts and Violent Times: A Comparative Approach to Postwar Homicide Rates," *American Sociology Review* 41, no. 6 (1976): 937–63. The study demonstrates continued contagion even when a war is over; in two-thirds of the cases, homicide rates stayed the same or increased.

Eric F. Dubow et al., "Exposure to Conflict and Violence Across Contexts: Relations to Adjustment Among Palestinian Children," *Journal of Clinical Child and Adolescent Psychology* 39, no. 1 (2010): 103–16. The study shows that exposure to the violence of war leads to violence at home (in the community and in the family). In other words, the enemy is gone, but the contagion continues in the brain and crosses into other syndromes.

Exposure to War and Mass Shootings

Kristen L. Rouse, "Recent Mass Shootings May Highlight a Critical Veteran Mental Health Care Shortage," MSNBC, September 30, 2025, https://www.msnbc.com/opinion/msnbc-opinion/michigan-north-carolina-shootings-veterans-mental-health-rcna234788.

Iraq and Syria Reports

G. Slutkin et al., "The CeaseFire Method Applied to Iraq: Changing Thinking and Reducing Violence" in *Beyond Suppression: Global Perspectives on Youth Violence*, ed. J. S. Hoffman et al. (ABC-CLIO, 2011): 69–80.

New Strategies for Health and Peace in Syria: Final Report, Bill and Melinda Gates Foundation, October 19, 2019.

Religion and Violence

Addressing the Social and Cultural Norms that Underlie the Acceptance of Violence (National Academies Press, April 2018). This report is an excellent overview on norms, including the effect of religion on norms and thus susceptibility. In particular see the section "The Role of Religion in Influencing Social and Cultural Norms: An Overview of the Intersection of Religion and Social Norms and How Those Norms Affect Gender Equality."

"Ayatollah Sistani: Much More Than a 'Guide' for Iraqis," in *Religion, Violence, and the State of Iraq* (Crown Center for Middle East Studies, October 2019).

Christopher P. Salas-Wright et al., "Religiosity and Violence Among Adolescents in the United States: Findings from the National Survey on Drug Use and Health 2006–2010," *Journal of Interpersonal Violence* 29, no. 7 (2014): 1178–200.

Sarah Demmrich and Paul H. P. Hanel, "The Relative Role of Religiosity in Radicalization: How Orthodox and Fundamentalist Religiosity Are Linked to Violence Acceptance," *Frontiers in Social Psychology* 2 (2024).

Charles Kimball, *When Religion Becomes Evil* (Harper San Francisco, 2002).

Stories, Violence, and War

Yuval Noah Harari, *Nexus: A Brief History of Information Networks from the Stone Age to AI* (Random House, 2024).

Nuclear War

Scott Horsley, "President Donald Trump to U.N.: North Korea's 'Rocket Man' Kim Jong Un on a Suicide Mission," NPR, September 19, 2017.

"North Korea Says It Successfully Tested Hydrogen Bomb, Marking Sixth Nuclear Test Since 2006," ABC News, September 2, 2017, updated September 3, 2017, abc.net.au/news/2017-09-03/north-korea-says-it-successfully-tested-hydrogen-bomb/8867568.

William Ury, *Possible: How We Survive (and Thrive) in an Age of Conflict* (Harper Business, 2024); see pages 199–201 for a discussion of the photo proposed and an iconic photo of the summit.

EPILOGUE
Scientific Revolutions and Paradigm Shifts

Thomas S. Kuhn, *The Structure of Scientific Revolutions*, 2nd ed. (University of Chicago Press, 1970).

Steven Pinker, *The Better Angels of Our Nature: Why Violence Has Declined* (Viking, 2011). This is the most complete book to date on the trends of violence across the world since earliest times. Through over one hundred graphs and timelines, Pinker, one of the world's leading cognitive scientists and thinkers, shows how violence has trended down over the centuries and discusses why and how our species' norms have changed. Though epidemic disease outbreaks can emerge and trends can reverse, Dr. Pinker's book is a must read.

Disease Elimination

Donald R. Hopkins, "Disease Eradication," *New England Journal of Medicine* 368, no. 1 (January 3, 2013): 54–63, https://www.nejm.org/doi/full/10.1056/NEJMra1200391.

Donald R. Hopkins, *Elimination and Eradication of Diseases, with Special Reference to Measles and Tuberculosis* (World Health Organization, Regional Office for the Eastern Mediterranean, June 1997), https://applications.emro.who.int/docs/em_rc44_7_en.pdf.

Walter R. Dowdle, "The Principles of Disease Elimination and Eradication" (Centers for Disease Control and Prevention) *Morbidity and Mortality Weekly Report* 48 (Supplement SU01, 1999): 23–27, "https://www.cdc.gov/mmwr/preview/mmwrhtml/su48a7.htm?utm_source=chatgpt.com"https://www.cdc.gov/mmwr/preview/mmwrhtml/su48a7.htm

Global Peace Index

Global Peace Index 2025: Measuring Peace in a Complex World (Institute for Economics and Peace, IEP, 2025).

Global Epidemic-Control Efforts

AIDS, Crisis and the Power to Transform: UNAIDS Global Aids Update 2025 (Joint United Nations Programme on HIV/AIDS, 2025).

D. A. Henderson, "Principles and Lessons from the Smallpox Eradication Programme," *Bulletin of the World Health Organization* 65, no. 4 (1987): 535–46.

"Malaria," Global Fund, September 10, 2025, theglobalfund.org/en/malaria/.

"Polio Global Eradication Initiative," Polio Eradication, updated October 2, 2025, polioeradication.org.

Richard Jolly, ed., *Jim Grant: UNICEF Visionary* (UNICEF Innocenti Research Centre, 2001).

"The United States President's Emergency Plan for AIDS Relief," PEPFAR, US Department of State, state.gov/pepfar.

Gary Slutkin, "Global AIDS 1981–1999: The Response," *International Journal of Tuberculosis and Lung Disease* 4, no. 2 (2000): S24–33.

Harry F. Dowling, *Fighting Infection: Conquests of the Twentieth Century* (Harvard University Press, 1977).

"Tuberculosis Elimination Priorities," National Center for HIV, Viral Hepatitis, STD, and Tuberculosis Prevention, CDC, November 21, 2024, cdc.gov/nchhstp/priorities/tuberculosis-elimination.html.

"The End TB Strategy," Global Programme on Tuberculosis and Lung Health, World Health Organization, who.int/teams/global-programme-on-tuberculosis-and-lung-health/the-end-tb-strategy.

International Systems, Networks, and Infrastructure

First Global Ministerial Conference on Ending Violence Against Children, Bogotá, Colombia, November 7–8, 2024, who.int/teams/social-determinants-of-health/violence-prevention/1st-global-ministerial-conference-on-ending-violence-against-children.

"Foundation for Global Governance and Sustainability," FOGGS, foggs.org.

"Integrated Management of Childhood Illness," Child Health and Development, World Health Organization, who.int/teams/maternal-newborn-child-adolescent-health-and-ageing/child-health/integrated-management-of-childhood-illness.

"Member States," ECOWAS CEDEAO, updated April 6, 2021, ecowas.int/member-states.

"Our Founder," Inter Mediate, accessed October 1, 2025, inter-mediate.org/aboutus/our-founder.

Paul van Tongeren, "Creating Infrastructures for Peace—Experiences at Three Continents," *Pensamiento Propio* 45, no. 55 (2012): 91–128.

"Programs," Integrated Management of Adult Illness (IMAI) Alliance, accessed October 5, 2025, imaialliance.org/programs.

"Search for Common Ground," SFCG, accessed October 1, 2025, sfcg.org.

"United Religious Initiative," URI, accessed October 1, 2025, uri.org.

Regional Economic Communities and Peacebuilding in Africa: Lessons from ECOWAS and IGAD (Routledge, 2021).

"William Ury: Possibilist," William Ury, accessed October 1, 2025, williamury.com.

Human Universals

Donald E. Brown, "Human Universals and Their Implications," in *Being Humans: Anthropological Universality and Particularity in Transdisciplinary Perspectives*, ed. Neil Roughley (De Gruyter, 2012).

SOLUTIONS BY VIOLENCE SYNDROME

What Works and Violence Syndromes (International)
Alexander Butchart and Susan Hills, *INSPIRE: Seven Strategies for Ending Violence Against Children* (World Health Organization, 2016). Although labeled as strategies for ending violence against children, this has a much broader scope. Since November 2024, over one hundred countries have pledged to address violence using the public health approach and the INSPIRE framework.

Ending Violence Against Children: Six Strategies for Action (New York: UNICEF, 2014), https://www.unicef.org/media/56121/file.

"What Works to Prevent Violence Against Women and Girls," What Works to Prevent Violence, https://ww2preventvawg.org/.

Global Study on Homicide, 4th ed. (United Nations Office on Drugs and Crime, 2019).

"Preventing Youth Violence," Youth Violence Prevention, CDC, October 29, 2024, cdc.gov/youth-violence/prevention/index.html.

Behavior Change for Public Health
People misunderstand why there has been a decline in tuberculosis, attributing it to modern medicine rather than to public health measures. For the decline in tuberculosis with behavior change alone, see the following articles:

Hannah Ritchie and Fiona Spooner, "Once a Leading Killer, Tuberculosis Is Now Rare in Rich Countries — Here's How It Happened," Our World in Data, June 1, 2025, ourworldindata.org/tuberculosis-history-decline.

Gary Slutkin et al., "How Uganda Reversed Its HIV Epidemic," *AIDS and Behavior* 10, no. 4 (2006): 351–60.

Community Violence Interventions
There are now over twenty-five studies and evaluations on the effectiveness of the epidemic-control approach under dozens of organizations, with many additional elements that increased the success rates. Over ninety cities in the United States are now using some form of this approach, and its success can be seen in the number of cities that now have thirty- to forty-year lows in rates and numbers of killings. Some of these cities have more police cooperation than others, but the basic elements are the same everywhere: case finding, outreach, credible messengers, case management with care, support, behavior change, and follow-up, the leadership of community organizations, and a structure that includes mayors and health departments. Groups working in this area are listed at the end of this section.

Domestic Violence Interventions
Claire Goudreau, "Domestic Violence: Looking Back at the Violence Against Women Act After 30 Years of Protection," *Hub* (blog), John Hopkins University, September 27, 2024. Rates of domestic violence dropped by 67 percent between 1992 and 2022, which is

attributable to the multidimensional Violence Against Women Act as well as to hotlines and norm-changing supporting laws.

Jacquelyn C. Campbell, "Risk Factors for Femicide in Abusive Relationships: Results from a Multisite Case Control Study," *American Journal of Public Health* 93, no. 7 (2003): 1089–97.

"National Domestic Violence Hotline," National Domestic Violence Hotline, accessed October 6, 2025, thehotline.org.

"Violence Against Women Act (AWA)," US Department of Housing and Urban Development, accessed October 6, 2025, https://www.hud.gov/vawa#close.

Gender-Based Violence

"Reducing Violence and Preventing Femicides in Honduran Communities," UNICEF Honduras, August 15, 2024, unicef.org/honduras/historias/reducing-violence-and-preventing-femicides-honduran-communities.

"Trained Violence Interrupters Avert Femicide in Honduras," Spotlight Initiative, October 18, 2021, spotlightinitiative.org/news/trained-violence-interrupters-avert-femicide-honduras.

Treatment for Domestic Violence Perpetrators

Derrik R. Tollefson et al., "A Mind-Body Approach to Domestic Violence Perpetrator Treatment: Program Overview and Preliminary Outcomes," *Journal of Aggression, Maltreatment and Trauma* 18, no. 1 (2007): 17–45.

Derrik R. Tollefson, "A Mind-Body Bridging Treatment Program for Domestic Violence Offenders: Program Overview and Evaluation Results," *Journal of Family Violence* 30, no. 7 (2015): 783–94. Although it is generally thought nearly impossible to change the behavior of perpetrators of domestic violence, this study and others have shown otherwise. (This was just a six-week intervention; results could likely improve with greater duration and follow-up.)

Reducing Sexual or Physical Adolescent Violence

"Reduce Sexual or Physical Adolescent Dating Violence," Office of Disease Prevention and Health Promotion, revised in 2024, odphp.health.gov/healthypeople/objectives-and-data/browse-objectives/violence-prevention/reduce-sexual-or-physical-adolescent-dating-violence-ivp-18.

Francis B. Annor et al., "Changes in Prevalence of Violence and Risk Factors for Violence and HIV Among Children and Young People in Kenya: A Comparison of the 2010 and 2019 Kenya Violence Against Children and Youth Surveys," *Lancet Global Health* 10, no. 1 (January 2022): e124-e133, doi:10.1016/S2214-109X(21)00457-5.

"Ring the Bell," Breakthrough, accessed October 6, 2025, letsbreakthrough.org/ringthebell.

Bullying Solutions

Olweus Bullying Prevention Program, Center for Schools and Communities, clemsonolweus.org/documents/Why%20the%20OBPP%20Works.pdf. This program produced a 50 percent drop in bullying through a comprehensive program that included active case finding, rapid responses, public education, and norm changes.

M. M. Ttofi et al., "Effectiveness of Programs to Reduce Bullying," Swedish National Council for Crime Prevention, 2008.

M. M. Ttofi and D. P. Farrington, "What Works in Preventing Bullying: Effective Elements of Anti-Bullying Programmes," *Journal of Aggression, Conflict and Peace Research* 1 (2009): 13–24.

Dan Olweus and Susan P. Limber, "Bullying in School: Evaluation and Dissemination of the Olweus Bullying Prevention Program," *American Journal of Orthopsychiatry* 80 (2010), 124–34.

Preventing Bullying Through Science, Policy, and Practice (National Academies Press, 2016).

"Tracy Vaillancourt, Ph.D.," Stop Bullying, accessed October 6, 2025, stopbullying.gov/blog/authors/tracy-vaillancourt-phd.

Susan Kelley, "Cornell Formalizes How It Assesses Disturbing Behavior," *Cornell Chronicle*, September 22, 2009, news.cornell.edu/stories/2009/09/look-cornells-threat-assessment-protocol.

Prison-Violence Reduction

Charles Ransford et al., "*Cure Violence Model Adaptation for Reducing Prison Violence*," Cure Violence, November 2016. The study showed 90 percent fewer violent attacks in prison when credible messengers were used.

James Gilligan and Bandy Lee, "The Resolve to Stop the Violence Project: Reducing Violence in the Community Through a Jail-Based Initiative," *Journal of Public Health* 27, no. 2 (2005): 143–48.

Violent Recruitment Interruption

"Moonshot," Moonshot: End Online Abuse, Terrorism, and Violence, accessed October 6, 2025, moonshotteam.com/. Originally based on the Cure Violence approach, Moonshot has built an online violence-prevention model to identify and interrupt violent recruitment, child sexual exploitation, and human trafficking, among other forms of abuse and violence.

Election-Violence Interruption

Seema Shah and Rachel Brown, *Programming for Peace: Sisi Ni Amani Kenya and the 2013 Election* (Center for Global Communication Studies, University of Pennsylvania, December 2014). The study showed a "total change from the 2008 to 2013 election" due to massive case finding, interruption, and norm-changing intervention throughout Kenya.

N. Githaiga, "When Institutionalization Threatens Peacebuilding: The Case of Kenya's Infrastructure for Peace," *Journal of Peacebuilding and Development* 15, no. 3 (2020): 316–30, https://doi.org/10.1177/1542316620945681.

Prisca Kamungi, Florence N. Mpaayei, and Thania Paffenholz, "Rethinking Peace Processes: Preventing Electoral Crisis in Kenya," *Accord* 29 (September 2020): 1–5.

Mass Shooting Prevention

Gary Slutkin, "Let's Treat These Mass Shootings Like the Public Health Crisis That They Are," *Hill*, February 21, 2018. Just under 67 percent of the interrupted plots were due to early detection through community reporting.

John S. Hollywood et al., "Mass Attacks Defense Toolkit," RAND Corporation, https://www.rand.org/pubs/tools/TLA1613-1.html.

John S. Hollywood, "Advance Detection and Reporting Are Key to Preventing Attacks," RAND Corporation: Commentary, July 18, 2024, https://www.rand.org/pubs/commentary/2024/07/advance-detection-and-reporting-are-key-to-preventing.html.

"Five Things About Protecting Against Mass Attacks," National Institute of Justice, October 30, 2023, https://nij.ojp.gov/topics/articles/five-things-about-protecting-against-mass-attacks.

Jillian Peterson and James A. Densley, *The Violence Project: How to Stop a Mass Shooting Epidemic* (Abrams Press, 2021).

S. J. Blumenthal and D. J. Kupfer, "Overview of Early Detection and Treatment Strategies for Suicidal Behavior in Young People," *Journal of Youth and Adolescence* 17, no. 1 (1988): 1–23.

Dewey Cornell et al., "A Retrospective Study of School Safety Conditions in High Schools Using the Virginia Threat Assessment Guidelines Versus Alternative Approaches," *School Psychology Quarterly* 24, no. 2 (June 2009): 119–29.

"Behavioral Threat Assessment and Intervention in Schools," *School Administrator* (March 2023), https://www.aasa.org/resources/resource/behavioral-threat-assessment-intervention-schools.

Child Abuse Reduction

Health-worker outreach to high-risk mothers, which involved active case finding by credible health workers, reduced child abuse by 56 to 79 percent. Follow-up studies showed the effects to be dose-responsive to amount of intervention, and the effect on reduced violent behavior lasted fifteen years.

David L. Olds et al., "Long-Term Effects of Home Visitation on Maternal Life Course and Child Abuse and Neglect: Fifteen-Year Follow-Up of a Randomized Trial," *JAMA* 278, no. 8 (1997): 637–43. The program reduced state-verified cases of child abuse and neglect in children from birth through age fifteen by 79 percent among mothers who were poor and unmarried.

David L. Olds et al., "Preventing Child Abuse and Neglect: A Randomized Trial of Nurse Home Visitation, *Pediatrics* 78 (1986): 65–78. In the second year of life (age thirteen to twenty-four months), nurse-visited children had 56 percent fewer visits to an emergency room for injuries and ingestions than children not receiving nurse home visits.

Margaret L. Holland et al., "Visit Attendance Patterns in Nurse-Family Partnership Community Sites," *Prevention Science* 19, no. 2 (2017): 1–12.

Parent Training

Cynthia Cupit Swenson et al., "Multisystemic Therapy for Child Abuse and Neglect: A Randomized Effectiveness Trial," *Journal of Family Psychology* 24, no. 4 (2010): 497–507.

Mark Chaffin et al., "Parent-Child Interaction Therapy with Physically Abusive Parents: Efficacy for Reducing Future Abuse Reports," *Journal of Consulting and Clinical Psychology* 72, no. 3: 500–510.

"WHO Guidelines and Handbook on Parenting Interventions to Prevent Maltreatment and Enhance Parent-Child Relationships with Children Aged 0–17 Years," World Health Organization, last updated July 18, 2024, who.int/teams/social-determinants-of-health/violence-prevention/parenting-guidelines. "Laws can reduce the use of violent punishment against children, change attitudes towards the use of such punishment.... Findings from a study comparing five European countries—three of which had bans on corporal punishment and two of which did not—report that nearly all forms of corporal punishment were used less commonly in countries with legal bans than in those without such bans. Furthermore, acceptance of corporal punishment was lower in countries with bans on corporal punishment... By 2016, nearly 50 countries had prohibited all violent punishment of children, and another 52 had committed to doing so."

Political Violence

Thomas S. Warrick and Mick Mulroy, "How to Put Out the Fires of Violent Political Extremism," *New Atlanticist* (blog), Atlantic Council, August 15, 2023, atlanticcouncil.org/blogs/new-atlanticist/how-to-put-out-the-fires-of-violent-political-extremism.

Rachel Kleinfeld and Nicole Bibbins Sedaca, "How to Prevent Political Violence," *Journal of Democracy* 35 (October 2024), https://www.journalofdemocracy.org/articles/how-to-prevent-political-violence/.

Catherine Kim, "An Expert on Political Violence Sees a Way Out of America's Crisis," *Politico Magazine*, July 14, 2024.

Wars and Civil Wars

When wars or civil wars are actively stopped it is by active case finding, outreach, and interruption; however, the process has been usually started late or taken years to accomplish, resulting in relapse rates of 20 to 25 percent for wars and 40 to 60 percent for civil wars. Violence within the country continues or worsens after the war ends. Hope can be found in the experiences of a few highly successful and persistent practitioners, including William Ury's Possibilist Network, the Harvard Negotiation Project, Inter-Mediate, Search for Common Ground, the work of John Paul Lederach, and others.

Suicide Interruption

Studies show 30 to 45 percent reductions in suicide attempts as a result of health-care-initiated intervention, early detection by family and community, and referrals from hotlines (more than twelve million calls are made to hotlines in the United States every year). Suicide attempts may be reduced by 50 percent by laws and by means restriction.

Doctors in primary care and nonpsychiatric-care settings see 45 percent of future suicide decedents in the thirty days prior to suicide, and 77 percent in the twelve months prior to suicide, about double the rate of consulting mental-health professionals.

Barbara H. Stanley et al., "Comparison of the Safety Planning Intervention with Follow-Up vs. Usual Care of Suicidal Patients Treated in the Emergency Department," *JAMA Psychiatry* 75, no. 9 (September 2018): 894–900, https://doi.org/10.1001/jamapsychiatry.2018.1776.

Stephanie K. Doupnik et al., "Association of Suicide Prevention Interventions with Subsequent Suicide Attempts, Linkage to Follow-Up Care, and Depression Symptoms for Acute Care Settings: A Systematic Review and Meta-analysis," *JAMA Psychiatry* 77, no. 10 (October 2020): 1021–30, https://doi.org/10.1001/jamapsychiatry.2020.1586.

Kevin J. Volpe et al., "Evaluation of the Effectiveness of a Suicide Deterrent System at the Golden Gate Bridge," *Injury Prevention* 30, no. 2 (April 2024): 159–64, https://doi.org/10.1136/ip-2023-045070.

A review of 20,234 articles, including ninety-seven randomized controlled trials, show suicidal behavior or ideation can be decreased by limiting access to lethal means, antidepressant treatment, training of primary care physicians (depression recognition and treatment), and educating youth on depression and suicidal behavior. Active outreach to psychiatric patients after discharge or crisis prevents suicidal behavior; antidepressants prevent attempts; and ketamine reduces suicidal ideation. CBT with dialectical behavior therapy also prevents suicidal behavior. Active screening for ideation has not proved to have better outcomes than screening for depression.

J. John Mann et al., "Improving Suicide Prevention Through Evidence-Based Strategies: A Systematic Review," *American Journal of Psychiatry* 178, no. 7 (2021): 611–24.

"Brief Interventions for Managing Suicidal Crises," American Foundation for Suicide Prevention, accessed October 3, 2025, afsp.org/brief-interventions-for-managing-suicidal-crises.

R. Büscher et al., "Internet-Based Cognitive Behavioral Therapy to Reduce Suicidal Ideation: A Systematic Review and Meta-Analysis," *JAMA Network Open* 3 (2020): e203933, doi: 10.1001/jamanetworkopen.2020.3933.

Laura Cramm, "New Study Finds That Countries with Corporal Punishment Bans Have Lower Rates of Adolescent Suicide, with Effects Peaking Around 12-13 Years After Prohibition Enacted," End Corporal Punishment of Children, October 21, 2024, https:

//endcorporalpunishment.org/loweradolsuicide. Compared to the countries that had a full ban of corporal punishment, countries that did not ban corporal punishment in any setting reported twice the rate of suicide in females age fifteen to nineteen.

"CDC Suicide Prevention for Action," Suicide Prevention, CDC, June 4, 2024, cdc.gov/suicide/resources/prevention.html.

Jason Cherkis, "What I Heard on a Suicide Hotline for Trans Kids," Opinion, *New York Times*, July 2, 2025.

Kellie R. Lynch et al., "Intent vs. Impact: A Qualitative Investigation of Domestic Violence and Extreme Risk Protective Order Gun Prohibitions in Two States," *Journal of Family Violence* (2024).

"Suicide Prevention," National Institute of Mental Health (NIMH), last reviewed August 2025, nimh.nih.gov/health/topics/suicide-prevention.

"Suicide Prevention Resource Center," SPRC, accessed October 2, 2025, sprc.org.

S. J. Blumenthal and D. J. Kupfer, "Overview of Early Detection and Treatment Strategies for Suicidal Behavior in Young People," *Journal of Youth and Adolescence* 17 (1988): 1–23, doi: 10.1007/BF01538721.

Personality Disorders (Including Psychopathy)

David P. Bernstein et al., "Schema Therapy for Violent PD Offenders: A Randomized Clinical Trial," *Psychological Medicine* 53, no. 1 (2023): 88–102.

Tori DeAngelis, "A Broader View of Psychopathy: New Findings Show That People with Psychopathy Have Varying Degrees and Types of the Condition," *Monitor on Psychology* 53, no. 2 (March 1, 2022).

Changing Norms (International — Human Rights, Public Health, Focused on Protecting Children)

Susan Bissell and A. K. Shiva Kumar, eds., *Protecting the World's Children: Public Health, Human Rights, Capabilities* (Oxford University Press, 2025).

Norm Change (Community Level)

Adam J. Milam et al., "Changes in Attitudes Toward Guns and Shootings Following Implementation of the Baltimore Safe Streets Intervention," *Journal of Urban Health* 93, no. 4 (2016): 609–26, https://doi.org/10.1007/s11524-016-0060-y. There was a 43 percent change in attitudes against violence (compared to 13 percent in controls) among high-risk persons in Baltimore Safe Streets interventions.

Daniel W. Webster et al., "Evaluation of Baltimore's Safe Streets Program: Effects on Attitudes, Participants' Experiences, and Gun Violence," Johns Hopkins Center for the Prevention of Youth Violence, 2012, https://www.jhsph.edu/research/centers-and-institutes/center-for-prevention-of-youth-violence/publications/Evaluation_of_Baltimore's_Safe_Streets_Program.pdf.

Sheyla A. Delgado et al., "Young Men in Neighborhoods with Cure Violence Programs Adopt Attitudes Less Supportive of Violence," John Jay College Research and Evaluation Center, March 16, 2017, https://johnjayrec.nyc/2017/03/16/databit201701/. "Young men living in neighborhoods with Cure Violence programs reported significant reductions in their willingness to use violence compared with men in similar areas without programs."

Jeffrey A. Butts and Sheyla A. Delgado, "Repairing Trust: Young Men in Neighborhoods with Cure Violence Programs Report Growing Confidence in Police," John Jay College Research and Evaluation Center, 2017, https://academicworks.cuny.edu/jj_pubs/418/.

Norm Change (International and Country Level)

S. Shreemoyee, "Women's Attitudes Towards Physical Intimate Partner Violence in India: Evidence from NFHS-3 to NFHS-5," *eClinicalMedicine* (2025), https://pmc.ncbi.nlm.nih.gov/articles/PMC12051491/.

M. R. Pradhan et al., "Men's Attitude Towards Wife-Beating: Understanding the Acceptance of IPV in India Using NFHS-3, NFHS-4, and NFHS-5," *BMC Public Health* (2024), https://pmc.ncbi.nlm.nih.gov/articles/PMC10829205/.

R. K. Biswas et al., "Women's Opinion on the Justification of Physical Spousal Violence in Bangladesh: Trends from 2007–2014," *PLOS One* 12, no. 11 (2017): e0187884, https://journals.plos.org/plosone/article?id=10.1371/journal.pone.0187884.

V. P. Patil et al., "Trends in Attitudinal Acceptance of Wife-Beating, Domestic Violence, and Help-Seeking Among Married Women in Nepal," *Journal of Biosocial Science* (2023), https://www.cambridge.org/core/journals/journal-of-biosocial-science/article/trends-in-attitudinal-acceptance-of-wifebeating-domestic-violence-and-helpseeking-among-married-women-in-nepal/A0F20FED956432A50995BD4669C6E526.

N. Asfaw et al., "Women's Empowerment in Ethiopia: A Trend Analysis Using DHS 2005–2016," *Open Journal of Women's Studies* 1, no. 2 (2018): 17–28, https://sryahwapublications.com/open-journal-of-womens-studies/pdf/v1-i2/3.pdf.

I. S. Speizer et al., "Gender Relations and Reproductive Health: Recent Evidence from Uganda," *Studies in Family Planning* 41, no. 1 (2010): 25–38, https://cdr.lib.unc.edu/downloads/th83m594h.

D. T. Kadengye et al., "Effect of Justification of Wife-Beating on Experiences of Intimate Partner Violence among Men and Women in Uganda: A Propensity-Score Matched Analysis of the 2016 DHS," *PLOS One* 18, no. 4 (2023): e0276025, https://journals.plos.org/plosone/article?id=10.1371/journal.pone.0276025.

I. Bergenfeld et al., "Global Trends in Men's and Women's Acceptance of Intimate Partner Violence: Analyses from 83 Countries, 1999–2022," *eClinicalMedicine* 76 (2025): 103072, https://www.thelancet.com/journals/eclinm/article/PIIS2589-5370(25)00131-2/fulltext.

INDIVIDUAL-LEVEL CASE MANAGEMENT

The use of CBT for community violence and postwar conflict syndromes yielded a 40 to 65 percent reduction in violence. The interventions involved individual and group management of people with active or high-level disease. (Note these are not community-wide interventions but they do focus on the highest risk.)

CBT and Related: Community Violence and Post-Conflict

Cali, Colombia: C. E. M. León et al., "Informe Final de la Evaluación de Impacto del Programa Abriendo Caminos de la Fundación Alvaralice," 2020, https://www.alvaralice.org/wp-content/uploads/2020/12/Informe-Final-de-la-Evaluaci%C3%B3n-de-Impacto-del-Programa-Abriendo-Caminos-de-la-Fundaci%C3%B3n.pdf.

Culiacán, Mexico: "Más Vida," *Informe Anual* (2023), https://cvg.org/wp-content/uploads/2023/11/Culiacan-final-report-2022.pdf.

Juarez, Mexico: Y. E. I. Gonzalez Martanez, "Barrio a la Comunidad: Informe Digital," Observatorio Ciudadano de Prevención, Seguridad y Justicia de Juárez, 2025. https://cvg.org/wp-content/uploads/2025/05/Digital-Barrioalacomunidad.pdf.

Trinidad and Tobago: Edward R. Maguire et al., *Evaluating Cure Violence in Trinidad and Tobago* (Washington, DC: Inter-American Development Bank, 2018), https://publications.iadb.org/publications/english/document/Evaluating-Cure-Violence-in-Trinidad-and-Tobago.pdf.

Sara B. Heller et al., "Thinking, Fast and Slow? Some Field Experiments to Reduce Crime and Dropout in Chicago," *Quarterly Journal of Economics* 132, no. 1 (2017): 1–54. Total arrests during the intervention period were reduced by 28 to 35 percent; violent-crime arrests were reduced by 45 to 50 percent.

Sarah Fleming, "Breaking the Cycle: Addressing Community Gun Violence with Evidence-Informed Solutions," *CBT Insights* (blog), Beck Institute, October 3, 2024.

"Rapid Deployment and Development Initiative (READI) Chicago," University of Chicago, Crime Lab, 2025, crimelab.uchicago.edu/projects/readi.

Monica P. Bhatt et al., "Predicting and Preventing Gun Violence: An Experimental Evaluation of READI Chicago," *Quarterly Journal of Economics* 139, no. 1 (2024): 1–56.

ROCA: https://www.abtglobal.com/files/Projects/PDFs/2021/final-report_abt-associates_roca-implementation-evaluation.pdf

See also Motivational Interviewing and Mind Body Approaches.

Hospital-Based

E. Bollman et al., "Recidivism Among Young Gunshot Victims: Analysis of Outcomes from CeaseFire New Orleans," *Annals of Emergency Medicine* 72, no. 4 (2018): S145, https://www.annemergmed.com/article/S0196-0644(18)31110-7/fulltext. "Recidivism rates among the 3 groups were roughly similar in the time period studied. Further analysis revealed that the CeaseFire participant group trended towards higher rates of GSWs suffered before the study index visit when compared to other groups, but following their CeaseFire enrollment, recidivism rates decreased to the overall group mean. Furthermore, participants had a mean of 805 days (67 months) until a recidivism event if it occurred, compared with 682 days for those who declined the intervention and 693 days for those not offered the intervention (both 57 months)."

Daniel Webster et al., "Research on the Effects of Hospital-Based Violence Intervention Programs: Observations and Recommendations," *Annals of the American Academy of Political and Social Science* 704, no. 1 (2022): 137–57.

Carnell Cooper et al., "Hospital-Based Violence Intervention Programs Work," *Journal of Trauma and Acute Care Surgery* 61, no. 3 (2006): 534–40.

Teresa Bell et al., "Long-Term Evaluation of a Hospital-Based Violence Intervention Program Using a Regional Health Information Exchange," *Journal of Trauma and Acute Care Surgery* 84, no. 1 (2018): 175–82.

Bethany L. Strong et al., "The Effects of Health Care–Based Violence Intervention Programs on Injury Recidivism and Costs: A Systematic Review," *Journal of Trauma and Acute Care Surgery* 81, no. 5 (2016): 961–70.

Erin McVey et al., "Operation CeaseFire–New Orleans: An Infectious Disease Model for Addressing Community Recidivism from Penetrating Trauma," *Journal of Trauma and Acute Care Surgery* 77, no. 1 (2014): 123–28.

Catherine Juillard et al., "Saving Lives and Saving Money: Hospital-Based Violence Intervention Is Cost-Effective," *Journal of Trauma and Acute Care Surgery* 78, no. 2 (2015): 252–58.

Leslie S. Zun et al., "The Effectiveness of an ED-Based Violence Prevention Program," *American Journal of Emergency Medicine* 24, no. 1 (2006): 8–13.

Randi Smith et al., "Hospital-Based Violence Intervention: Risk Reduction Resources That Are Essential for Success," *Journal of Trauma and Acute Care Surgery* 74, no. 4 (2013): 976–82.

Tina L. Cheng et al., "Effectiveness of a Mentor-Implemented, Violence Prevention Intervention for Assault-Injured Youths Presenting to the Emergency Department: Results of a Randomized Trial," *Pediatrics* 122, no. 5 (2008): 938–46.

Chicago-Based Community Violence Interventions (CVI)

"Chicago CRED: A Nonprofit for Reducing Gun Violence in Chicago," Chicago CRED, 2025, chicagocred.org.

"Institute for Nonviolence Chicago: Community Violence Intervention," Institute for Nonviolence Chicago, accessed October 4, 2025, nonviolencechicago.org.

"Metropolitan Family Services," Metropolitan Family Services, 2025, metrofamily.org.

US-Based Community Violence Intervention (CVI)

"Advance Peace: Believe in America Without Urban Gun Violence," Advance Peace, 2017, advancepeace.org.

"About: Who We Are," BUILD Program, 2025, buildprogram.org.

"CAPS Initiative," Coalition to Advance Public Safety (CAPS), accessed October 4, 2025, capsinitiative.org.

"Cities United," Cities United, 2025, citiesunited.org.

"Common Justice," Common Justice, 2025, commonjustice.org.

"Community-Based Public Safety," CBPS Collective, accessed October 4, 2025, cbpscollective.org.

"CVI Leadership Academy," Crime Lab, University of Chicago, 2025, crimelab.uchicago.edu/projects/community-violence-intervention-leadership-academy.

"Health Alliance for Violence Intervention: HAVI," HAVI, 2025, thehavi.org.

"Live Free," Live Free USA, 2025, livefreeusa.org.

"Local Initiatives Support Corporation (LISC)," LISC, 2025, lisc.org.

National Alliance of Trauma Recovery Centers," NATRC, 2025, nationalallianceoftraumarecoverycenters.org.

"National Institute of Criminal Justice Reform," NICJR, accessed October 4, 2025, nicjr.org.

US, Latin America, and Global

Cure Violence Global www.cvg.org

United Religious Initiative https://www.uri.org/

ADDITIONAL REFERENCES BY CITY AND COUNTRY

See text and notes for Chapters 6–8 for more complete references on communities discussed in book.

For reviews of all cities and countries, see Charles Ransford, Monique Williams, and Gary Slutkin, "A Systematic Review on the Effectiveness of the Cure Violence Approach," *Inquiry: The Journal of Health Care Organization, Provision, and Financing* 62 (2025): 1–12, https://doi.org/10.1177/00469580251366142 and cvg.org/impact.

BALTIMORE, MARYLAND

Alex MacGillis, "When Law Enforcement Alone Can't Stop The Violence," *New Yorker*, January 30, 2023.

Andrew Zaleski, "Can These Former Felons Save Freddie Gray's Violent Neighborhood," *Washington Post*, July 15, 2016.

Barry Simms, "Safe Streets Celebrates Over a Year of No Homicides in Penn-North," WBAL-TV, March 6, 2024.

Brandon M. Scott, "Safe Streets Brooklyn Achieves Over 365 Days with No Homicides," City of Baltimore press release, November 13, 2024.

Dan Rodricks, "Rodricks: Baltimore Needs to Expand Safe Streets Effort," *Baltimore Sun*, June 6, 2017.

Daniel W. Webster et al., *Estimating the Effects of Safe Streets Baltimore on Gun Violence: 2007–2022* (Center for Gun Violence Solutions, Johns Hopkins, Bloomberg School of Public Health, 2023).

Daniel W. Webster et al., *Evaluation of Baltimore's Safe Streets Program: Effects on Attitudes, Participants' Experiences, and Gun Violence* (Center for Gun Policy and Research, Johns Hopkins Bloomberg School of Public Health, 2012).

Daniel W. Webster, Jon S. Vernick, and Jennifer Mendel, "Interim Evaluation of Baltimore's Safe Streets Program," Center for the Prevention of Youth Violence, Johns Hopkins Bloomberg School of Public Health, January 7, 2009.

Darcy Costello, "Three Baltimore Safe Streets Sites Reach One Year Without a Homicide: 'I Can Go Outside,'" *Baltimore Sun*, September 6, 2024.

Fawn Johnson, "What Role Can Ex-Convicts Play in Curbing Violence?," *Atlantic*, October 31, 2014.

Stephon Dingle, "Baltimore Community Hits Major Milestone in Reducing Gun Violence, 400 Days Without a Homicide," CBS, November 12, 2024.

CHICAGO, ILLINOIS

Alex Kotlowitz, "Blocking the Transmission of Violence," *New York Times*, May 4, 2008.

Ana Lucia Gonzales, "Crossing Divides: Where Shootings Have Become 'Normal' for Teens," *Washington Post*, 2018.

"A Worthy Investment to Stop the Shooting," editorial, *Chicago Sun-Times*, 2004.

CeaseFire Final Report: An Evaluation of Gun and Non-Gun Violence in 47 Chicago Police Beats: 1999–2009 (Cure Violence, 2012), https://cvg.org/wp-content/uploads/2025/05/2012-CeaseFire-Final-Report_Thuy-Tran.pdf.

Charlie Ransford et al., "An Examination of the Role of CeaseFire, the Chicago Police, Project Safe Neighborhoods, and Displacement in the Reduction in Homicide in Chicago in 2004," in *Youth Gangs and Community Intervention: Research, Practice, and Evidence*, ed. Robert J. Chaskin (Columbia University Press, 2010).

"Chip and Lil' Tony," *Chicago Tribune*, December 10, 2004, updated August 19, 2021.

Clarence Page, "A Cure for Urban Violence Right Under Our Noses," *Chicago Tribune*, August 17, 2018.

Damian Whitworth, "Street Violence Is an Infection. I Can Cure It," *Times*, July 2, 2008, thetimes.com/best-law-firms/profile-legal/article/street-violence-is-an-infection-i-can-cure-it-j7g0gxttj76.

Frank Main, "Treating Gun Crime Like Disease Shows Results: CeaseFire Program May Cut Shootings by as Much as 67%," *Chicago Sun-Times*, 2002.

James O'Shea, "Get Behind CeaseFire to Reduce Chicago Violence," Opinion, *Chicago Sun-Times*, August 5, 2016.

Jamie Friedlander, "When I Was in the Line of Fire," *Success*, March 21, 2017.

Nancy Pompilio, "Chicago Program Treats Violence as Health Issue: CeaseFire Helped Slayings Fall 25 Percent," *Philadelphia Inquirer*, 2005.

"Negotiating a Cease-Fire," editorial, *Chicago Tribune*, 2002.

Samira Shackle, "Should We Treat Crime as Something to Be Cured Rather Than Punished?," *Guardian*, July 24, 2018.

Tina Rosenberg, "Fighting Street Gun Violence as if It Were a Contagion," Opinion, *New York Times*, May 8, 2018.

Tina Rosenberg, "Want to Quit the Gang Life? Try This Job On," Opinion, *New York Times*, May 15, 2018.

MAYWOOD, ILLINOIS

"CeaseFire Returns to Grateful Maywood," *Chicago Tribune*, January 1, 2009, updated August 22, 2021.

"Murder-Free Maywood Marks an Awkward Anniversary," *Chicago Tribune*, June 14, 2010, updated August 23, 2021.

NEW YORK CITY

Greg Berman and Emily Gold, *From Chicago to Brooklyn: A Case Study in Program Replication* (Center for Court Innovation, 2011).

Jeffrey A. Butts et al., "Effectiveness of the Cure Violence Model in New York City," John Jay College of Criminal Justice, CUNY, 2015.

Jim Dwyer, "Six Blocks, 96 Buildings, Zero Shootings: New Recipe at the Queensbridge Houses," *New York Times*, January 19, 2017.

Rachel Avram et al., "Do Cure Violence Programs Reduce Gun Violence? Evidence from New York City," Cornell University arXiv, submitted June 4, 2024, arxiv.org/html/2406.02459v1.

Samar Khurshid, "Why Does Crime Keep Falling in New York City?," *Gotham Gazette*, January 8, 2018.

Sarah Picard-Fritsche and Lenore Cerniglia, *Testing a Public Health Approach to Gun Violence: An Evaluation of Crown Heights Save Our Streets, a Replication of the Cure Violence*

Model (Center for Court Innovation, 2012), innovatingjustice.org/wp-content/uploads/2013/01/SOS_Evaluation.pdf.

The Cure for Crisis: The Power and Potential of Community Violence Intervention (Office of the New York City Comptroller, March 2025).

PHILADELPHIA, PENNSYLVANIA
Caterina G. Roman et al., *Philadelphia CeaseFire: Findings from the Impact Evaluation* (Temple University, January 2017).

YONKERS, NEW YORK
John Klofas et al., SNUG Evaluation (Center for Public Safety Initiatives, Rochester Institute of Technology, July 2013), rit.edu/liberalarts/sites/rit.edu.liberalarts/files/documents/our-work/2013-10.pdf.

IRAQ (BASRA AND SADR CITY)
Ambassadors for Peace — Iraq: Final Report (December 10, 2010–December 31, 2013), American Islamic Congress, 2013.

SOUTH AFRICA (CAPE TOWN)
CeaseFire — Hanover Park, First Six Months (First Community Resource Centre, 2013).
CeaseFire — Hanover Park, Second Six Months (First Community Resource Centre, 2014).
Sophia M. Newman, "The Secret Life of a Violence Interrupter," *Narratively*, April 8, 2015, narratively.com/p/the-secret-life-of-a-violence-interrupter.

WHAT HAPPENED IN THESE PLACES: 2025 UPDATES
In 2025, the US had historic drops in killings in many cities, to fifty-to-sixty-year record lows. This followed the expansion of the work of cities using the epidemic approach including "credible messengers," "violence interrupters," and focusing on the highest risk. In 2021, the US government provided hundreds of millions of dollars to the approach, now called Community Violence Intervention (CVI) and by dozens of other local names in over ninety cities. City and state governments and local foundations and business leaders added. This included support to police involved approaches with a similar focus. https://bidenwhitehouse.archives.gov/briefing-room/statements-releases/2021/04/07/fact-sheet-biden-harris-administration-announces-initial-actions-to-address-the-gun-violence-public-health-epidemic.

Baltimore:
In 2025, killings in Baltimore declined furthest and fastest in the country and was on pace to a sixty year low; the lowest since 1965. Further, more than a dozen Baltimore communities were poised to end 2025 without a single homicide for the whole year. https://mayor.baltimorecity.gov/news/press-releases/2026-01-01-joint-statement-historic-public-safety-progress-2025; https://www.thebanner.com/community/criminal-justice/baltimore-homicides-decline-48-year-low-U3UFWCQOUNHTHIUECCX3JK2KYY/.

Chicago:
Following the initial seven years in Chicago, government investment slowed but increased in the last four years as federal and local investment allowed expansion to nearly half of Chicago's seventy-seven neighborhoods. In 2025, Chicago recorded its fewest killings in sixty years: Mayor Johnson hailed this as "one of the most transformative years in violence

reduction in our city's history...pointing to the influx of investment in violence prevention." https://www.chicagotribune.com/2025/12/10/opinion-chicago-community-violence-intervention-crime/; https://blockclubchicago.org/2026/01/02/chicago-recorded-fewest-murders-in-60-years-in-2025-bucking-trumps-murder-capital-insult/.

LA:
Although final totals were not available as of this writing, the first half year showed LA being on pace to its lowest number of killings in sixty years. https://www.police1.com/lapd/l-a-on-pace-to-see-lowest-homicide-total-in-nearly-60-years-as-killings-plummet.

NYC:
2025 was the safest year in Brooklyn's history and record lows in shootings were reported for NYC as a whole. From November–December, 2025, New York City went twelve consecutive days without a single homicide throughout the entire city, matching the longest stretch without a murder in the city's recorded history. https://brooklynda.org/2025/12/31/brooklyn-finishes-2025-with-fewest-murders-shootings-shooting-victims-and-shooting-homicides-in-recorded-history/; https://www.nyc.gov/site/nypd/news/pr018/nypd-record-low-shooting-incidents-shooting-victims-the-first-11-months-the.

San Pedro Sula, Honduras:
San Pedro Sula, which in 2012 was the most violent city in the world, with killings now still down 79%, has dropped from the first to the forty-third most violent city in 2024. https://www.lawg.org/san-pedro-sula-honduras-nearly-a-war-zone/; https://en.wikipedia.org/wiki/List_of_cities_by_homicide_rate.

BIBLIOGRAPHY AND FURTHER READING

BIOLOGY, PHYSIOLOGY, AND MEDICINE
J. Larry Jameson et al., *Harrison's Principles of Internal Medicine*, 20th ed. (McGraw-Hill Education, 2018).
Michael Ruse, *Philosophy of Biology* (Prometheus, 2007).
Robert Ames and Philip Siegelman, eds., *The Idea of Evolution: Readings in Evolutionary Theory and Its Influence* (University of Minnesota, 1959).
Robert Lanza, *Biocentrism: How Life and Consciousness Are the Keys to Understanding the True Nature of the Universe* (BenBella Books, 2010).
William F. Ganong, *Review of Medical Physiology*, 21st ed. (McGraw-Hill, 2001).

INFECTIOUS DISEASE DYNAMICS
Major C. Greenwood, *Epidemics and Crowd Disease: An Introduction to the Study of Epidemiology* (Macmillan, 1935).

INFECTIOUS DISEASE CONTROL
Alexandra M. Levitt, *Deadly Outbreaks: How Medical Detectives Save Lives Threatened by Killer Pandemics, Exotic Viruses, and Drug-Resistant Parasites* (Skyhorse, 2013).
David L. Heymann, ed., *Control of Communicable Diseases Manual*, 18th ed. (American Public Health Association, 2004).
L. Khawar et al., "Elimination and Eradication Goals for Communicable Diseases: A Systematic Review," *Bulletin of the World Health Organization* 101 (2023): 649–65, doi: 10.2471/BLT.23.289676.
Michael H. Merson et al., *Global Health: Diseases, Programs, Systems, and Policies*, 3rd ed. (Jones & Bartlett Learning, 2012).
Richard Conniff, *Ending Epidemics: A History of Escape from Contagion* (MIT Press, 2023).

TUBERCULOSIS
Gareth M. Green et al., eds., *Koch Centennial Memorial: 1882–1982* (American Philosophical Society Press, 1982).
"Tuberculosis," special issue, *Clinics in Chest Medicine* 24, no. 3 (2003).

HIV/AIDS
Michael Merson and Stephen Inrig, *The AIDS Pandemic: Searching for a Global Response* (Springer, 2018).

SMALLPOX
D. A. Henderson, *Smallpox: The Death of a Disease* (Prometheus Books, 2009).

SCIENTIFIC REVOLUTIONS

Kay Herel, *Darwin's Love of Life* (Columbia University Press, 2022).
Charles Darwin, *On the Origin of Species by Means of Natural Selection, or the Preservation of Favoured Races in the Struggle for Life* (London, 1859).
Charles Van Doren, *A History of Knowledge: Past, Present, and Future* (Ballantine Books, 1991).
Karen Magnuson Beil, *What Linnaeus Saw: A Scientist's Quest to Name Every Living Thing* (Norton Young Readers, 2019).
Thomas S. Kuhn, *The Structure of Scientific Revolutions*, 2nd ed. (University of Chicago Press, 1970).

THE BRAIN

Chris Frith, *Making Up the Mind: How the Brain Creates Our Mental World* (Blackwell, 2007).
Daniel Kahneman, *Thinking, Fast and Slow* (Farrar, Straus and Giroux, 2011).
David Eagleman, *Incognito: The Secret Lives of the Brain* (Pantheon, 2011).
Sara E. Gorman and Jack M. Gorman, *Denying to the Grave: Why We Ignore the Facts That Will Save Us* (Oxford University Press, 2016).
Wilder Penfield and Theodore Rasmussen, *The Cerebral Cortex of Man* (Macmillan, 1950).

ADOLESCENTS

Frances E. Jensen, *The Teenage Brain: A Neuroscientist's Survival Guide to Raising Adolescents and Young Adults* (Harper, 2015).
Linda Spear, *The Behavioral Neuroscience of Adolescence* (W. W. Norton, 2010).

EXPOSURE

Eye
Richard L. Gregory, *Eye and Brain: The Psychology of Seeing* (Princeton University Press, 1997).

Mirroring
Marco Iacoboni, *Mirroring People: The New Science of How We Connect with Others* (Farrar, Straus and Giroux, 2008).

Copying
Albert Bandura, *Social Learning and Personality Development* (Holt, Rinehart and Winston, 1963).
Leonard Berkowitz, *Causes and Consequences of Feelings* (Cambridge University Press, 2000).

Dopamine and Belonging
Alain de Botton, *Status Anxiety* (Vintage International, 2005).
David J. Linden, *The Accidental Mind: How Brain Evolution Has Given Us Love, Memory, Dreams, and God* (Belknap Press, 2008).

SUSCEPTIBILITY

Grievance and Pain
Frank Bruni, *The Age of Grievance* (Avid Reader Press, 2024).
James Kimmel Jr., *The Science of Revenge: Understanding the World's Deadliest Addiction — and How to Overcome It* (Harmony, 2025).

BIBLIOGRAPHY AND FURTHER READING 317

INTERRUPTION
Behavior Change
Aaron T. Beck, *Prisoners of Hate: The Cognitive Basis of Anger, Hostility, and Violence* (HarperCollins, 1999).

Isaac Levi, *The Fixation of Belief and Its Undoing: Changing Beliefs Through Inquiry* (Cambridge University Press, 1991).

Robert Cialdini, *Influence: The Psychology of Persuasion* (Harper Business, 2006).

Robert Cialdini, *Pre-Suasion: A Revolutionary Way to Influence and Persuade* (Simon & Schuster, 2016).

NORMS
Bronislaw Malinowski, *A Scientific Theory of Culture and Other Essays* (University of North Carolina Press, 1990).

Cristina Bicchieri, *The Grammar of Society: The Nature and Dynamics of Social Norms* (Cambridge University Press, 2006).

Everett M. Rogers, *Diffusion of Innovations*, 5th ed. (Free Press, 2003).

John R. Zaller, *The Nature and Origins of Mass Opinion* (Cambridge University Press, 1992).

Leandro Herrero, *Viral Change: The Alternative to Slow, Painful and Unsuccessful Management of Change in Organizations*, 2nd ed. (Meetingminds, 2008).

Lee Ross and Richard E. Nisbett, *The Person and the Situation: Perspectives of Social Psychology* (McGraw-Hill, 1991).

Malcolm Gladwell, *The Tipping Point: How Little Things Can Make a Big Difference* (Little, Brown, 2000).

Michele Gelfand, *Rule Makers, Rule Breakers: How Tight and Loose Cultures Wire Our World* (Scribner, 2018).

Community Violence
Cobe Williams and Josh Gryniewicz, *Interrupting Violence: One Man's Journey to Heal the Streets and Redeem Himself* (Rowman & Littlefield, 2024).

Jens Ludwig, *Unforgiving Places: The Unexpected Origins of American Gun Violence* (University of Chicago Press, 2025).

Randolph Roth, *American Homicide* (Harvard University Press, 2012).

Thomas Abt, *Bleeding Out: The Devastating Consequences of Urban Violence — and a Bold New Plan for Peace in the Streets* (Basic Books, 2019).

Tio Hardiman, *Interrupting Gun Violence: The Public Health Approach* (Violence Interrupters, 2023).

INFECTIONS OF THE STATE
Tribes, Political Division, and Violence
George Lakoff, *The Political Mind: Why You Can't Understand 21st-Century Politics with an 18th-Century Brain* (Viking, 2008).

Joshua Greene, *Moral Tribes: Emotion, Reason, and the Gap Between Us and Them* (Penguin, 2013).

Marc D. Hauser, *Moral Minds: The Nature of Right and Wrong* (Ecco, 2006).

Seth Godin, *Tribes: We Need You to Lead Us* (Portfolio, 2008).

Race, Policing, Punishment, and Incarceration
Mark Mauer, *Invisible Punishment: The Collateral Consequences of Mass Imprisonment* (New Press, 2006).

Mark Mauer, *Race to Incarcerate: The Sentencing Project* (New Press, 1999).
Richard Rothstein, *The Color of Law: A Forgotten History of How Our Government Segregated America* (Liveright, 2017).
Ta-Nehisi Coates, *Between the World and Me* (Spiegel & Grau, 2015).

Holocaust

Aly Götz, *Europe Against the Jews, 1880–1945* (Metropolitan Books, 2020).
Daniel Jonah Goldhagen, *The Devil That Never Dies: The Rise and Threat of Global Antisemitism* (Little, Brown, 2013).
Daniel Jonah Goldhagen, *Hitler's Willing Executioners: Ordinary Germans and the Holocaust* (Alfred A. Knopf, 1996).
Martin A. Lee, *The Beast Reawakens: Fascism's Resurgence from Hitler's Spymasters to Today's Neo-Nazi Groups and Right-Wing Extremists* (Little, Brown, 1997).
Peter Hayes, ed., *How Was It Possible? A Holocaust Reader* (University of Nebraska Press, 2015).
Steven T. Katz, *The Holocaust in Historical Context*, vol. 1, *The Holocaust and Mass Death Before the Modern Age* (Oxford University Press, 1994).
Viktor E. Frankl, *Man's Search for Meaning* (Beacon Press, 2006).

Genocide

Daniel Jonah Goldhagen, *Worse Than War: Genocide, Eliminationism, and the Ongoing Assault on Humanity* (PublicAffairs, 2009).
David A. Hamburg, *Preventing Genocide: Practical Steps Toward Early Detection and Effective Action* (Routledge, 2008).
David McKean, *Watching Darkness Fall: FDR, His Ambassadors, and the Rise of Adolf Hitler* (St. Martin's Press, 2021).
Dennis Prager and Joseph Telushkin, *Why the Jews? The Reason for Antisemitism* (Touchstone, 1983).
Paul Weindling, *Epidemics and Genocide in Eastern Europe, 1890–1945* (Oxford University Press, 2000).
Peter Hayes, *Why? Explaining the Holocaust* (W. W. Norton, 2017).
Robert Jay Lifton, *Losing Reality: On Cults, Cultism, and the Mindset of Political and Religious Zealotry* (New Press, 2019).
Robert Jay Lifton, *The Nazi Doctors: Medical Killing and the Psychology of Genocide* (Basic Books, 1986).
Samantha Power, *"A Problem from Hell": America and the Age of Genocide* (Basic Books, 2002).

Stories

Mark Buchanan, *Nexus: Small Worlds and the Groundbreaking Science of Networks* (W. W. Norton, 2003).

Beliefs

Andrew Newberg and Mark Robert Waldman, *Why We Believe What We Believe: Uncovering Our Biological Need for Meaning, Spirituality, and Truth* (Free Press, 2006).
Grof Stanislav, ed., *Human Survival and Consciousness Evolution* (SUNY Press, 1988).
Mel Ash, *Shaving the Inside of Your Skull: Crazy Wisdom for Discovering Who You Really Are* (Tarcher, 1997).

BIBLIOGRAPHY AND FURTHER READING

AUTHORITARIAN VIOLENCE DISORDER
Power and Empathy
Brian Klaas, *Corruptible: Who Gets Power and How It Changes Us* (Scribner, 2021).

Propaganda and Lies
Annalee Newitz, *Stories Are Weapons: Psychological Warfare and the American Mind* (W. W. Norton, 2024).
Barbara McQuade, *Attack from Within: How Disinformation Is Sabotaging America* (Seven Stories Press, 2024).
Edward Bernays, *Crystallizing Public Opinion* (Boni and Liveright, 1923).
Federico Finkelstein, *A Brief History of Fascist Lies* (University of California Press, 2022).
Harry G. Frankfurt, *On Bullshit* (Princeton University Press, 2005).
Peter Pomerantsev, *How to Win the Information War: The Propagandist Who Outwitted Hitler* (PublicAffairs, 2024).
Renée DiResta, *Invisible Rulers: The People Who Turn Lies into Reality* (PublicAffairs, 2024).

Cruelty
Roy F. Baumeister, *Evil: Inside Human Violence and Cruelty* (W. H. Freeman, 1997).
Simon Baron-Cohen, *The Science of Evil: On Empathy and the Origins of Cruelty* (Basic Books, 2011).

Fascism, Tyranny, AVD
Adam Serwer, *The Cruelty Is the Point: The Past, Present, and Future of Trump's America* (One World, 2021).
Alice Miller, *Banished Knowledge: Facing Childhood Injuries* (Doubleday, 1990).
Anne Applebaum, *Autocracy, Inc.: The Dictators Who Want to Run the World* (Doubleday, 2024).
Anne Applebaum, *Twilight of Democracy: The Seductive Lure of Authoritarianism* (Doubleday, 2020).
Bandy Lee, *The Dangerous Case of Donald Trump: 27 Psychiatrists and Mental Health Experts Assess a President* (Thomas Dunne Books, 2017).
Erich Fromm, *The Anatomy of Human Destructiveness* (Holt, Rinehart and Winston, 1973).
Erich Fromm, *Escape from Freedom* (Holt, Rinehart and Winston, 1941).
George Lakoff, *Whose Freedom? The Battle Over America's Most Important Idea* (Farrar, Straus and Giroux, 2006).
John W. Dean and Bob Altemeyer, *Authoritarian Nightmare: Trump and His Followers* (Melville House, 2020).
Jason Stanley, *Erasing History: How Fascists Rewrite the Past to Control the Future* (One Signal Publishers, 2024).
Jason Stanley, *How Fascism Works: The Politics of Us and Them* (Random House, 2018).
Jason Stanley, *How Propaganda Works* (Princeton University Press, 2015).
Jerrold M. Post, *Dangerous Charisma: The Political Psychology of Donald Trump and His Followers* (Pegasus Books, 2020).
Jerrold M. Post, *Leaders and Their Followers in a Dangerous World: The Psychology of Political Behavior* (Cornell University Press, 2004).
Jerrold M. Post, *Narcissism and Politics: Dreams of Glory* (Cambridge University Press, 2014).
Karen Stenner, *The Authoritarian Dynamic* (Cambridge University Press, 2005).
Malcolm Nance, *The Plot to Destroy Democracy: How Putin and His Spies Are Undermining America and Dismantling the West* (Hachette Books, 2018).

Malcolm Nance, *They Want to Kill Americans: The Militias, Terrorists, and Deranged Ideology of the Trump Insurgency* (St. Martin's Press, 2022).
Marcel Dirsus, *How Tyrants Fall: And How Nations Survive* (John Murray Publishers, 2024).
Matthew C. MacWilliams, *On Fascism: 12 Lessons from American History* (St. Martin's Griffin, 2020).
Nassir Ghaemi, *A First-Rate Madness: Uncovering the Links Between Leadership and Mental Illness* (Penguin Press, 2011).
Paul Mason, *How to Stop Fascism: History, Ideology, Resistance* (Allen Lane, 2021).
Peter Ackerman and Jack DuVall, *A Force More Powerful: A Century of Nonviolent Conflict* (St. Martin's Griffin, 2000).
Peter Turchin, *Ages of Discord: A Structural-Demographic Analysis of American History* (Beresta Books, 2016).
Richard J. Bernstein, *Why Read Hannah Arendt Now* (Polity Press, 2018).
Robert Jay Lifton, *Thought Reform and the Psychology of Totalism: A Study of 'Brainwashing' in China* (University of North Carolina Press, 1989).
Ruth Ben-Ghiat, *Strongmen: Mussolini to the Present* (W. W. Norton, 2021).
Shane Burley, *Fascism Today: What It Is and How to End It* (AK Press, 2017).
Theo Horesh, *The Fascism This Time: And the Global Future of Democracy* (Cosmopolis, 2020).
Timothy Snyder, *Black Earth: The Holocaust as History and Warning* (Tim Duggan Books, 2015).
Timothy Snyder, *On Tyranny: Twenty Lessons from the Twentieth Century* (Crown, 2025).
Timothy Snyder, *The Road to Unfreedom: Russia, Europe, America* (Crown, 2018).

War and Civil War

Alexander B. Downes, *Targeting Civilians in War* (Cornell University Press, 2012).
Andreas Wimmer, *Waves of War: Nationalism, State Formation, and Ethnic Exclusion in the Modern World* (Cambridge University Press, 2013).
Barbara F. Walter, *How Civil Wars Start: And How to Stop Them* (Crown, 2022).
Barbara F. Walter and Jack Snyder, eds., *Civil Wars, Insecurity, and Intervention* (Columbia University Press, 1999).
Barbara W. Tuchman, *The March of Folly: From Troy to Vietnam* (Random House, 1985).
Christopher Blattman, *Why We Fight: The Roots of War and the Paths to Peace* (Viking, 2022).
Daniel Muñoz-Rojas and Jean-Jacques Frésard, *Roots of Behaviour in War: A Survey of the Literature* (International Committee of the Red Cross, 2004).
Gustave Le Bon, *The Psychology of Revolution*, trans. Bernard Miall (Macmillan, 1916).
Jack Snyder, *From Voting to Violence: Democratization and Nationalist Conflict* (W. W. Norton, 2000).
Jonathan Blitzer, *Everyone Who Is Gone Is Here: The United States, Central America, and the Making of a Crisis* (Penguin Press, 2024).
Jonathan Powell, *Terrorists at the Table: Why Negotiating Is the Only Way to Peace* (St. Martin's Press, 2015).
Louis Fitzgibbon, *The Betrayal of the Somalis* (Africa Book Centre, 1982).
Oliver Kaplan, *Resisting War: How Communities Protect Themselves* (Cambridge University Press, 2017).
Paul Collier et al., *Breaking the Conflict Trap: Civil War and Development Policy* (World Bank, 2003).
Peter Turchin, *War and Peace and War: The Rise and Fall of Empires* (Plume, 2007).
Robert Pape, *Dying to Win: The Strategic Logic of Suicide Terrorism* (Random House, 2005).

Scott Atran, *Talking to the Enemy: Faith, Brotherhood, and the (Un)Making of Terrorists* (Ecco, 2011).

William Ury, *The Third Side: Why We Fight and How We Can Stop* (Penguin Books, 2000).

Poverty, Inequity, and Mistrust in Government

James Gilligan, *Why Some Politicians Are More Dangerous Than Others* (Polity, 2011).

Richard Wilkinson and Kate Pickett, *The Spirit Level: Why Greater Equality Makes Societies Stronger* (Bloomsbury, 2011).

Trauma and Healing

Bessel van der Kolk, *The Body Keeps the Score: Brain, Mind, and Body in the Healing of Trauma* (Penguin Books, 2014).

Gabor Maté and Daniel Maté, *The Myth of Normal: Trauma, Illness and Healing in a Toxic Culture* (Avery, 2022).

Judith L. Herman, *Trauma and Recovery: The Aftermath of Violence—from Domestic Abuse to Political Terror* (Basic Books, 1992).

Judith L. Herman, *Truth and Repair: How Trauma Survivors Envision Justice* (Nation Books, 2023).

Peter A. Levine, *Waking the Tiger: Healing Trauma* (North Atlantic Books, 1997).

Richard C. Schwartz, *No Bad Parts: Healing Trauma and Restoring Wholeness with the Internal Family Systems Model* (Sounds True, 2021).

Miscellaneous and Compelling

Albert Einstein, *Ideas and Opinions* (Crown Publishers, 1954).

Andrew Boyd, *I Want a Better Catastrophe: Navigating the Climate Crisis with Grief, Hope, and Gallows Humor* (New Society Publishers, 2023).

Gad Saad, *The Parasitic Mind: How Infectious Ideas Are Killing Common Sense* (Regnery Publishing, 2020).

James J. Heckman and Alan B. Krueger, *Inequality in America: What Role for Human Capital Policies?* (MIT Press, 2003).

Jeremy Rifkin, *The Empathic Civilization: The Race to Global Consciousness in a World in Crisis* (Tarcher, 2009).

Robert M. Sapolsky, *Determined: A Science of Life Without Free Will* (Penguin Press, 2023).

Sogyal Rinpoche, *The Tibetan Book of Living and Dying* (Harper San Francisco, 1992).

INDEX

A

acceptance, sense of and need for, 53, 55, 57, 77, 93–96, 201–204
ACE (adverse childhood event) scores, 100
ACLED (Armed Conflict Location & Event Data), 208
ACTH, 88
Action Plan, 275–281
   being prepared to respond to conflicts to prevent escalation, 277–278
   educating others, 275–276
   educating yourself, 275
   getting involved in community and more broadly, 278–279
   helping people in need, 278
   remembering that violence is not inevitable and is stoppable, 280
   speaking out and protesting peacefully, 276–277
   starting community groups or community-led movements, 279–280
   taking care of yourself, 280
active case finding, 79–81, 100–101, 119–121, 245
   active cases, defined, 269
   authoritarian violence disorder, 219
   defined, 22
   following up on active cases, 22
   interrupting transmission and reducing exposure, 63, 66
   limited number of active cases, 79
   manpower and social connection required, 101
   outreach workers and systems, 101–102
   public education and training, 119
   syndromes benefiting from, 247
adenylate cyclase, 43
adolescent violence, 70–71, 77–78, 302. *See also* gangs
Advancement Project, 172
adverse childhood event (ACE) scores, 100
affective process, 57
agents of disease, 26, 31, 33, 41–43, 86–87, 269
AI, 64
AIDS. *See* HIV/AIDS
alcohol, 90, 126, 291
Allen, Susan, 67
Alliance of Local Service Organizations, 231
Alma (gang kidnapping victim), 186
Alma (violence interrupter), 133
Ambassadors for Peace (AFP), 233–234
American Islamic Congress, 233
amygdala, 88, 98, 138, 269
Angelica (case finder), 114–115, 120
Annan, Kofi, 227
anterior insula, 56
"Anthem" (Cohen), 111
Anthony (gang member), 153
Armed Conflict Location & Event Data (ACLED), 208
Assad, Bashar al-, 237–238
assessment. *See also* contact tracing; diagnosis
   asking questions about violence, 12–14
   of epidemic situations, 11
   of exposure, 81
   need for data about violence, 15–16
   of risk factors, 100

INDEX

authoritarian violence disorder (AVD), 213–222, *215*
  active case finding, 219
  authoritarian personality tendencies, 216–217
  authoritarianism, defined, 269
  changing the story, 220–221
  community responses, 220
  contagion pathways, 214
  defined, 269
  epidemic-control approach, 217–222
  intergenerational transmission of violence, 216
  interruption of spread, 219
  isolation and containment, 221–222
  outreach workers and systems, 219–220
  providing an off-ramp, 221
  public education and training, 217–219

B

Ban Ki-Moon, 227
Bandura, Albert, 46
Barre, Mohamed Siad, 34, 211
Barrio 18 gang, 176–177, 179
Beck, Charlie, 173
Beer, Francis A., 229
belief systems, 90. *See also* religiosity
belonging, sense of and need for, 53, 93, 142, 179, 201–202, 209, 233
Benton, Marjorie Craig, 156
Bethel New Life, 102, 126
biology, 269. *See also* disease
Bloomberg, Michael, 171
Bobo inflatable clown toy, 46
Bolland, John Michael, 70
Bottom Billion, The (Collier), 27
Braggs, Tony, 123
brain and neurology
  amygdala, 88, 98, 138, 269
  anterior insula, 56
  dopamine and dopamine pathways, 53–55
  dorsal anterior cingulate cortex, 56
  frontal lobe, 90, 93, 98–102, 138, 291
  functional/structural changes to, 42–44
  hypothalamus, 51, 88
  mirror neurons, 48–51, 272
  mirroring, 47–50, *47, 50*
  optic nerve, 44–45
  pain network, 55–56, *56*
  pituitary gland, 88
  prefrontal cortex, 49, 89
  premotor cortex, 48–49
  reward network, 53–55, *54*
  script acquisition, 51–52
  social pain, 55–56, *56*
  social reward, 54–55, *54*
  switchboard model, 49
  visual cortex, 45
Bratton, Bill, 172
bullying
  active case finding, 247
  authoritarian violence disorder, 214
  community responses and norms, 249
  defined, 269
  exposure within and between syndromes, 81, *81*
  public education and training, 251
  solutions for, 302–303
  state violence, 222
Bunyan, John, 1
Bush, Laura, 231–232

C

Camilo (violence interrupter), 111–115, 120–121
cAMP (cyclic AMP), 43
Carlsson, Arvid, 53
carriers, 34, 269
cartels, 112, 175–177, 180–181, 307
case management
  solutions involving, 307–309
  syndromes benefiting from, 248–249
CeaseFire. *See* Cure Violence Global
Centers for Disease Control and Prevention (CDC)
  data collection, 16–17
  funding from, 102, 156
  males and violence, 98
  predicting future risk of violence, 100

refugee health system in Somalia, 157
tuberculosis, 120
Cespedes, Guillermo, 172
Charleston mass shooting, 100
chatbots, 64
Chekhov, Anton, 21
Chicago Community Trust, 156
Chicago Project for Violence Prevention, 68
Chicago Sun-Times, 125, 145
Chicago Tribune, 4
chicken pox, 53
child abuse
  active case finding, 247
  community responses and norms, 250
  exposure within and between syndromes, 81–82, 82
  outreach workers and systems, 247
  solutions for, 304
  state violence, 222, 224
China Joe (violence interrupter), 129, 136–137
cholera, 2, 23, 34
  catching up and pulling ahead of, 243
  dirty water, 217, 284
  hijacking intestinal function, 43
  identifying contagion from observable signs, 42
  infectious agent, 42
  public education and behavior change, 116, 117
Chris (gang member), 153
Chris (peer pressure victim), 91–93
Christoffel, Kathy, 61–62
CHWs (community health workers), 100–101, 119, 149, 155, 269. *See also* outreach workers and systems
clinical screening score development, 291
closeness in space/time/relationship, 74
clusters and clustering, 18–19, 19, 29, 62, 229, 269
CNN, 146
Cohen, Leonard, 111
Collier, Paul, 27
Columbine school shooting, 83–85, 94–96

communicable diseases, 128, 251, 269
community health workers (CHWs), 100–101, 119, 149, 155, 269. *See also* outreach workers and systems
community violence
  active case finding, 246
  case management, 247
  community responses and norms, 248–250
  defined, 269
  exposure within and between syndromes, 80–82
  isolation and containment, 251
  outreach workers and systems, 246
  social networks, 77
  solutions for, 300, 307–309
  state violence, 221, 223, 226, 231
  using gang infrastructure, 181
community violence interventions (CVIs), 148, 308–309. *See also* violence interruption
community-level strategies and responses, 17, 23, 66, 101–107, 249–250
connection, sense of and need for, 53, 96, 179
conspiracy theories, 204–205, 251
contact tracing
  contacts, defined, 270
  defined, 270
  index cases, 210
  interrupting transmission and reducing exposure, 63, 66
  outreach workers and systems, 105, 119, 166
  in prisons, 35
  violence as predictable product of proximity and dose, 80
contagion. *See also* disease; epidemics
  barriers to, 86–87
  defined, 270
  dose, 72
  elimination of, 8
  state violence, 209–210, 214, 229
contagion accelerators, 208–209, 270
"Contagion of Great Power Behavior, The" (Levy), 229

Contagion of Violence, 50
contagious disease. *See also* disease; epidemics
  borderless, 223
  cause and effect, 62
  cumulative dose, 74
  defined, 270
  dose, 72–73
  epidemic sequence, 59–60
  etiologic agents, 41
  gender and risk, 98
  proximity, 73–74
  replication, 44
  susceptibility, 86
  violence as, 7–8, 23, 37, 61–62, *61*
  war as, 229–230
Cook County Hospital, 171
Cookham Wood Prison, 35
cortisol, 88
COVID
  crisis-management infrastructure, 171
  determining who is at risk, 97
  epidemic-control systems, 228
  exposure, 60
  factors affecting susceptibility, 87
  isolation and containment, 252
  marker of success, 118
  politics, 196
  public education and behavior change, *116*, 117
  susceptibility, 86
Crime Bill (Violent Crime Control and Law Enforcement Act of 1994), 15, 283
Cruz, Frankie, 141–143
Cruz, Guadalupe "Lupe," 141–145, 175, 182, 185, 188, 250
Cruz, Sergio, 141
culture. *See also* norms
  acceptance of violence in US, 99
  adapting to, 148, 234
  changing, 245–246
  defined, 270
  males and violence, 98
  state violence, 208–209

Cure PNW, 204, 208
Cure Violence Global (formerly, CeaseFire), 7, 24, 78. *See also* violence interruption
  city investment and adoption of methods, 165–166
  community responses, 122–124
  expansion of, 154–155, 157–159, 169–170
  extremism and hate groups, 205–206, 208
  flyers and posters, 121–124, *122*, *123*, 154
  funding, 102, 149
  gang summit, 150–154
  gender-based violence and femicide, 186
  hospitals and health systems, 171–172
  international efforts, 174–175, 176–187
  origins of, 67–69
  police support, 167–168
  prison pilot program, 35
  public health outreach workers, 102–107
  violence reduction results, 124–125, *125*, 160, 292–293, 295
  war, 232–240
CVIs (community violence interventions), 148, 308–309. *See also* violence interruption
cyclic AMP (cAMP), 43

D
DAYS WITHOUT A KILLING signs, 187–188
de Blasio, Bill, 171
DeAndre (gang member), 153
Decker, Brent, 176–178, 179, 182, 188
dehumanization, 151, 154, 208, 210, 214, 217–220, 227, 229
democide, 214
Department of Criminal Justice, 170
Department of Health and Human Services (HHS), 15
Department of Justice (DOJ), 16, 102, 146, 156, 292

INDEX

diagnosis, 11–20
  asking questions about violence, 12–14
  certainty without sufficient investigation, 11
  clustering, 18–19, 19
  lack of agreement on what to do about violence, 12–15
  misdiagnosis, 2, 11, 243
  need for data about violence, 15–16
  observable signs versus isolating the agent, 42
  policing, punishing, or moralizing versus, 8
  rethinking diagnoses, 36–37
  understanding the disease, 8, 11–12, 17, 23
  wave pattern, 17–19, 18
directly observed therapy (DOTS), 120
Dirsus, Marcel, 222
disease. *See also* contagious disease; epidemics
  barriers to infection, 86–87
  borderless, 223
  cause and effect, 62
  communicable, 128, 251, 269
  cumulative dose, 74
  defined, 270
  degrees of exposure, 72
  determining who is at risk, 97
  dormancy/latency and susceptibility changes, 52, 52
  dose, 72–73
  dose-response relationship, 287
  elimination of, 242
  epidemic sequence, 7, 59–60
  etiologic agents, 41–43
  factors affecting susceptibility, 87–88
  functional/structural changes to body, 42–44
  gender and risk, 98
  greater exposure = greater risk, 60
  identifying contagion from observable signs, 42
  infection through exposure, 62–63, 63
  interrupting transmission, 128
  markers of success, 118
  myopic thinking, 36
  open wounds or sores, 96–97
  proximity to infection, 72–74
  replication, 44
  susceptibility, 86
  understanding people's perception and fear of, 150–151
  violence as, 7–8, 23, 37, 61–62, 61
  viral load, 73
  war as contagious disease, 229–230
DOJ (Department of Justice), 16, 102, 146, 156, 292
domestic violence
  active case finding, 247
  case management, 249
  community responses and norms, 249–250
  early exposure to, 51, 70
  exposure within and between syndromes, 81
  isolation, 252
  public education and training, 251
  solutions for, 301–302
Donaldson, Kristen, 171
DON'T SHOOT, I WANT TO GROW UP posters, 122, 123
dopamine and dopamine pathways
  addiction to, 216
  anticipatory nature of dopamine release, 53–55
  authoritarian violence disorder, 216, 220
  defined, 270
  enjoyment of violence, 75
  reward network, 53–55, 54
  social reward, 57, 93, 210, 211
Dorland's Illustrated Medical Dictionary, 43
dormancy/latency
  carriers, 34
  defined, 270, 272
  immunity, 91
  infection and script acquisition, 44–45, 51–53, 52, 89–90
  war, 226–228
dorsal anterior cingulate cortex, 56

dose, 71–73, 77–80, *80*
  cumulative, 74
  defined, 270
  dose dependency, 71
  dose-response relationship, 287
DOTS (directly observed therapy), 120
Dowling, Harry F., 34–35
drugs and substance abuse, 14, 66–67, 112–113, 123, 126, 135, 142, 158, 180

E
Ebola, *116*, 246, 257
Economist, 146
education. *See* public education and training
Edwards, Chip, 127–129
Egal, Qassim Aden, 94, 157
Einstein, Albert, 11
Eisenberger, Naomi, 57
El Salvador, 225
election violence, 247, 303
elimination of disease, 8, 242, 270
Elkamel, Farag, 218, 251
Emanuel African Methodist Episcopal Church, 100
empathy disorders, 218–219
endemic, 74, 80, 211, 213, 226, 245, 270
epicenters, 174, 225, 228–229, 270
epidemic fatigue, 213
epidemic waves, 17–19, *18*, 226, 271
epidemics, 1–2. *See also* disease
  assessment of, 11
  blaming the afflicted, 151, 154
  catching up and pulling ahead of, 243
  clustering, 18–19, *19*
  continuing to ask questions, 11–12
  defined, 270
  dehumanizing the afflicted, 151, 154
  epidemic diseases, defined, 271
  epidemic fatigue, 213
  epidemic sequence, 7, 59–60
  epidemic-control approach, 7–8, 21–23, 67–69, 78, 164–166, *167*, 217–222, 242–243
  lack of progress against, 2
  politics, 196
  success spurring other successes, 187–188
  understanding people's perception and fear of, 150–151
  wave pattern, 17–19, *18*
"Epidemiology of Peace and War, The" (Beer), 229
eradication, 8, 69, 242, 257, 271
etiologic agents, 41–43
exposure
  defined, 271
  degrees of, 71–74, *71*, *72*
  epidemic sequence, 7, 59–60
  greater exposure = greater risk, 60
  infection through, 42–44, 62–63, *63*, 70–71, *71*, *72*
  reduction of, 22, 64–67
  social networks, 78–80, *80*
  types of, 75–78
  understanding to make different choices, 106–107
  vicarious, 78, 288
  within and between syndromes, 80–82, *81*, *82*

F
Faber, Jan, 229
Faruq, Leon, 159–160, 188
Feinstein, Dianne, 30
femicide, 185–186, 302
fight-flee-or-freeze response, 88
Fighting Infection (Dowling), 35
Fine, Catherine, 158–160
Fitzgerald, David "MooMoo" (violence interrupter), 161–163
Fonzo (violence interrupter), 129
Ford, Glyn, 239–240
forever wars, 226
Foundation for Global Governance and Sustainability, 227
Fox, Jonathan, 230
Frith, Charles, 48
frontal lobe, 90, 93, 98–102, 138, 291

G

gangs, 4, 15–16, 71, 126–128, 132, 144, 164, 173
  case management, 248–249
  gang network analysis, 146
  gang summit, 150–154, 181
  gender-based violence, 186
  in Latin America, 112–113, 115, 141–142, 176–177, 179–185
  not wanting violence, 123
  similarity to tribes, 233
  social networks, 78
  splintering off, 227
  war, 225
Gani, Mohammed Hashi, 34, 177
Gates Foundation, 238
gender-based violence, 186, 234, 302
genocide, 175, 194–195, 197, 211, 213, 222, 227, 250, 271
George, Francis, 122, 230–231
Giardi (priest and school principal), 199–200
grandmother test, 161
Gray, Freddie, 228
Gugenheim, Ada Mary, 156

H

Harari, Yuval Noah, 230
Hardiman, Tio, 90, 126–127, 129–130, 135–136
Harris, Eric, 83–85, 94–95
hate speech, 194, 271
Henriquez, Freddy, 183–184
Henriquez, Lourdes, 178–188, 250
herd immunity, 271
HHS (Department of Health and Human Services), 15
Hillard, Terry, 125
Hitler, Adolf, 215–216
HIV/AIDS, 2–4, 28–31
  active case finding, 119
  catching up and pulling ahead of, 243
  categories of professional and paraprofessional workers, 128
  changing norms, 245
  dormancy/latency and susceptibility changes, 52
  epidemic-control approach, 23
  exposure reduction, 65–67
  infectious agent, 31, 42
  lack of national system to combat in US, 155–156
  needle program, 65–67
  normalization of, 211–212
  open wounds or sores, 96, 290
  politics, 196
  public education and training, 116, 117, 218, 244–245
  refugees, 241
  testing programs and contact tracing, 35
  therapy development, 128
Hoffer, Eric, 59
Holocaust, 201, 205, 215
Hopewell, Phil, 28–29
hospital-based case management, 308–309
host factors, 85–87, 270
hosts, 26, 44, 87, 271
Houweling, Henk W., 229
How Tyrants Fall (Dirsus), 222
Huesmann, Rowell, 51
Hussein, Saddam, 191–194
hypothalamus, 51, 88

I

Iacoboni, Marco, 49–51
Icke, David, 204
IDB (Inter-American Development Bank), 174
immune system, 31, 52, 86–87, 91, 95, 97
immunity. *See also* susceptibility
  contributors to, 93
  defined, 271
  herd, 271
  social and cultural norms, 90, 106
  susceptibility versus, 91
incubation period, 34, 271
index cases
  authoritarian violence disorder, 216, 219, 221
  defined, 209–210, 271

infection. *See also* infection of the state
    asking questions about violence, 12–14
    assessment of epidemics, 11
    barriers to, 86–87
    clustering, 18–19, *19*
    continuing to ask questions, 11–12
    cumulative dose, 74, 77
    defined, 271
    dose, 72–73, *73*, 77–78, 79–80, *80*
    epidemic sequence, 7, 59–60
    epidemic-control approach, 21–23
    lack of agreement on what to do about violence, 12–15
    misdiagnosing, 11
    myopic thinking, 36
    need for data about violence, 15–16
    open wounds or sores, 96, 290
    proximity, 72–74, *73*–74, 77–78, 78–80, *80*
    rethinking diagnoses, 35–36
    through exposure, 42–44, 62–63, *63*, 70–71, *71*, 72
    wave pattern, 17–19, 18–19, *18*
infection of the state, 196–198, *198*
    authoritarian violence disorder, 213–222, *215*
    building pilot systems, 237–238
    contagion by recruitment, 201–203
    infected authoritarian leaders and mass-contagion pathways, 209–212
    interrupting extremism, 201–208
    moral disengagement and dopamine highs, 215–217
    nuclear war, 238–240
    state violence against those within the state, 197, 208–217
    state-on-state violence, 197, 222–235
    violence against and within the state, 197, 199–208
infectious agents, 26, 31, 33, 41–43, 86–87, 271
infectivity, 72, 96, 119, 219, 272, 290
Institute for Democracy and Electoral Assistance, 211
Institute of Medicine, 50

Inter-American Development Bank (IDB), 174
International Association of Chiefs of Police, 173
International Classification of Diseases, 7
international mediation, 298
Interrupters, The (documentary), 146
interruption. *See* violence interruption
Iraq, 191–194, 198, 230–232
isolation and containment, 35, 42, 244, 248
    authoritarian violence disorder, 221
    defined, 272
    syndromes benefiting from, 251–252
Israel-Hamas war, 228–230

J
James "Monster" (violence interrupter), 129–132
January 6 Capitol riot, 208–209
Jerron (gang member), 152
John Jay Center, 170
Johns Hopkins Bloomberg School of Public Health, 168
Johns Hopkins Center for Gun Violence Solutions, 160
Joubert, Donny, 173

K
Kalyvas, Stathis, 197
Kane, Candice, 172
Kenya, 5, 196
Kerr, Norman Livingston, 150
Kim Jong Un, 238–239
Klebold, Dylan, 83–85, 94–96
Klebold, Susan, 94
Klebold, Tom, 94
Koch, Robert, 33–34
Kostakos, Georgios, 227–228

L
LA Gang Reduction and Youth Development program, 172–173
latency. *See* dormancy/latency
leapfrog technique, 206–207
Lee, Bennie, 150–152

Leo XIV, 231
leprosy, 69
Levy, Jack, 229
Life After Hate, 207
Living Classrooms, 160
Lloyd, Susan, 156
Longfellow, Henry Wadsworth, 191
longitudinal care, 140
love, 84, 95–96, 132, 144, 201
Lurie Children's Hospital of Chicago, 61

M
macaque monkeys, 48–49
MacArthur Foundation, 156
MacWilliams, Matthew, 217
malaria, 2, 26, 211
Malawi, 211
Mandela, Nelson, 241
markers of success, 118
mass shootings, 83–85, 94–98, 100, 290, 303–304
Max (violence interrupter), 133
Mayor's Office of Neighborhood Safety and Engagement (MONSE), 165
McAleer, Tony, 199–203, 207–209
measles, 118, 248
Mendoza, Susana, 24
Merkel, Angela, 236
midnight basketball program, 15–16
Mika, Elizabeth, 218
Milgram, Stanley, 216
Milk, Harvey, 30
mirror neurons, 48–51, 272
mirroring, 47–50, *47, 50*
misinformation, 196, 210, 251
Monahan, Kathleen, 67–69, 121
MONSE (Mayor's Office of Neighborhood Safety and Engagement), 165
moral disengagement, 210, 215–217, 272
morbidity, 43, 210, 272
mortality, 43, 210, 272
Moscone, George, 30
Mother's Reckoning, A (Klebold), 94
MS-13 gang, 176–177, 179, 183
Mussolini, Benito, 215

mutations, 11, 213, 224, 272
mycobacteria, 33
Mycobacterium tuberculosis, 42

N
Nakade, Ryan, 204–207
National Research Council, 50
Natural Born Killers (NBK), 85
Nelson, Mary, 102
neurology. *See* brain and neurology
New Shape (New Strategies for Health and Peace), 237
New York Times Magazine, 146
Nexus (Harari), 230
Norm (staff member), 103, 124
norms
 changing, 22, 124, 161, 164, 183–185, 306–307
 defined, 272
 hospitals and health systems, 171
 influence of, 90, *91*
 quantifiable change, 168
 susceptibility, 90, *91*, 99
 syndromes benefiting from changes in, 249–250
 understanding local, 180–181
North Korea, 238–240
Northwestern University Feinberg School of Medicine, 61
Note-Book of Anton Chekhov (Chekhov), 21
nuclear doomsday clock, 224–225

O
obedience, 90, 216–217
observational learning, 46–47, *47*
Olweus Bullying Prevention Program, 251
optic nerve, 44–45
organized crime and violence, 197, 307. *See also* cartels; gangs
outreach workers and systems
 active case finding, 119
 authoritarian violence disorder, 219–220
 in Baltimore, 165–166
 confidentiality and trust, 134

outreach workers and systems *(cont.)*
    deep underlying caring, 188–189
    epidemic-control approach, 22, 66
    in Honduras, 179–180
    hospitals and health systems, 171–172
    paying for, 149
    public health approach, 102
    roles of, 105, 166
    syndromes benefiting from, 247–248
    violence interrupters versus, 127–128

P
pain network, 55–56, 56
pandemics
    COVID, 87
    defined, 272
    ending, 8, 252
    epicenters, 174
    interruption, 199
    taking over politics, 196
    tuberculosis, 32–33
    war, 215, 224, 226, 229
Papachristos, Andrew, 78
Paracelsus, 33
parent training, 304. *See also* public education and training
Passionate State of Mind, The (Hoffer), 59
Pat (nurse), 127
pathogenesis, 29, 272
PBS, 146
peer pressure, 91–94, 232
Perez, Frank, 176, 179
personality disorders, 306
Philadelphia Inquirer, 146
Picket, Tony, 127–129
Pickford, Marilyn, 103–104
pituitary gland, 88
plague, 8, 42, 69
plasmodia, 26
polio, 48, 69
political violence, 101, 111, 195–197, 251, 303–305
Powell, Jonathan, 239–240
prefrontal cortex, 49, 89
premotor cortex, 48–49

prions, 41
prisons and incarceration
    active case finding, 247
    case management, 248–249
    exposure scenario, 75, 77
    incubators of violence, 34–35
    outreach workers and systems, 247
    pilot program, 35
    solutions for prison violence, 303
Pritzker, Gigi, 156
propaganda, 272
Prose Works of Henry Wadsworth Longfellow (Longfellow), 191
protective factors, 272
Proud Boys, 204
public education and training
    active case finding, 119–121
    authoritarian violence disorder, 217–219
    behavior change, 116–118, *116*
    community responses, 121–124
    epidemic-control approach, 22, 146, 250–251
    HIV/AIDS, 66
    outreach workers and public health department, 166
    reasons for optimism, 244–245
    recognizing exposed and susceptible people, 105
    risk awareness and reduction, 74
    syndromes benefiting from, 250–251
Pucker, Michael, 156
Putin, Vladimir, 216, 221, 224, 236

Q
Quintana, Elena, 171

R
Redmond, LaDonna, 68–69, 150–152
Reed, Jackie, 14
relapses, 81, 117, 140, 224, 272, 305
religiosity, 90, 178
    religious wars and conflicts, 197, 214, 221, 225, 230
    role in interruption of violence, 230–231, 233–234

remission, 272
replication, 41, 43–44, 52, 272
reservoirs, 272–273
resistance. *See* immunity; susceptibility
reward network, 53–55, *54*
Rice, Connie, 172, 173
risk factors, 97–102, 147
  alcohol, 291
  assessment of, 100
  contagious disease, 62
  culture, 98–99
  defined, 273
  exposure within and between syndromes, 82
  gender, 98
  greater exposure = greater risk, 60
  risk awareness and reduction, 74
  youth, 98
Rivera, Craig, 70
Rizzolatti, Giacomo, 48–49, 51
Robert Wood Johnson Foundation, 102, 156
Rocky (trauma surgeon), 171
Roof, Dylann, 100
Rose City Nationalists, 204
Russia-Ukraine war, 226, 236
Rwanda, 5, 67, 227

S
Safe Streets, 157–161, 228
  current management of, 165
  grandmother test, 161
  origins of, 157–159
  violence reduction results, 161, 164, 293–294
Salaad, Abdikamal Ali, 94
Sally (nurse), 127
San Francisco General Hospital (SFGH), 1, 16–17, 28, 90
Sandifer, Robert "Yummy," 4–7, 57
Save Our Streets (SOS), 170, 295
saving face, 91–94, 152–153, 233, 239
Schwarzenegger, Arnold, 95
Scott, Brandon, *147*, 165
script acquisition, 44–45, 51–52, *52*, 89–90, 210–211

September 11 attacks, 191, 198
sexual violence, 133, 302
SFGH (San Francisco General Hospital), 1, 16–17, 28, 90
Shah, Nirao, 51
shingles, 53
Siccama, Jan G., 229
signs, 8, 43, 105, 273
Silverman, Mervin, 30
SIPRI (Stockholm International Peace Research Institute), 237
Sistani, Ali al-, 231, 233
skinheads (white supremacy), 199–203, 205, 207
smallpox, 8, 18, *18*, 69
Snow, John, 217
social media, 22, 64, 74, 203, 218–219
social networks, 78–80
social pain, 55–57, *56*, 287
social proximity, 73–74
social reward, 54–55, *54*, 74, 93, 210
Social Science and Medicine, 78
Somalia, 1–3, 5–6, 23
  authoritarian violence, 211
  catching up and pulling ahead of cholera, 243
  community healthcare system, 101–102, 155, 157
  hiring recognized people, 135
  reputation and face saving, 93–94
  Somalia-Ethiopia war, 226, 241
  stuck thinking, 34–35
  therapy and relapses, 117
SOS (Save Our Streets), 170, 295
Spano, Richard, 70–72, 77–78
"sponge-y" style of learning, 46–47, *47*
spread. *See also* violence interruption
  defined, 273
  wave pattern, 17–19, *18*
Stalin, Joseph, 215
Stanford University, 46, 51
state infection. *See* infection of the state
Stockholm International Peace Research Institute (SIPRI), 237
Stone, Oliver, 85

STOP. KILLING. PEOPLE. posters, 122, 122, *123*, 124
stress and stress response, 88–89
substance abuse. *See* drugs and substance abuse
suicidality
    active case finding, 247
    chatbots, 64
    exposure within and between syndromes, 81–82
    gender and risk, 98
    mass shootings, 97–98
    public education and training, 251
    solutions for, 305–306
    state violence, 222, 224
susceptibility, 51–53, 86–107
    belonging, attention, and social status, 93
    clinical screening score development, 100–101
    culture and risk, 98–99
    defined, 273
    determining who is at risk, 98–102
    dormancy/latency, 51–53, *52*, 89
    factors affecting, 87–88
    gender and risk, 98
    grievances, 94–97
    host factors, 86–87, *88*
    loneliness, 94–96
    norms, 90, *91*, 99
    pain, 94–97
    peer pressure, 92–94
    racist/sexist ideologies, harmful beliefs, and distorted stories, 99–100
    resistance or immunity versus, 91
    saving face, 91–94
    stress, 88–89
    youth and risk, 98
Suwaij, Hamid al-, 191
Suwaij, Zainab al-, 191–194, 198, 232–235
switchboard model, 49
symptoms, 8, 12, 17, 28–29, 43–44, 273
syndromes of violence, 8
    effect of war on other syndromes, 222–225, *223*
    exposure within and between, 80–82, *82*
    one disease with multiple syndromes, *82*, 185, 195, 223
    solutions for, 301–309
    variety of syndromes with singular pattern, 31
Syria, 237–238
systematizing public health, 149–150, 155–156
    community, 168–169
    four pillars of, *167*, 168–174, 294
    government, 169–171
    hospitals and health systems, 171–172
    integrating systems, 164–168, *167*
    lack of existing infrastructure, 175–178, 237
    police support, 167–168, 172–174

T

Tanzania, 2, 290
Tarantola, Daniel, 2, 156
TB. *See* tuberculosis
Terminator (film), 95
Tibetan Book of Living and Dying, The, 3
Tingirides, Phil, 173
Toles, Linda, 102–103, 132
Towers, Shery, 96
training. *See* public education and training
transmission. *See also* brain and neurology; exposure; susceptibility; violence interruption
    defined, 273
    epidemic sequence, 7, 59–60
treatment
    defined, 273
    of every act of violence, 124
    understanding the disease, 8, 11–12, 17, 23
Truman, Harry, 235
Trump, Donald, 238–240
Trump, Ivanka, 239
tuberculosis (TB), 1–2, 16–17, 23, 32–34
    active case finding, 119–120, *120*, 245
    case management, 248
    crowding, 284

determining who is at risk, 97
dormancy/latency and susceptibility changes, 52
dose, 73
early, erroneous theories about, 33
greatest predictor of, 62–63
identifying contagion from observable signs, 42
infectious agent, 33, 42
interrupting transmission, 128
isolation and containment, 251
Koch's scientific discoveries about, 33–34
marker of success, 118
outreach workers and systems, 119–120, *120*, 127, 245
public education and behavior change, 117, *117*–118, 244
refugees, 241
rethinking diagnoses, 36
susceptibility, 52, 86
testing programs and contact tracing, 35, 63
therapy and relapses, 117
Two-Six gang, 142–143

U
UCLA, 57
Uganda, 23, 52, 119, 121, 211, 245
UNICEF, 95, 122, 174, 186, 218, 251
United Nations (UN), 227–228, 235
University of Chicago, 5
University of Colorado, 229
University of Illinois Chicago (UIC), 67–69, 121, 130
University of Michigan, 100
University of Texas, 229
Ury, William, 228, 238–240
US Attorney General's Office, 146
US Conference of Mayors, 146
US State Department, 232
USAID, 174–175

V
vectors, 273
vertical transmission, 228, 273

veterans, 98, 290
Vibrio cholerae, 42
vicarious exposure, 78, 288
Vice Lords gang, 150–152
violence. *See also* violence interruption
  acceptance of in US, 99, 211–212
  active case finding, 79–81, 100–101, 120–121
  asking questions about, 12–14
  in Baltimore, 160, 164, 293–294
  blaming the afflicted, 151, 154
  cause and effect, 62–63
  in Chicago, 4–6, 23–25, 78, 124–125, *125*, 145–148, *147*, 293
  chronic vicarious victimization, 78
  clinical screening score development, 100–101
  clustering, 18–19, *19*
  community education and training, 105–106
  community-level strategies for, 17, 23, 101–107
  conjuring alternative explanations, 85, 94
  contact tracing, 80–81
  as contagious disease, 7–8, 23, 37, 61–62, *61*
  cumulative dosage, 74, 77
  defined, 211, 253, 273
  degrees of exposure, 71–74, *71, 72*
  dehumanizing the afflicted, 151, 154
  dopamine and reward network, 54
  dormancy/latency and susceptibility changes, 51–53
  dose, 73, 77–78, 79–80, *80*
  dose dependency, 71
  economic development and, 27
  enjoyment of, 75, 113
  epidemic language, 253
  epidemic sequence, 7, 59–60
  epidemic waves in, 17–19, *18*
  epidemic-control approach, 7–8, 67–69, 78, 164–166, *167*, 242–243
  as everything problem, 28
  exposure reduction, 64–67

violence *(cont.)*
   exposure within and between syndromes, 80–82, *81*, *82*
   fictional versus real, 63–64
   fighting violence as nonjudgmental act, 123–124
   functional/structural changes to brain and body, 42–44
   global growth in, 252
   grandmother test, 161
   greater exposure = greater risk, 60
   greatest predictor of, 61–62
   host factors, 86–87
   inequity and mistrust in government, 284
   infection through exposure, 42–44, 62–63, *63*, 70–71, *71*, *72*
   intergenerational transmission of, 216
   lack of agreement on what to do about, 12–15
   lack of data about, 15–16
   laser focus on violence itself, 23, 123
   in Latin America and the Caribbean, 175–176, 185–187, *187*
   limited understanding and solutions that worsen, 34–35
   in Los Angeles, 173, *174*
   marker of success, 118
   mirror neurons, 50–51
   misdiagnosing, 26–27, 243
   in Mobile, 70–71
   myopic thinking, 36
   in New York, 170–171, 188, 295
   normalization of, 64, 74, 100, 113, 153, 181, 210, 211–213
   not a human universal, 245–246
   one disease with multiple presentations/syndromes, 82, 185, 195, *223*
   outreach workers and systems, 120–122, 127–128
   proximity to, 73–74, 77–80, *80*
   public education and training, 116–118, *116*, 120–122
   public health outreach worker approach, 102–105
   punitive measures, 13
   reasons for optimism, 244–246
   rethinking diagnoses, 36–37
   script acquisition, 51–52, 89–90, 210–211
   senseless, 25–26
   as social disorder or moral problem, 7, 26
   social networks and exposure, 78–80, *80*
   stress, 88–89
   systematizing public health, 149–150, 155–157
   treatment for perpetrators, 302
   types of exposure scenarios, 75–78
   understanding people's perception and fear of, 150–151
   variety of syndromes with singular pattern, 31
   visual experience of, 43–45, *45*, 51, 73
violence interruption, 24, 78, 111–148
   agreements, 139
   buying time, 138
   catalyzing a perspective shift, 139–140
   confidentiality and trust, 134
   cooling down, 138, 140
   deep underlying caring, 188–189
   defined, 273
   ensuring physical and social safety, 138–139
   extremism and hate groups, 206–207
   follow-up, 140
   goal of, 134
   hospitals and health systems, 171
   international efforts, 178–187
   interruption, defined, 272
   mothers and grandmothers as, 132–133
   need for information, 134
   nonjudgmental listening, 137
   police support, 167–168
   principles of, 137–140
   recognized people as, 130, 134–135
   role in system of epidemic control, 166
   successes of, 146–148
   validation, 137–138
   women as, 133
Violence Project, 96, 98

violent extremism, 90, 196, 201, 204, 247, 273
violent media, 63–64, 289
viral load, 60, 73
visual cortex, 45
Volker, Karen, 231, 237

W

war, 222–235
  addressing fears of leaders, 236, 240
  chains of transmission, 225–226
  as contagious disease, 229–230
  defined, 273
  effect on civilians, 223
  effect on other syndromes, 222–225, 223
  in El Salvador, 225
  existing mediation systems, 227–228
  forever wars, 226
  interruption of spread, 227–228
  obstacles to fast intervention, 235
  postwar homicide rates, 224
  principal cause of, 229
  role of stories, 230
  solutions for, 305
Webster, Daniel, 160, 164, 168
Wen, Leana, 147
Westside Health Authority (WHA), 14–15, 67–68, 152, 181
white supremacy (skinheads), 199–203, 205, 207
Wiebel, Wayne, 65–67, 135
Wiley, Mildred, 102
Wooten, Kathy, 173
World Bank, 27
World Health Organization (WHO), 2–3, 13, 20, 21, 65, 67, 188, 211, 213, 218, 250
  alcohol, 291
  assessing epidemics, 11
  Global Programme on AIDS, 243
  political violence, 196
  systematizing public health, 155–157
  violent media, 95
World War I, 225–226
World War II, 226

Y

Yale University, 191

Z

Zelaya, Manuel, 176
"Zero Grazing" slogan, 121
Zimbardo, Philip, 216

ABOUT THE AUTHOR

Dr. Gary Slutkin is a physician and epidemiologist and innovator in violence reduction. As the founder and former CEO of Cure Violence Global, he is widely recognized for pioneering the epidemic-control approach to violence prevention.

Formerly the director of interventions at the World Health Organization, Dr. Slutkin guided efforts to combat epidemics of tuberculosis, cholera, and AIDS in over twenty countries in Africa and Asia. Dr. Slutkin has presented his solution-oriented understanding of the violence epidemic to the World Bank, the World Economic Forum, the US State Department, Harvard Law School, the Institute of Medicine, MIT, the US Congress, and the National Intelligence Council.

His work has been featured in the *New York Times*, *Wall Street Journal*, *Financial Times*, the *Economist*, CNN, BBC, and in the award-winning film *The Interrupters*.